D1563456

# RUNNING
## ALL OVER THE
# WORLD

OUR RACE AGAINST EARLY-ONSET ALZHEIMER'S

Todd
Thanks for your support
So glad we had our time
together, you thought
me so much.
Enjoy the fruits of your
labor
              Tony + Cat

Anthony Copeland-Parker

NEWMAN SPRINGS PUBLISHING
320 Broad Street
Red Bank, NJ 07701

First originally published by Newman Springs Publishing 2021

ISBN 978-1-63692-193-8 (Paperback)
ISBN 978-1-63692-194-5 (Hardcover)
ISBN 978-1-63692-195-2 (Digital)

Printed in the United States of America

To all the people we met while we ran all over the world. I appreciate all the encouragement you gave me to write this book and your votes of confidence throughout this process.

To the Alzheimer's Association, which has given us the support and much-needed reference materials as Catherine and I have adjusted to the new normal of her early-onset Alzheimer's.

# ACKNOWLEDGMENTS

I'd like to thank Christopher Piehler for his editing work. He was able to transform my somewhat disjointed blog, PlayHard-HaveFun.com, into a descriptive and informative mosaic of what it was like to be nomads who carried everything we owned in our suitcases.

# CONTENTS

# FOREWORD

Like many older siblings, when my baby brother, Tony, was first born, I didn't pay much attention to him. To my five-year-old self, he was a mere curiosity, a miniature human who seemed to have only one or two tricks: crying, eating, and kicking his legs in a fun way. When he became an active toddler, he occasionally became a playmate, but I still did not take his measure as a person in his own right. However, I distinctly remember the moment he first impressed me, where I saw something nascent in him that I would return to again and again, as an early harbinger of the man he would become.

It was sometime before Christmas. Each Christmas our parents would give me and Tony and my older brother Garrett money to pick out presents for our extended family. We would shop and carefully craft our Christmas tags—to Aunt Ginn, love Gwennie Mac one of mine might read. But Tony—five years my junior—announced when he was seven that he would not be accepting this money. He logically pointed out that the presents were not really from him if he had not paid for them, and since none of us kids had any money of our own, he would work before Christmas to earn money to buy his own presents.

He had a red wagon that he took around the neighborhood collecting bottles and cans to return for the deposits. He also raked leaves and did other odd job errands. I was stunned by this decision—with one fell swoop he had surpassed both me and my older brother in measures I hadn't even considered yet—namely maturity and independence, a desire to stand on his own two feet and make his own way in the world. I suddenly saw him as someone with a very strong ethic that had grown quietly all on his own and then sprung, full-grown, like a tree someone might have secretly seeded in their basement till it was ready to meet the sun, sturdy trunk, leaves, and all.

I saw that same sturdy young man when, after two years in college, he decided that college was not for him and instead left to enroll in flight school. I recognized him when he drove his three children, all young elite soccer players, all weekend long to away games in their motor home, snacks and sodas and lunches and uniforms and schoolbooks—all meticulously packed the night before, supervising schoolwork for one while the other played, covering hundreds of miles in a weekend so that they could all participate in sports at their highest level, then back to the full-time job that often took him away from home for days at a time. And I saw that man years ago when he took care of our mother in a way that allowed her to want for nothing, and to maintain her independence until the last three weeks of her life.

You'll meet that uncommon man in these pages. A man of unusual grit and determination and unfathomable love. He describes himself as a man who was not particularly good at anything, who succeeded in life by turning what he called his C-plus skills into something more with his A-plus effort. I won't weigh in on the skills he denigrates (our family's emphasis on grades might have had something to do with that given the dyslexia that made school difficult for him); instead, I will say that when judging my brother, any sensible person would say that character counts, ethics count, commitment counts, and in all those ways his measure is extraordinary.

This book is an account of his last five-plus years on the road as he and his partner ran all over the world after his partner Catherine's diagnosis of early-onset Alzheimer's and Tony's open-heart surgery. If you are a runner, you will recognize the focus on one step at a time, pushing past pain, setting and meeting goals. If you are a traveler, you will revel in adventures and monuments and exotic locales vicariously experienced. And if you are a spouse or other loved one to a person with Alzheimer's, whether early-onset or diagnosed at a later stage, you will recognize the daily challenges, the commitment to being the best partner one can be to someone who was facing a loss on a daily basis. Yet despite this looming specter of loss, Tony was committed to an additive model. Neither he nor Catherine focused on or were deterred by the stumbles, the falls, the broken ankle, the leaky heart valve; instead, every day, every step they took was animated by—what can we add? What new people can we meet? What new goal can we conquer? What new vista can we experience?

If you take this journey with Tony and Catherine, you can share in their determination that turns obstacles into challenges, their openness that transforms strangers into, as Tony puts it, new best friends, and the zest for life that embraces new experiences and the horizon beyond measure.

Tony says he is a vista junkie, driven to climb mountains, steep winding roads, and treacherous paths all in order to see a dazzling novel view—a heretofore yet seen a vision as the world opens in a new and glorious way. Despite whatever hardships you may be facing, this attitude says, there is always a new way of viewing and experiencing your life if you just keep going till you find that new perspective.

You can join Tony and Catherine in experiencing these new worlds, and you don't even have to get off your couch—just open these pages, and take that first step.

Gwendolyn M. Parker
Author, *These Same Long Bones*, Houghton Mifflin, 1994
and *Trespassing: My Sojourn in the Halls of
Privilege*, Houghton Mifflin, 1997

# CHAPTER
# 1

## Refusing to Act Normal

You don't stop running because you're old. You
get old because you stop running.
—Christopher McDougall

This is the story of our five-year journey to run all over the world after my open-heart surgery and my life partner Catherine's diagnosis of early-onset dementia. We refused to act normal under these circumstances. We both retired, we sold our home, and we began a journey to create memories that would last a lifetime—since neither knew how long that would be.

I was a commercial management pilot at UPS, and Catherine was working for the Transportation Security Administration (TSA) when a routine exam discovered I had a leaky aortic valve. I was running marathons at the time and thought my pace was getting slower because I was getting older. Two years later, the fall race season was in full swing when my surgeon and I picked a date between two races on my schedule. My surgeon, who was also a triathlete, and I felt it was best to put in an artificial valve, something that could handle my level of exercise.

The decision to give up our careers and travel the world wasn't etched in stone until we learned about Catherine's reason for her forgetfulness at the age of fifty-three. I had noticed something was wrong the year prior, but it wasn't until her job performance started to suffer that we had to find out what the problem was before she was fired.

Exhaustive testing confirmed our fears with a diagnosis of early-onset Alzheimer's. We managed to get her six months' severance and have her put on disability with both the government and Social Security.

I struggled with the thought of retirement, but the decision was made for us. In December 2014, I was informed that my seventeenth different job at UPS would be one that I had done before for five years. I really wasn't looking forward to doing it again, so I made the decision to simply retire at the age of fifty-nine.

At the same time, our condo in Indiana was on the market. I got a call from my realtor saying that she had an offer, but there was a catch. A sweet lady who had just lost her husband needed something smaller. She had cash from the sale of their home and wanted to close in two weeks. The price was right, so we sold the condo—and I gave my boss my resignation.

We had some races on the schedule, so the thought was for us to travel for a while from race to race and see if we could find some place to call home. We figured we could fill the time between races with side trips to places I had always wanted to visit—not as a pilot on an eight- or sixteen-hour layover, but as a tourist.

Off we went, right after the closing, with what we would need for the next few weeks. Since you can fly nonstop on Delta from Atlanta to just about everywhere, we sold our cars, loaded up our motor home, and made our way to Atlanta. We didn't see ourselves living in a motor home, so we put it in storage there. Most of our household goods went into storage in our hometown of Jeffersonville, Indiana, and the rest still resides in a five-by-five storage unit near the Atlanta airport.

We didn't know at the time that this journey was to last five years (and counting) and take us through ever-changing landscapes as we completed race after race in far-flung locations, such as Madagascar, Bhutan, and Antarctica. We've both completed a race on all seven continents and finished the six world major marathons: New York, Chicago, Boston, London, Tokyo, and Berlin.

Of course, along the way, we've had our share of what I call "the blue days." I can't say I always have the perfect solution for Catherine. Simply saying "I love you" will not always work since, from her point of view, she can be a burden.

I recorded a voice memo for Catherine to listen to on those blue days and have our song, "You and Me" by the Dave Matthews Band, playing in the background. Two lines in this song set the tone for us: "When we get to the ocean, going to take a boat, to the end of the world, all the way to the end of the world. You and me together, we can do anything."

# CHAPTER
# 2

# The Hospital Endurathon

Aspire to inspire before you expire.

—Eugene Bell Jr.

In June 2014, during the lead-up to my open-heart surgery to replace my aortic valve with a mechanical valve, one of the thoughts that always came to mind was, "Why me?" Was there something that I could have done differently?

One thought was that I had an aneurysm in my descending aorta, which might have caused the problem with the aortic valve. A closer look by the folks at the Cleveland Clinic found that for my size, 6'6", that might be normal for me. Due to my height and the fact that I am often referred to as lanky, they put me through a battery of test for Marfan syndrome. Those tests came back negative.

When I did the Iron Man competition in Louisville, the swim portion was in the Ohio River, and three months later, I noticed a sore on my scalp that was later diagnosed as a MRSA skin infection. Infections have been known to cause valve problems, but we have no direct proof that was the cause, even though my doctor first noticed my heart murmur five months later.

Last but not least was the number of endurance events I had participated in. Was I merely blowing out my valve? No one told me to stop running before the surgery, so I took part in a challenge where a group of us decided to exercise for at least thirty minutes each day for one hundred days. I had no symptoms, but I obsessed over my condition and was on a downward spiral mentally.

Even when one hundred days were up, I decided to keep exercising every day until the day of my operation. Physically, I felt great, and eventually, I decided that the question "Why me?" might not ever be answered.

A little more than six weeks before the surgery, I finished my fifty-second marathon. Some people might have called me crazy, but running was actually what kept me sane. The stresses from work and surgery seemed to melt away when I was out breathing the fresh air and watching the world go by, step by step.

I had seen people with one leg, cancer survivors, and even one guy in a traditional wheelchair at running events. I had a chance to speak to the gentleman in the wheelchair at the finish, and I mentioned that he was such an inspiration. He turned the tables and said that mere fact keeps him going. I would have never thought of it that way.

Time seemed to stand still when I was waiting for my surgery date. I made lists of plans on the postoperative side of the calendar. I worried about germs more than usual. I understood that the operation could be postponed for a simple cold, so I found myself washing my hands with sanitizer several times a day.

I remember reading an article in *Runner's World* magazine where they compared running a marathon to an open-heart surgery. In both cases, no one wants to hear the gory details. I saw some other similarities too. I feel that completing a marathon is 90 percent mental. Your preparation, training, and planning are essential. During the race, your body is working in every way to tell you to stop, but your mind must convince your body to continue. I approached the operation like I would a marathon and decided to come out of it stronger and better than before. I would use modern medicine to help fight off the disadvantage of getting older.

We all know that as time marches on, cells don't replicate as they used to, but I was replacing a faulty valve with a brand-new one that would easily outlive me. I imagined what I could accomplish without the distraction of worrying about my heart.

Still, during the week before surgery, I didn't get much sleep. I found myself thinking about my mother, who I had the honor and privilege of taking care of for nine years before she passed away in July 2013. During her many hospital stays, she never complained and always tried to bring a smile to the face of everyone she had contact with. I resolved to keep her attitude close to my heart for my very first overnight stay at a hospital. My plan was to be out of the hospital four days after the surgery, and I knew that the only way to make that happen was to do what my doctors and nurses said and to try to brighten their days.

The morning of my surgery, I had a great three-mile walk. I knew it might be awhile before I could get back to walking that distance. With two hours remaining before the operation (and 107 days until the Berlin Marathon), I had prepared myself as best as humanly possible.

When I woke up from the surgery, I had no pain. This was sort of worrisome since I expected it to creep up on me as the drug dosage decreased. To help myself learn to be a patient patient, I took a ten-minute walk around the area.

One thing I hadn't prepared for was how difficult it was to get a good night's sleep in my hospital room. I'm a light sleeper, and it didn't help that this was my nightly routine:

10:00 p.m.: Oral medication plus a stick to the belly
11:00 p.m.: Vitals check
12:00 a.m.: More meds through an intravenous line
1:00 a.m.: Someone sticks their head in and asks how I'm doing
3:00 a.m.: Vitals check
4:00 a.m.: Someone sticks their head in and asks how I'm doing
5:00 a.m.: Blood draw
6:00 a.m.: More meds through an intravenous line
7:00 a.m.: Vitals check
8:00 a.m.: More oral meds plus a shot to the belly

Before the surgery, I could only sleep on my right side since my murmur had gotten so loud it would reverberate off my ribs and keep me awake—or wake me up if I turned that way. I didn't know that when you're hooked up to IVs in a hospital bed, sleeping on your back is a required skill.

I also underestimated how the lack of endorphins was going to affect me. I thought that if I was able to get out and walk the halls a dozen times a day for a total of an hour or so, I would be okay.

With the lack of sleep, lack of endorphins, and a headache that wouldn't go away, I was not my totally positive self. For the hospital to release me, I had to have an INR (International Normalized Ratio) of at least 2.5, meaning that my blood was thin enough that it wouldn't clog my new artificial valve.

On the fourth day after surgery, my INR still wasn't in the safe range, so I wouldn't be going home. I told myself that what I was going through was temporary and somewhat out of my control. I focused on what I could control more, which included walking with my favorite running shoes on.

Early that morning, the manager of the floor saw me out walking and suggested that I go to the rehab facility near my room. They didn't open until ten, so I was like a kid waiting for my parents to wake up on Christmas morning. With my vitals up on a screen for the folks to review and my blood pressure taken every five minutes, I was able to get in a slow walk for twenty minutes straight. I covered around .6 miles. I now had a new goal for the next day: Do a little bit better.

The icing on the cake was an afternoon walk on the rooftop lounge. It didn't matter that it was ninety degrees outside—the fresh air was worth its weight in gold. When a chopper landed nearby, I imagined they had dropped in to pick me up and get me out on the day that I had originally hoped. While I was on the roof, I also decided to name my scar MZ for Mini Zipper. My positive attitude was back in full bloom.

During my time in the hospital, I learned a number of things I never thought I would:

- How sweet the words "wake up" can sound
- How to snap and tie a hospital gown with one arm hooked up to an IV

- How to ask for more hospital food
- That I could lose ten pounds in a week without dieting
- Over a dozen ways to tell someone that what was going to happen was going to hurt
- What INR stands for and how its movement varies widely from person to person
- That the surgeon you have is always the best one on staff—thanks, Gosta Pettersson, MD, PhD!
- That a new heart valve costs about $150,000
- That pain is truly temporary
- How great the sound of two beeps after hitting the pain pump in ICU is
- That your heart is pretty smart; after surgery, it knows that it's time to get some rest all by itself
- That it's quicker to go from fully dressed to ready for open-heart surgery than to go from hospital gown to your car on discharge

Seven days after surgery, my INR was in the target range, and I completed the hospital endurathon. Usually, I got a medal and a T-shirt at the end of such endurance events. In this case, my heart pillow was substituted for the T-shirt, and my brand-new On-X #27-29 mechanical valve was my medal.

# CHAPTER
# 3

# Why We Run

Travel is more than the seeing of sights; it is a change that
goes on, deep and permanent, in the ideas of living.
—Marty Ritter Beard

Our favorite commercial is a straightforward ad for ALZ.org
where they talk about their belief that the first person who will be
cured of this dreaded disease is alive today. We both feel Catherine is
that person. For that to be the case, though, we have to preserve what
she can do as long as possible. I'm pretty sure that the initial cure will
be for a specific subset of sufferers, and we want to make sure she is
part of that subset.

It was in 2013 that I began to notice that something was wrong
with Catherine. Back then, I would talk for hours about work, running, or our travel plans; and I started to notice that, from time to
time, Catherine would ask me a question that seemed a bit odd. I
just chalked it up to my big mouth. There I was running off at the
mouth, and all she was hearing was "blah, blah, blah." But that was
the first clue.

I had taken a job that required me to travel more than usual, so
when we were together, I felt compelled to bring her up to date on
everything that had happened while we were apart. She would listen,
but more and more, she would ask questions to which I was sure she
knew the answers.

Just before my heart-valve surgery, Catherine got a new boss who was a very shake-things-up type of guy. Her routine was her cornerstone, so stress at work went way up. Over time, we became increasingly convinced that she might lose her job—her boss had put her on probation and entered her into an employee improvement program. That is when we started going to doctors to try to figure out what was going on.

While I was in the hospital for my surgery, I noticed something serious: Catherine was staying at a nearby hotel, and sometimes she would forget to call me when she arrived at the hotel or would take several hours to get back to the hospital. She could recall things in the distant past way better than I could, but what happened earlier that day was unavailable for instant recall.

After my surgery, it slowly became a reality that Catherine was going to lose her job one way or another. Luckily, we had quite a bit of documentation concerning her condition. Since she was fifty-three at the time, the diagnosis was "younger-onset Alzheimer's or like condition." Doctors use that term since the diagnosis can only be confirmed by an autopsy.

There might be folks around you who have this condition, but you might never know it, especially in the early stages. We hope that our story will find its way to someone who would find this information useful since we firmly believe that the sooner, the better, is the best policy. As in Catherine's case, documentation can protect one from losing their job. Like many other disabilities, there are benefits available; but first, you have to prove that such a disability exists.

There are treatments and drugs that can reduce the symptoms of dementia, but there is presently no cure. That being said, through our experience, we've found a number of habits that have made a difference for Catherine.

*Social engagement.* As time goes on, people with Alzheimer's tend to withdraw socially, but we have found that social interaction helps to make stronger connections and, in turn, stronger memories. Catherine loves telling others about our adventures, and I fill in the details when asked questions to which she may not know the answer.

Large groups can be problematic, though since multiple conversations can come in as merely white noise.

*Dedicated support.* As a partner, you have to be all in and realize that you probably will be together 24-7. Leaving the affected person home alone only accelerates the progression of the disease, and in such cases, you won't be there to see the signs until it is too late.

Additionally, the affected person may need assistance financially, with work, and with medication: I have seen that there is a difference when Catherine misses a dose or two of her medication, and this is when I've needed to take an active role. Furthermore, it is good to have someone to encourage social involvement when the affected person wants to withdraw.

I have gone online several times looking for support groups, and I know they can be helpful, but frankly, we've been too busy enjoying life to take advantage of them!

*Having new experiences.* We feel that exciting new experiences go into the long-term memory unaffected by the condition, at first. When an individual sees the same thing every day, these experiences go into the short-term memory part of the brain and disappear. Their partner comes home and asks, "What did you do today?" and the answer is, "I can't remember." The frustration begins for both.

Don't get me wrong. I'm not suggesting that everyone should aim to run marathons on all seven continents. It can merely be a 5K in a nearby city or a visit to a monument or museum. The premise is that exercise, coupled with a memorable experience, is the key.

*Exercise and sleep.* We try our best to get some form of exercise every day, as it stimulates the brain, and the sense of accomplishment goes a long way when other things in life might not be going as planned.

Sleep is also important. With younger-onset Alzheimer's, deposits of beta-amyloid protein fragments (plaques) and tau protein strands (tangles) form in the brain, causing nerve cell damage. While Catherine sleeps, however, some of these plaques and tangles are removed, so I try my best to make sure she can get eight to nine hours of sleep a night.

Given Catherine's condition, why are we running all over the world? We've decided to see as much of the world for as long as we can and stay fit at the same time. We both found running as a refuge from our pain that also gave us concrete goals we could aspire to.

Catherine began long-distance running right after she lost her husband to cancer at a very young age. She was only thirty, and her big brother, Tommy, saw her spiraling down the drain of despair, so he suggested that she train to run a marathon. Catherine ran track in high school, so this was a great idea for her to keep her mind off her recent loss.

They started with 5Ks and 10Ks, building their way to half-marathons and eventually the Chicago Marathon in 1997 and 1998. If you're only going to run one marathon in your life, the Chicago Marathon is the one. It's flat as a pancake, and millions come out to cheer you along. If you try to quit, they will literally push you back on the course.

So far Catherine has completed eighty marathons, one ultra-marathon, one Iron Man, and numerous triathlons and shorter races of various distances. When we set out to run all over the world, we set the goal for her to complete marathons in all fifty states plus DC, and she's on track to achieve that goal this year if all goes well.

As for me, I was on the cross-country team in high school. I was always in the last heat and remember hating the sport and the pain in my legs after practice. I started running as an adult when I was going through a separation. I needed something to grasp hold of to keep my mind on track so I wouldn't obsess over the current situation. It forced me to keep a disciplined lifestyle.

I started back with a nine-mile race, the Gil Clark Memorial in Louisville in the spring of 2000. I don't think I had ever run a mile as an adult without stopping. I didn't train at all, but I finished the race at 1:36:30, an average pace of 10:37 a mile. Another thing I like about running is that you can set goals for every day and for your lifetime.

As a midpack runner, I compete against myself and I always win. Each day that I head out the door, either for a training run or a race, I set a goal and have always been able to achieve that goal. When I turned fifty, I set out to run a fifty-mile race. Even though I was one of the last finishers, mentally I won, since I was able to achieve that goal.

Together, Catherine and I have done at least a half-marathon in thirty-one different countries and, so far, have visited eighty-one countries, some multiple times. Training with all our traveling can be a challenge, but I'm at my best when I'm solving problems one day at a time. We train when we can, and rest when it's a travel day.

As I tell Catherine all the time, if she shows up at the start, she will finish. I just need to get her to the starting line confident that she has put in the work necessary to finish in the six to eight hours allotted.

I see running all over the world as a way for Catherine to have some part of her independence back. Running is something she can do without my help. It gives her a sense of satisfaction she needs. Endorphins will be in overdrive. Last but not least, it gives her a way to get the intensive level of exercise that research says can positively affect her brain. (More on that later.)

As I prepared to run my first postsurgery marathon, I remembered the first mile of that first nine-miler. I was amazed that I ran the whole thing without walking but quickly realized that if I was going to finish, I would have to walk some. I had two goals that day: to finish and not to die after crossing the finish line.

I didn't die, but the soreness in my legs I remembered from high school was there in full bloom. So why go through that pain again twenty-five years later? Simply put, because I can. I set the goal to achieve, and I achieved that goal. Nobody can take that away from me.

Catherine and I run because it has taken us places we have never been before, both mentally and physically. A few years back, I ran the Missoula Montana Marathon. I needed the state in my quest to complete races in all fifty states, but the experience of the city will stay with me for a lifetime.

# CHAPTER

# 4

## Where the Rubber Meets the Road

Life should not be a journey to the grave with the intention of
arriving safely in a pretty and well-preserved body, but rather
to skid in broadside in a cloud of smoke, thoroughly used up,
totally worn out, and loudly proclaiming "Wow! What a Ride!"
—Hunter S. Thompson

The rubber met the road in 2014. In this case, the rubber of our
running shoes on the road in Berlin, Germany. Throughout my
recovery, I had focused on achieving my goal of running a marathon
mere months after open-heart surgery. I had prepared myself as best
I could. I knew what it took to run 26.2 miles, and I put a recupera-
tion and training program together to achieve my goal.

In my mind, the hard part was behind me. This was my third
marathon of the year. I felt very in tune with my body. I planned
on starting really slow and slowing down all the way to the finish. I
wanted to be able to keep my head up, enjoy the tour of the city on
foot, and try my best to keep a smile on my face.

The weather was perfect, and the course was flat and lined with
over a million folks cheering us on the entire way. Not only did my
heart perform just as I had hoped, but the rest of my body parts
cooperated. That is not always the case when trying to cover 26.2
miles by foot.

There were miles where I second-guessed myself. I doubted my abilities, and every part of my body begged me to stop. It was Berlin, so I was sure there would be cold beer at the end. When I would have usually hit the wall, at mile 20, I started taking pictures and waving at all the well-wishers. I felt great. I used every fiber of my being to cross the finish line. Catherine told me later that it was a walk in the park for her.

Modern medicine is amazing. Only 108 days after open-heart surgery, I was able to run my fifty-third marathon. I must credit the skilled surgeons and team at the Cleveland Clinic. We had planned all along for me to be in a position to run this marathon. I followed their rehab instructions to the "T" and was so grateful to them for helping me achieve my goal.

The mini zipper scar from my surgery was quickly fading away but would always be there to remind me of what had transpired over the two-and-a-half years since my general practitioner first mentioned to me, "Do you know you have a heart murmur?" My life had forever changed—in my opinion for the better.

One of the things I hope will always stay with me is patience. I used to be a type "A" personality, someone who had never spent a day in the hospital. During every race, I used to look at my watch and try to improve my times, but in Berlin, I told myself to be patient and enjoy each and every moment.

Time flies when you're having fun. It also goes by pretty fast as you get older, but I must admit that it hauls ass when you retire.

In December 2014, I offered my resignation, and we started a new chapter in our life. I had been working steadily since I started delivering papers at fourteen. I decided that forty-five years was long enough, and I had enough vacation days banked that I would still get paid until March 2015. I had been blessed with an outstanding career in aviation, but there was so much of the world I wanted to see and experience, and I was not told how long I would be on this earth.

I became a pilot to travel and see the world, but after thirty-seven years, I noticed that I was always going places that my employer requested. Being in management I did have the opportunity to pick and choose the destinations, but still, we were always told when and for how long. Now, I would have to wait for six months or more to get my FAA medical clearance back, so I would be flying a desk for the foreseeable future.

I have heard it said that the filter between your mouth and your brain tends to malfunction from time to time after open-heart surgery. I was pretty outspoken beforehand, so there was no telling what was in store. I tried my best to think before I opened my mouth and sometimes found those thoughts taking the form of poems.

Retirement
You save and spend
not knowing
which is enough
or
too much
You just hope and pray
before the end
that you get to see that day
Will your body and mind
survive
or did you just play it safe
only enough just to stay
alive
I tried to live each day
as if it was my last
no regrets
no do-overs
so they say
I hope to continue
till the very last day
The average black male lives
until 74
my dad left us at 94
so how many days do I have
left
time will tell

# RUNNING ALL OVER THE WORLD

Did my open-heart surgery give me
more or less
I was an aviator
a manager
I am a motivator
and marathoner
none of this is factored in
Just our genes
they say
but who are they
Does it all matter
on judgment day
time now to play the actuary game
this where I only collect my pension
for 5 years
they hope
my plan is to take after my dad
and make them pay and pay
I have lived to start my
new chapter in my life
so many have or will not
they will work till
they die
not I
I often say
I worked too damn hard and long
not to see this day
and not have it be the one that got
away
I lived my dream as a pilot
to see the world
but now
on my own terms
to come and go
as I see fit
and not wonder if I did not

stay in one place
long enough
you can't do and see it all
But as I slide into home plate
all bruised and weathered
I will at least know that
I had one hell of a ride
nothing to hide
This is not the road to the end
but a new beginning that
has no end
I might either find that I did not
save enough
or
spent too much
but one thing is for sure
I will never say
I did not enjoy
my stay

After the excitement of Berlin (and my fifty-fourth marathon in Boise, Idaho), we went on our very first Windstar Cruises in the Caribbean. Then we met up with family in St. Kitts for a week, then headed to Fort Lauderdale, where we embarked on the eastern Caribbean with Marathon Expeditions. The concept is to put around 150 runners/walkers on a cruise ship and, at each stop, have the local running group set up a road/trail/beach race for the group. We've made five trips with them: two to the Caribbean, one to Alaska, a river cruise along the Danube, and a land-based running event in Florence, Italy.

This cruise was out to sea for two days as we made our way to St. Maarten. The first event was a three-mile night deck run. The winds across the bow made for an exciting event, and the winner was the one who predicted the time, with no timing devices were allowed during the run.

When we made land on the third day, we did a six-mile run. There was some beach running involved, but mostly we were along the walking path. The winner of this event was the fastest. A small group of us rented a catamaran for some sun and snorkeling. We all had a lot of fun—so much fun that we almost missed the cruise ship.

We headed back to St. Kitts where we met up with the Hash House Harriers. They're a running group with a drinking problem—or maybe it's the other way around. We set out on a six-mile, somewhat well-marked trail run, parts of which were through the rain forest. It was a very hilly course, so not much running was done there.

We pulled up anchor and were off for San Juan where we dressed up as pirates and invaded the port area in a six-mile Amazing Race-type adventure. A small group of us decided to turn it into a pub crawl near the end since it was apparent we were not going to win. Many of us met at the notorious Senior Frogs to celebrate.

From there we were off to Labadee, Haiti, where we met a group of homeless young men through a local nonprofit called Street Hearts. We brought shoes and the like for them so they could join us in an eight-mile relay race. The runners from the cruise also ended up donating $10,000 to help fund a new home for them.

In Haiti, we also rode the longest overwater zip line in the world. It's half a mile long. We started up at five hundred feet and ended down on the beach going more than sixty miles an hour, where the sand brings you to a pretty abrupt stop. During the course of the cruise, we ran a bit over 26.2 miles, so our marathon expedition lived up to its name.

With the cruise over, we headed back to Atlanta and then on to Tokyo, where I finished my fifty-fifth marathon. Having completed New York, Chicago, London, Berlin, and Tokyo, I only needed to finish Boston to complete the top 6 world major marathon series.

There are two ways to get to run Boston. Most folks, like Catherine, qualify, which means you must run another marathon within a certain time based on age and gender—I'll never run fast enough to get in that way. The other way is to donate to selected charities to earn a "charity spot." I have spent a pretty penny to run the first five majors, so at least I'll be giving to a good cause to complete the series.

Over the years, many people have asked me how I have been able to run so many marathons for so many years, and I tell people that I don't run if it hurts. That was not true of the Tokyo marathon. My calf gave me a warning sign on the twelve-hour flight over, but I didn't listen to my body. The calf screamed and cried right from the start of the marathon, and I just kept running. After much research, I discovered that this was a side effect of a new blood pressure medication I have started taking. It also gave me a nasty cough. Strangely, neither of these side effects was brought up by my doctor when he prescribed them.

The race in Tokyo was fantastically organized. It had to be great for me to want to keep running with all that pain. It was a very organized event with one volunteer to every three runners. They cheered you on while doing whatever job they were assigned. I've never experienced anything like that at another marathon.

This next leg of our nomad lifestyle was some R and R so I could nurse my calf injury with a plan to run Rome in twenty-one days. Using the RICE (Rest, Ice, Compression, and Elevation) method, I hoped to be ready to go by then. For the R and R, we went to Malaysia for six nights, and then three nights in Singapore.

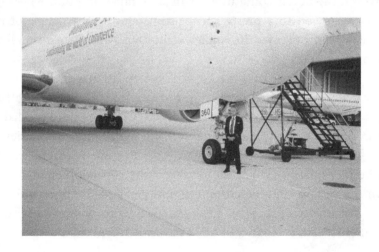

While we were waiting for our flight in Kansai airport in Osaka, I was surprised to notice a UPS B747 taking off right out the gate's window. What a pretty sight. With the help of my friends, I was able to find out it was flight 80 headed to Shanghai. I sent the Captain and First Officer an email about our chance encounter. The Captain wrote me back wishing me well, which was fitting because that day was February 28, my official last day at UPS.

In Johor Bahru, Malaysia, we stayed at the Marriott Renaissance for six days. Their slogan is "Live life to discover," which summed up the first part of my retirement. The Malaysian people really go all out to make you feel at home. It was a great place to start my rehab. I was able to take it easy and take care of my sore leg and swollen ankle. In Malaysia, Singapore, and Bangkok, I was able to walk when I wanted, swim when I wanted, and lift weights to build up my core while the lower parts continued to heal.

They say Singapore is the most expensive place to live in the world, and they are not exaggerating. I haven't experienced anything like that in my short life. Everything in excess. I am sure whoever invented the expression "shop till you drop" had this place in mind.

We took what we usually call the "big red bus" tour of the city and learned some exciting facts. One is why there are no old cars on the road. Because of registration and taxes, it's cheaper to buy a new vehicle than to keep the one that is perfectly fine past four years. Because of this, Singapore is the largest exporter of used cars in the world. They have no traffic problems. All roads have electronic tolls, and they change the fares depending on how many vehicles are on that particular road at the time.

Bangkok was a different story. Everything was cheap there: food, transportation, hotel, entertainment. Not only that, the people bend over backward to make sure you are happy. Every meeting is with hands together, a big smile, and a bow. How could anyone be in a bad mood after a greeting like that?

People in Bangkok are serious about their food. Every street was full of carts selling anything to eat. The malls had just about an equal number of stores and places to eat—and no fast food is allowed. Our favorite was where you would walk in and get a card. They had food from around the world. You filled up your tray with what you wanted and took your first-class seat to enjoy. When you finished, they would scan your card so you could pay on the way out. On the other end of the spectrum, I fell in love with an Irish beer called Kilkenny. It came in handy on St. Patty's day.

We had another "it's a small world" moment when I got a message from an old friend, Walter. We used to fly together back in the '80s at a tiny commuter airline, Wheeler Airlines. He now flies for Federal Express, and we've only seen each briefly a couple of times since our Wheeler days. While we were in Bangkok, he posted a short video of how he was going to be flying there to see a friend, and we ended meeting for dinner a few days later.

His friend there was a singer, Deborah, who he brought to join us for dinner. To make the world even smaller, it turns out we had just seen Deborah perform at a nearby hotel two days earlier. We often cry about how technology has taken over our lives, but to be sitting at dinner in a setting like that because of a social media tool is excellent in my book.

Seeing old friends and making new friends was great, but now that neither Catherine nor I were getting paychecks, I had also started keeping track of pretty much every penny we spent. As I got better over time, I figured we might be able to keep this up for seven to ten years—if our hearts and heads hold up.

# CHAPTER
# 5

## Does Exercising Your Brain Do Any Good?

*The joy of life comes from our encounters with new experiences,*
*and hence there is no greater joy than to have an endlessly*
*changing horizon, for each day to have a new and different sun.*
*—Christopher McCandless*

These days, a lot of people will tell you, "I do puzzles to keep my brain sharp." But have you ever wondered if those endless crosswords and Sudoku actually make a difference in reducing "senior moments" and possibly even dementia?

Research from Tel Aviv University has proven that exercising your brain can truly make a difference in preventing Alzheimer's disease. But the way it works might surprise you!

Alzheimer's disease develops when certain types of proteins (called amyloid-betas) aggregate into plaques. These plaques build up between the nerve cells responsible for the brain's electrical communication, causing the classic signs of dementia such as slow speech and memory loss.

However, just as there are two types of cholesterol—one healthy and one dangerous—the same is true for amyloid proteins. Scientists now believe that a high level of amyloid-beta 40 is healthy while amyloid-beta 42 is dangerous because it's more likely to accumulate into plaques. If you have a high ratio of 40 to 42, you're likely to be in good neurological shape.

So how does exercising your brain make a difference? Here's how it works, according to Nature Neuroscience. Dr. Inna Slutsky and her team have shown that by using high frequency "bursts" of electricity in the animal hippocampus—the center of learning—they could increase the production of amyloid-beta 40.

This led the team to conclude that people who experience regular "bursts" of sensory experience can physically increase the level of amyloid-beta 40 in their brains. These kinds of bursts include environmental changes, new experiences, emotional reactions, and sessions of learning and focus (including completing crossword puzzles).

Scientists are even optimistic that this discovery could, someday, lead to a gentle electric treatment for Alzheimer's. But don't worry—it would be pain-free! Says neurologist Amos Kocyzn, also from Tel Aviv University, "Unlike crude electroshock treatments used in schizophrenia, we are talking about a very delicate, gentle, and highly focused electrical stimulation."

*How to create your own "bursts"*

Prevention is always the best medicine. There are many easy free ways to create the same types of electrical bursts in your own brain. Each of these activities forces your brain to adapt, think differently, and rewire your neural network in a process scientists call neuroplasticity.

Read every day, and not just your normal fare. If you always read the newspaper or technical journals, try fiction and vice versa. Even traveling as much as we do, Catherine does a lot of reading on her iPhone.

Do puzzles. Crossword puzzles, Sudoku, riddles, logic puzzles…anything that makes you stop and think for a period of time will do it.

Learn a new language. A study performed at the Swedish Armed Forces Interpreter Academy showed learning a language causes significant brain development in the hippocampus and three areas of the cerebral cortex. "There is a lot to suggest that learning languages is a great way to keep the brain in shape," said Johan Martensson, a psychology researcher at Lund University, Sweden.

Take an online course. Several universities offer free "open courses" with materials and lectures online. If you always meant to learn more about French culture or astrophysics, now is a great time to start!

When you perform "brain exercises" like these, you literally strengthen your brain, increasing the strength and connectivity of your neural networks, and you get the benefits of increasing your levels of healthy amyloid-beta 40 proteins.

Whatever you decide to do, it's my opinion that you should start soon. It's never too late to start fighting Alzheimer's disease. As for Catherine and me, we're doing our part by seeing and doing new things every day.

# CHAPTER

# 6

## Location, Location, Location

You don't have infinite money. Spend it on stuff
that research says makes you happy.

—Jay Cassano

After pulling my calf in Tokyo three weeks ago, I really thought my marathon days were behind me. A lot of cold baths—numerous with my feet over my head—and keeping active did the trick though. I knew that the R in RICE stands for "rest," but for some reason, my body responded better to staying active.

Surprisingly enough our marathon in Rome went rather well. They're never flawless: there was cold rain most of the day, and running on all the cobblestone streets really took a toll on my feet. My calf was a bit tight at the start, but I had no pain at all, and things got better by the mile.

By contrast with Tokyo, where every detail was well-organized and there was plenty of support, Rome had mass confusion all the way through, and the people watching us run didn't seem to care at all. I guess they were all more interested in getting into one of the many museums or cathedrals.

I did have a flashback during the race to an idea I had as I was preparing for my retirement. You hear stories all the time where the retiree gets a part-time job or starts a business, but I actually had come up with a running application that would describe what you are running by during the marathon. I scrapped the idea since it seemed too much like work, and with all our travel and training, I really didn't have time for that. As we were running by all the famous places I thought, what a great idea if I could hear something about these places as opposed to my feet hitting the cobblestones.

The day after the marathon, a group of us took a guided bus trip to our next destination, Florence. On the way, we stopped off at the best wine-tasting experience ever called Osteria. It started with a tour of where the wine was kept and a full description of the three wines we would be tasting. The owner started us off with some bruschetta and the youngest of the three wines. This was not the typical pour of a few drops. This was at least half a glass, and if you finished before the next wine was presented, he kept pouring. The food came out in waves and seemed to be endless.

We moved on to the next vintage until we got to the Reserve that had been sitting up waiting for us for at least six years. The meal included some of their own pasta that was made right there. The same pouring style held true, but we finally met our match with the dessert wine and biscotti, which we dipped for twenty seconds and then ate. Everyone left with at least two bottles of the Reserve, of course. The final leg of the bus trip was very quiet as we all slumped into our seats and took a well-deserved nap.

The next day a few of us took a train trip out to the Leaning Tower of Pisa. The walk up the stairs was well worth the eighteen euros. It actually was not that hard, and the views from the top were breathtaking. Or maybe it was the climb up the stairs that took my breath away. Everyone was taking pictures of them holding the tower up, but I decided to take a selfie where I pretended I was using my head. All along the streets of Italy, there were men every few feet selling selfie sticks if it was sunny and umbrella and ponchos if it was raining. I decided to be a smart-ass and told them that I didn't need a selfie stick since I had such long arms.

I also learned that Florence is famous for its T-bone steaks and wild boar. I wasn't going to eat anything with "wild" in its name, but I had to try one of the smaller T-bone steaks. When it arrived and was the size of my plate, I was happy that I went for the junior size and also decided to handle it like a marathon: one step (or, in this case, one bite) at a time. It was fantastic, and if that was not bad enough, I had to top it off with some gelato.

We stayed at a hotel called Plaza Lucchesi. We had been there before, when we did a Marathon Expeditions running event where we ran all over Venice, around all the famous statues, and through the Tuscan mountainsides. The hotel had been updated somewhat, but the church bells every fifteen minutes were a great reminder of a time gone by. They say that the three most important factors in selling a house are "location, location, location," and the same holds true for hotels—Plaza Lucchesi was mere blocks from the major square of Florence.

After Florence, we headed back to Atlanta for a quick trip to the storage unit near the airport to switch out our clothes for the next week and stop by the UPS store to get all the mail from the last thirty-six days. From there we were off to Reno to meet up with the kids and drive over to Lake Tahoe for my niece Kate's wedding. Then we flew to Denver to meet up with our Marathon Tour Coordinator, Jacqui, who lives in Boulder for dinner.

During the month of late March when there was a drought going on, Boulder seemed like a great place to live. As we ran all over the world. I saw many places that I could live in, but each one had a drawback—and it was mostly the location. Asia is great, but the location is just too far away from the USA where my kids presently live.

The downside of Boulder's location was a great deal of snow most of the year. I used to ski a lot as a kid, but now I've decided that I'd rather live someplace warm. I like running marathons in cool weather, but the rest of the time (including sleeping) I'd rather be warm, so Denver/Boulder didn't make my short list.

Another thought I've had was to move from one location to the next every three months and basically follow the sun year-round. We could rent a home or apartment and just keep moving. I do get bored easily, so I'm not sure how three months would work out. It would cut down on our daily cash burn rate since the airfare was our number 1 expense.

To keep running all over the world for the seven to ten years I was aiming for, we would have to get our cash burn rate down a bit. Everywhere we went on these trips had an admission charge or a per glass charge, if you know what I mean.

To save on airfare, I highly recommend a company called air-treks.com. I send them an email of where we want to go, and if there are at least four legs outside the USA they work a great deal for us. They send an email with the price and what airlines we would be using. After fifteen minutes of going over all the departure and arrival times on the phone, you pay for your trip online. You can even split the cost over several credit cards if need be. They set you up with your own website so you have all your flights booked with them in one place. They alert you to any schedule changes and the personal website then reflects the new itinerary. I have booked all my flights with them, and they even include postdeparture insurance so that if something happens after your trip starts, you're covered.

For predeparture insurance, I use roamright.com. The prices are great, and you can buy as you go. In other words, when you buy your airline tickets, you buy insurance to cover that, and as you add on to the trip with other items, you then buy insurance to cover that cost. They also cover you once the trip starts so you get double the coverage, but I did find out that if you pull your calf while running a marathon, they will not cover the doctor bills.

Our next destination was Belize for a week. I was really looking forward to it since I had heard so much about it, and a lot of expats call it home. It was our thirty-second destination in three-and-a-half months, and we found that, once again, location rules.

We had a great stay, but Belize City needs some work. They love their dogs there—or at least they all seemed to join in with a song each night, so Catherine was in heaven. We made a visit to San Pedro for the day, and it wasn't worth the extra ferry or flight, plus I heard that the rainy season lasts for six months. The Mayan ruins in Altun Ha were enormous, but the roads are rough, so the ride there and back was a bit much.

The food was amazing. I am a sucker for fish tacos, and since I like to eat, that was a plus. We also got some nice slow runs in along the water. I really do love to run anywhere where you can hear the water hitting the beach or rocks.

During a quick trip back to Atlanta, we hit the cleaners and the storage unit to switch out from beachwear to marathon clothes. Our next destination was Boise for my fifty-sixth marathon, the fourth since my surgery. I had five more marathons for the rest of the year, along with a twenty-one-miler and two half-marathons. I hoped the old body could hold out.

I could only imagine where running would take us in the future, both in fantastic destinations and in my mind. Where would marathon number 60 take place before I turned sixty in July, a mere 360 days away?

The world is so big. That was something I had to relearn. Growing up and looking at the map of the world, you know that the world is big, but you really don't fully understand the sheer size until you start to travel all over the world. As a pilot, I was in my own world, and each destination was tied to where I was departing. Now that I was going from place to place and trying to decide where to go next, I really started to understand how truly big the world is. I heard of places that I never knew before and wondered if there was enough time to actually get to see it all.

The marathon outside of Boise was spectacular. Even though Boise did not make the short list of where to live, it was still a nice visit. I broke down and bought a Jeff Galloway timer for this marathon. I'd seen him go by us many times with his walk/run regime and finally gave in and tried it. I set ours for two minutes of running and one minute of walking, and it worked well. I highly recommend it. Jeff actually qualified for Boston using this method, so maybe there was still hope for me. I had completed the last dozen marathons by running 4/10 of a mile then taking a walk break for a tenth. Near the end, I would always find myself walking more and running less, but I didn't have that problem with Jeff's timer.

The marathon was in the town of Nampa, Idaho, and we ran near and around Lake Lowell. We were mostly on roads facing oncoming traffic, which was a bit unnerving at first. I wasn't the last one to cross the finish line, but there were only one hundred folks running the marathon, so it was safe to say that there were not many behind me. It was a very strange experience after running the last two international marathons where there were tens of thousands of runners. The volunteers were helpful though, and I think there were two ladies who actually came out to cheer us on. Even when the race themselves aren't ideal, the people we've met while touring on our own or with Marathon Tours groups have always been memorable.

# CHAPTER
# 7

## It's the People, Stupid

One way to get the most out of life is to
look upon it as an adventure.

—William Feather

"It's the people, stupid" is a thought that keeps running around in my head. The trip to Monterey for the twenty-one-mile portion of the Big Sur Marathon was amazing. We chose the twenty-one-mile run because they had several races. We'd already run a marathon in California, and the half-marathon didn't include some of the most awe-inspiring views, so we chose the twenty-one-mile race. We met some extremely warm and friendly people, some new and some old. The race itself was one of the top ten races I have run so far. The views and vistas were out of this world: the waves splashing against the rocks below, and the vistas—as we achieved the top of each mountain we climbed—were breathtaking. The other part I loved was the sheer challenge of the race. There was one section where we climbed uphill for two miles. Each bend had its own surprise when it came to seeing the ocean on the left and the mountains on the right.

The people we met all seemed to enjoy living there, and as they put it, the weather was perfect running temperature year-round: midfifties to low sixties. That's a tad cool for me but would be perfect for running. They had a well-marked trail near the water that went for miles in either direction.

On a bus tour to nearby Pebble Beach and Carmel, we met a few other couples who were with Marathon Tours. It was always easy to start and continue a conversation when folks heard about what we had been up to this year. During our travels, we have met some very interesting people. Most of them say they would like to get in our suitcase and join us in our travels. The truth of the matter is that this lifestyle is not for everyone. Most would have problems giving up their things. Those items are who they are, whereas our experiences are who we are.

After Monterey, we headed south, down the coast to Malibu Beach. My sister Gwen works in LA, and her very close friend Wendy suggested we stay at the Malibu Beach Inn. It was a very nice hotel, and we had dinner on the deck overlooking the ocean at sunset. As the sun went down, the chill was in the air, and they provided blankets to keep us all warm. It was really cool how we all got together. Wendy lives nearby. Gwen was working on a project in LA, and my nephew's wife, Carla, traveled nearby for a conference, so for us all to meet there was very special. It doesn't get any better than that. Another example of how our travels have shown us that it's the people, stupid. No matter where we go, we seem to run into some old friends, new friends, or family.

For a complete change of pace, we flew off to Kentucky for the Derby. I've been in or around Louisville most of my twenty-seven years at UPS, and they do an outstanding job when it comes to the famous Kentucky Derby. It is a really big deal for the state, and they make it a weeklong event with something going on every day leading up to the grand event. We met up with Gwen, my sister-in-law Joan, and one of her very close friends for an all-out great time. I didn't win at the track. but figured that I did a great job stimulating the economy.

After a few days to recover in Atlanta, we were in the air again, headed for China. We were working on running at least a half-marathon on all seven continents. Having just run in Tokyo, there was no sense repeating Asia, so we opted to run half of the Great Wall of China Marathon. We also had a full marathon scheduled in Copenhagen eight days later, so there was no reason to totally abuse our bodies. The thousand or so steps along the Wall would be enough abuse.

I used to say that I didn't fly to Asia more while I was at UPS because I stuck out like a sore thumb, and if something were to happen at home while I was there, it would take a long time to get home. On this trip, the same principle would apply. It would take me a long time to get home.

It certainly took us a long time to get there. After the first leg to Amsterdam, we spent four hours on the ground before an eleven-hour flight to Hong Kong. We flew over Moscow at 33,000 feet, traveling at 579 mph. With a little over seven hours to go before our 10:00 a.m. local arrival time, this would have been a great time to take a nap. I had been up for twenty-four hours, but I've never been able to sleep on an airplane. I think it comes from all the years of flying planes myself.

For me, there's something unnatural about sleeping in an airplane. It wasn't a problem for our flight attendant on this flight: She slept all the way from when we left the gate to the top of our climb. I'm sure it was a bit unsettling for passengers around her, but I thought it was pretty funny to watch her head bobbing up and down just like everyone else's.

We spent three days in Hong Kong, and there was so much to learn that I did not know about the area. As part of our tour, we had a daylong bus tour, and our guide did a thorough job of giving us the inside scoop—with so much information for the group, he used his sense of humor to keep everyone interested. I've never seen so many overhead cable cars. They had them everywhere. I was surprised they didn't have one at the airport but did have one nearby. They really take advantage of all the surrounding mountains by putting them from one peak to the next.

A couple of things we were able to see were on the list of "500 things you should see before you die." The first was the largest nightly light show in the world. They used the sky as their background and coordinated music to make the light show come alive. Even though it was raining at the time, it was well worth the soaked shoes. Our hotel was on the Kowloon Peninsula, and they are noted for having the tallest building built on a landfill. Apparently they have doubled the land size by merely filling in the surrounding waterway. They have ferries going everywhere, both slow and high-speed, and some even out to the airport.

The second noted marvel in the area was the largest sitting Buddha in the world. This was not an easy trip, but it was well worth the effort. Unfortunately, one of the many cable cars was out of commission, so it was two subways and a bus ride up the mountain. Catherine and I marveled at the fact that so far we had seen many Buddhas in different settings, but few people could say that they had seen the largest sitting Buddha. Our concern was getting the best picture of it since it was so large.

I enjoyed the highly efficient subway ride and white-knuckle trip up and down the mountain. The road was one way in each direction, and I was surprised we managed to make all the turns without hitting someone going in the opposite direction. I can't seem to go and come to any place the same way, so on the way back, we opted for the two ferries to make it back to Kowloon, one fast and one slow. In between, while we were in Hong Kong, we had to experience the longest outdoor escalator/moving sidewalk in the world—almost half a mile, all uphill!

This is where I jump back to the idea that "it's the people, stupid." While we were making the trip up the mountain past all the shops, restaurants, and bars, there were often short places to walk as you transitioned from one escalator to the next. In one of those places, sitting in a restaurant was a fellow UPS pilot who was on a layover. He saw me first and came out to greet us. We were both very surprised to see each other halfway around the world. We talked about how you see another person and wonder at first if you actually know them, then from where, and many times as you get closer you realize that it was actually someone else. As we parted ways, I commented on how small the world is.

After reaching the top of the escalator system, we had to take a different route to get back down since the escalator only goes up during the day. They run it from the top to the bottom in the morning so people can get to work. We could have simply paralleled the system for the way back down, but of course, I had to find an alternate route, which turned out much better. It not nearly as many steps, and we were able to find a great wine bar to wet our whistle.

After a slow ferry back to Kowloon and a short walk to the hotel, I had one of the best steaks ever. The saying "you get what you pay for" definitely applied in this case. I guessed that to stay under budget, we were going to have to fast between one included breakfast in Hong Kong, and the next included breakfast at the JW Marriott in Beijing.

This portion of the trip was like a marathon and not a sprint. We were busy on tours from sunup to well past sundown, and each tour got better and better. It was overwhelming to be actually standing and touring Tiananmen Square, with all its rich history. Marathon Tours pulled out all the stops on this one. I will need some rest and relaxation after this tour.

In order to properly prepare ourselves for the Great Wall of China half-marathon, two days before the race we drove two-and-a-half hours to the start and walked the steps we would be trying to run. This gave everyone a good feel for what they would be up against.

The going up part was not that bad. It was trying to come down on the steps in some parts that really scared me. When there were handrails, I held on with both hands, for dear life. I was glad we decided to only do the half. We got the complete rundown on what to expect on race day, and off we were for the trip back to the hotel—and more tours. Some folks took time off from the tours, but I figured I came all this way so why not try to see it all, from the Chinese National Museum of Ethnology, which represents various cultures from around the world in exquisite and colorful detail, to the impressive China Central Television Tower.

There were people everywhere in Beijing, and I was surprised to learn that most of the tourists were Chinese. The air quality was not as bad as I thought it was going to be, but many on the trip ended up with bad coughs. The race itself was spectacular, and we took our time and enjoyed most of it. Catherine ended up tripping on some rocks around mile 10, which is after the wall, and cut her knee pretty badly. We were able to patch it up, and we ended up finishing but had to get it attended to right after the finish.

It turned out that the doctor who stitched her up had a clinic in Copenhagen. We were headed there in a few days, so she gave us her info so she could remove Catherine's stitches. Once again, what a small world it is!

The next day, off we went to Xian to view the world-famous terra cotta warriors. They said this was the eighth wonder of the world. I thought there were only seven, but what do I know? It was amazing to see and think about what was possible over two thousand years ago. The air quality was even worse in Xian, though, so we were glad to be headed to Copenhagen in a few days.

At the Copenhagen Marriott, the monitor in the elevator endlessly looped a commercial with the slogan:

> Every day is yours for the taking.
> There are adventures to be had,
> Challenges to face,
> Opportunities to do something great.

I had to agree. I've been trying all my life to think along the same lines. In retirement, it was all amplified. I was reading an article that said you should plan out your retirement. If you think you could play golf for thirty years, you will realize that you will be bored after six months. I'm not sure how you can plan for thirty years. I've learned that during retirement, you have to be flexible. You might think you know what you will be doing for the next year or two, but, in reality, shit happens and you have to bend and flex to those circumstances. You do need to do some financial planning and budget your expenses. I refused, however, to pay someone to invest my money. They had no skin in the game, so I would rather just spend it all until it was gone.

When I told people I was going to Copenhagen, everyone would say, "You have to rent a bike for a day and tour the city." I've ridden bikes a lot over my lifetime and have had two serious accidents on them, so I must admit I was somewhat reluctant. Copenhagen made it easy for me to resist the temptation. They are bike crazy there. The streets are laid out perfectly for bikes, but they are everywhere and come out of nowhere to try to run you down. Walkers are on the bottom end of the totem pole, with bikes on top.

They even let motor scooters in the bike lane, so you really have to be careful crossing through the bike lanes and must look in all directions at all times.

During the marathon, we ran all over the city and through some parts twice, so there was no need to tour the city by bike. The marathon itself was well-organized and really had a party feel to it. It kind of reminded me of London, with people shouting encourage-ment from the pubs. It was a very flat course, and it was easy to see why people fall in love with this place. They have parks everywhere, and with the weather in the '60s, everyone was out cheering us on.

Copenhagen has a fantastic mass transit system, but on two sep-arate days, I ended up renting a car. The first time was to drive out to the country to go to the clinic of the doctor who put in Catherine's stitches so she could remove them. It was a nice drive, but once again I had to get out of the way of all the bikes. The second time was to drive back out to the airport since mass transit would take several hours and trying to catch a cab at 4:00 a.m. did not look promising.

After Copenhagen, we were off to Amsterdam for six days. We were able to use mass transit to get to our apartment. Traveling like this is a learning experience. We got our train ticket at the airport and went down to the track for the train to Central Station. To my surprise, you really have to be careful getting on a train two minutes before the one you are supposed to get on departs. Needless to say, we got on the wrong train. Lucky for us, the man sitting next to us not only spoke English but also pulled up an app that gave us the information on how to get on the right train. Two stops later, we ran from one track to another, and lucky for us, the original train was one minute late and were now on our way to Central Station.

A tram ride and several minutes later, we were lugging all our bags up the steepest three flights of steps I had ever seen in my life. The great wall of China paled by comparison. The man from who we were renting the apartment gave us a tour of his incredible place, which included several very interesting displays concerning many of his travels. I had mentioned earlier about the terra cotta warriors, and he had a complete display concerning their exploits. It truly is a very small world.

If I were doing the advertising for Amsterdam, the catchphrase I would use is "ONLY IN AMSTERDAM." I'm sure many of you know some of what I'm talking about. There are hundreds of things you can only see and do in Amsterdam. I'll touch on two items here; the rest of them you'll just have to go and see for yourself.

The first one is diversity. I've covered millions of miles in my lifetime but have never seen so many different people in one city in my life. New York City is a close second. Every third person was someone from a different race and/or religion. There weren't very many African American males to be seen—many looked like me, but by listening to their speech, it was clear English wasn't their first language.

The second thing I couldn't help noticing was the lack of police presence. I'm sure they were somewhere, but they must have been in the shadows. For a tourist destination that was very surprising. I was overwhelmed by the sheer number of people who were walking around in bars and clubs as far as the eye could see, nearly everyone in some state of drunkenness, with not a single policeman or policewoman present. The only thing I could figure was that since the crowds were so diverse, no one felt that if they started something that they had someone to watch their back, so survival instincts took over and everyone kept to themselves.

In Amsterdam, the same folks who ran the canal boats and the Big Red Bus also had an organized pub crawl. About five hundred of us, very diverse in both age and ethnic makeup, met up at the first bar. We were split up into three groups, and for the next five hours, we went from bar/club to bar/club. It was all coordinated so that not more than one group ended up at the same place at the same time. Each group had three or four guides to make sure we got from one place to the other and that we had a great time. That was the best-organized chaos I had ever seen. I highly recommend it, especially if you want to experience the red-light district at arm's length.

Little did I know that the first Heineken brewery was in Amsterdam. We took the tour called "The Heineken Experience," which was like an interactive beer museum with beer at the end. Not as good as beer at the end of marathons but still worth the trip. In my experience, most marathons have a beer sponsor, and they usually give out beer in the food court area after you finish the race. It only takes a sip or two to get a buzz, and at that time, you need to replenish the carbs.

When we weren't drinking, we did a lot of running along Amsterdam's canals and visited my second favorite park in the world called Vondel Park. Of course we also did the canal boat tour, along with a hop-on/hop-off bus with an audio tour. Every time I did one of these audio tours, I thought back to my business idea of doing the same thing while running a marathon. You could listen to your playlist, and when you passed someplace famous, it would give you a full description. Once again, though, that sounded too much like work.

# CHAPTER
# 8

## You Can't Do and See it All

Traveling—it leaves you speechless,
then turns you into a storyteller

—Ibn Battuta

As the one-year anniversary of my open-heart surgery approached, we were preparing to go on a weeklong Windstar Cruises out of Tahiti.

I often joke that running a marathon is like childbirth. If it wasn't, no one would do it more than once. You only seem to remember the great parts of a marathon and not how much it sucks during the actual event. Having open-heart surgery is similar, and I chose a mechanical valve so that I wouldn't have to ever do it again. My doctors told me that a tissue valve would only last about fifteen years, and with my active lifestyle, I decided not to take the chance of blowing out another valve.

I have no regrets about that choice; but there have been downsides, the biggest being that, to prevent blood clots around the valve, I now have to take a blood thinner once a day. It really has been no big deal; at that time, I had to keep my INR between 2.5 and 1.5, so once a week, I took one drop of my blood from my finger and called the results in to my doctor. He would decide how to adjust my daily dosage of Warfarin, a blood-thinning drug that is actually rat poison. I was consistently eating well and taking my meds, and so far, so good. I noticed that running or at least staying active helped a lot too.

After the cruise, we planned to spend a month in Tahiti, and then on to Australia for the Outback Marathon—marathon number 59 for me and the seventh since my operation. I love to set goals, and that fact has kept me motivated over the years. I did a fifty-miler when I turned fifty and ran fifty-five miles in two days at fifty, so it seems fitting that my next goal was to have finished sixty marathons at the age of sixty. Open-heart surgery was not going to stop me. Marathon number 60 would be in Bordeaux, France, in September.

There was no telling what the next twenty or thirty years would be like, but I knew one thing for sure: I would not be the one sitting on the couch watching it go by.

However, when traveling the world is your lifestyle and you have a budget, you can't do or see it all. Many of the people we've met on our travels are able to see everything a place has to offer because they're on vacation for a week or so. If we had that same mentality, we'd be broke by now.

As we waited in Papeete, French Polynesia, for the gangplank of the Wind Spirit to open to our home for the next seven days, we were like kids on Christmas morning, waiting to open up our presents. This was our second trip on Windstar, and we couldn't wait for their signature "sail away."

The sail away music was played each time we left a port, and the sails were put up from front to rear. The song is called "1492," written by Vangelis for the movie Columbus. It's very dramatic, and everyone makes a point to come out to watch. The only problem is that when the sails are fully up, the ship tends to bob and weave a bit more. The environmental benefits of cruising this way made up for it in many ways.

Our trip on the Windspirit was a seven-night cruise. On the first day, Catherine broke her ankle going down a set of stairs. It was somewhat ironic that with all the training and racing miles on her feet, a simple slip and fall on the stairs took her out of commission. Windstar bent over backward to care for her while making sure we were able to enjoy all they had planned on this cruise. She got an X-ray on one island and a soft cast on another one.

We still laugh about when the doctor arrived to access her injury. He asked what her level of pain was in order to decide if she needed a shot to ease it. Catherine reminded him that she was a marathoner and that pain was relative.

In Taha'a, we had lunch on a private Motu (the local name for little islands that are privately owned but can be rented from time to time). They brought all the food and beverages off the ship and set up chairs and umbrellas so we could eat on the beach. From there, it was on to Raiatea for the day.

The highlight of our two days in Bora Bora was Windstar's private "Bora Bora Celebration Festival." It included a Tahitian-inspired dinner and authentic dancing and a fire show. All this took place on another private Motu. Our final stop was the island of Huanine, with an overnight trip back to Papeete where we had to get off the boat. I did manage to get two short runs during the cruise.

During the cruise, there were all sorts of ways to spend everyone's hard-earned cash. I enjoyed asking others what their plans were for the day. Listening to their various answers, I counted over seventy different excursions for the week.

But as I said earlier, you can't do or see it all. You can get sensory overload if you're not careful. The other problem is that you start to worry about how much money you're actually spending. I want this lifestyle to last as long as possible. I can't imagine anymore waking up in the same bed every day. I desire different stimuli to keep me going.

We transitioned from the ship to our new home, which was a fantastic apartment I found on Homeaway.com: one bedroom one bath, with a deck overlooking the pool and a full view of the sunset. The nice-size porch was perfect to enjoy breakfast and dinner and sunrise in the morning.

With Catherine in a cast, it was up to me to do the grocery shopping. We were up on a hill, and it was a great form of exercise to make the daily 2.5-mile roundtrip to the mall and grocery store. During our month in Tahiti, I was forced to understand the term "rest and relaxation." I had been carrying around a stack of magazines and books and was determined to read them all. It was hard work, but someone had to do it.

After a week in paradise, I was about halfway through the stack of books and magazines. The days seemed to fly by, even though we have pretty much nothing planned to do. I rented a car and did my usual self-guided tour of the island. It was great to go to the grocery store for once and not have to figure out how to get all the items in my backpack for the trip back up the hill to the apartment.

We went by the harbor for dinner and a few drinks and got to see the Wind Spirit pull out for another week. I thought I would wish I was on board, but not this time. We were really enjoying the easy life on the island of Papeete. A few minutes after the boat pulled off, I could see it heading back to port. An ambulance went down the street in that direction and my curiosity got the best of me. I had to go see what happened.

From what I understood, someone got injured and was helped into the ambulance with his family members in tow, and off they went to the hospital. A few minutes later, you could hear the Captain on the PA thanking everyone for their patience, and off they went into the darkness. I can only hope that the family had travel insurance.

With all this time on our hands, I was able to take some great time-lapse pictures of the sun rising in the morning and setting in the evening. I had never been someplace where I could see both from the same place. We opened up the sliding doors in the bedroom and living room and enjoyed the trade winds blowing through all day and night until it was time for bed.

Three weeks into our time in paradise I was reminded that there is a downside to everything in life, and that was no different in Papeete. The people were extremely friendly and helpful, but since just about everything arrived by plane or boat, prices were a bit high. The other downside was the number of stray dogs. They say you can tell a lot about the locals by how they treat their animals. The pluses outweighed the minuses big time, but I thought it was worth pointing out.

One of those pluses was that I got to spend my sixtieth birthday in Tahiti. I had planned where I wanted to spend the day for more than a year. Back when I came up with this harebrained scheme to run all over the world, I pieced the places together like it was a jigsaw puzzle.

I had always wanted to go to Tahiti, and the Windstar cruise was an easy fit. That left us with the question of what to do after the cruise and before the trip to Australia for the Outback Marathon. Why not just spend the month in Tahiti and enjoy my birthday there? The pieces fell together, and it was the perfect way to spend the big day. I enjoyed every minute of it, and since we were six hours behind the east coast, I actually started celebrating at 6:00 p.m. the night before and kept going until midnight Tahiti time, a whole thirty hours.

I was able to find some candles at the local store and blew them out in a big dish of fresh-cut pineapples, oranges, cherries, and mango. I figured for me to live another sixty years, I needed to cut back on the cake and such. Speaking of which, I decided to try a more Mediterranean diet and started working on the old midsection with some well-needed floor exercises.

It seems that on all these trips I learn life lessons. As we were winding down our last few days in Tahiti, things were going along just as planned. I went down the hill to rent another car for the last weekend there, and we went out to see some more sights and hit the beaches. We had a very nice lunch out over the water. I made a comment to myself that I hoped to get off the island without getting run down by one of the many motorcycles and scooters that frequent the island.

They're not required to travel in traffic lanes, so as you come to a stop at a light, they squeeze between the cars on both sides and get in the front of the line. My biggest fear was getting my side-view mirror taken off by one of them and having to explain what happened since the offender was probably just going to keep going. I think they call what happened next a self-fulfilling prophesy.

While going around a round-about on our way to the store for some last-minute items, I was T-boned by a motorcycle. I wasn't exactly sure how it happened since I was in my lane, and the motor-cycle ran into my side of the car. Within minutes, I found myself surrounded by not only the Tahiti police but also the French police for a total of six police officers. One of them asked me to blow into a breathalyzer.

At that very moment, I realized that they were all speaking French, including the man who hit me. I was outnumbered and very glad to know that I only had one glass of wine several hours ago. They did take the motorcycle driver off to the hospital for scrapes and scratches and maybe on to jail since I was not aware of how he did on the same test.

They were very efficient, and it only took an hour including me running by the airport to report the damage to Hertz. The rest of the evening was uneventful and off we were the next day for our next stop: Port Douglas, Australia, where we had another example of "you can't do and see it all."

We took Air Tahiti Nui to Auckland, New Zealand. The next flight was on to Brisbane, Australia, but we only had ninety minutes to collect our bags and make our way from the international to the domestic terminal for our Qantas flight to Cairns. (I learned that the R is silent.) Needless to say, when we returned to the gate in Brisbane for a faulty oven for thirty minutes, we were going to miss our flight.

By the time we made it by bus to the domestic terminal, our plane was long gone, but we were booked on the next flight two hours later. The journey didn't end there. From Cairns, we had a two-hour van ride to our hotel in Port Douglas, the majority of which was along a very winding road.

Even though I was very sleepy, I felt compelled to stay awake in case we went off the road. The time difference on this trip was twenty hours, which meant we arrived at 2:00 a.m. local time, but for my body, it was 6:00 a.m. the next day—twenty-four hours since I had gotten up. We lost an entire day in the process. The Great Barrier Reef all-day tour left at 8:00 a.m., but we had been up for twenty-four hours so we decided to sleep in and miss the tour. I guessed we'd have to Google "Great Barrier Reef" and look at the pictures.

What we really came to Australia to do was run the Outback Marathon in Ayers Rock, in the middle of the Great Sandy Desert. The course was mostly along red dirt trails, and with only about 150 of us running the marathon, I did the majority of it completely by myself.

Catherine and I usually start and finish races together and cross the finish hand in hand, but she was still in a boot, so she chose to walk the half-marathon.

We were only about two miles from the rock and did two large loops, so most of the time we had a great view of it. It was a very spiritual experience, but most of my body parts did not appreciate the foot slippage and uneven terrain. As luck would have it, it had rained the day before the marathon, firming up the ground, and there was cloud cover the entire race to keep the temperature nice and cool.

This was marathon number 59 for me, so I was closing in on my goal to have completed sixty marathons at the age of sixty. It was also my fourth continent, moving me closer to my other goal of running at least a half-marathon on all seven continents. And no, I'm not going to run one on the North Pole, even if others have.

This was the first time I had flown into an airport whose sole purpose was to bring folks to see two rock formations and was entirely supported by the self-contained resort. There was a multitude of tours, so it was impossible to do them all. You could watch the sun rise and set on different tours. You could take helicopter rides, jump out of airplanes or—my favorite—take the sunrise camel ride tour.

We stayed at the Sails in the Desert, one of the four different hotel options. Right down the road was the Pioneer, which had an outdoor restaurant and bar where you got to cook your own meat or seafood and sample from the salad bar—all at a very reasonable price.

A truly unique experience was the Sounds of Silence dinner. They bussed five hundred of us out to a remote area where you could watch the sunset while sipping champagne or your favorite beverage then have a buffet-style dinner from soup to nuts. You could stare at the stars overhead during dinner, and then an astronomer came out and gave a very informative talk about all the constellations in the area.

The last leg on this fifty-one-night venture took us to Sydney. The hotel was right on the harbor, so we could see the Opera House and Sydney Harbor Bridge from the rooftop bar on the thirty-sixth floor. While we were being given a tour of the Opera House, they actually had an orchestra performance going on for some local school kids. That was a very impressive structure, and they definitely got what they paid for.

The original estimate was $10 million, with the final price tag coming in at $100 million and many years behind schedule. Our tour guide said that, based on the original drawings from the architect, it took engineers several years just to figure out how to keep the building from not collapsing on its own weight.

The most elaborate of the tours I have been on so far was climbing the outside of the Sydney Harbor Bridge at night. It took us over an hour to get all the safety equipment on, and then we climbed around the bridge for another two full hours, including many opportunities for pictures.

Not everything in Sydney was very expensive. Food and beverages seemed reasonable; however, I heard that home prices are out of this world. There were way too many cars for the roads, but everyone there seemed in good spirits.

We took several tours with a bus driver/tour guide. I had never had a bus driver/tour guide before. He was very opinionated and had a very dry sense of humor that cracked himself up.

We visited an interactive zoo called Featherdale Park where we were able to get up and personal with some of the local animals. Our bus driver/tour guide also took us out to the Blue Mountains where the Three Sister rock formation is located. He explained in great detail that it was similar to our Grand Canyon only a lot older and with trees.

After Sydney, we headed eastbound from Australia past Tahiti on our way back to Atlanta via Dallas. It was my first ever flight on the A380. Next time I'll pay the extra fare for economy comfort seats so I can experience it from the upper deck. This time it was

Groundhog Day for us: we left Sydney at 1:00 p.m. and arrived in Dallas at 1:30 p.m. the same day.

To add some spice to the very long trip to Atlanta, we ended up missing our flight in Dallas. It seemed like it took forever to get all the bags off the A380, and the ninety-minute connection time was simply not long enough. As the Aussies say, "No worries." This was a continual learning experience for me. Note to self: Pay the extra for Economy Comfort since their bags come off first.

The next leg of our trip would consist of numerous trips in the states until the 9th of September, where we were headed to Bordeaux, France, for the big sixty at Le Marathon du Medoc. It's a run through twenty-some vineyards, and they have both water and wine-tasting stops. My plan was to hold off on the wine until I was sure I could make the six-hour-and-thirty-minute cutoff.

We got a lot accomplished on this leg of our running all over the world tour, but there was plenty more to do. Most times, the cost was the limiting factor, but in some cases, we simply wanted some downtime to catch our breath.

# CHAPTER
# 9

## Thoughts on Pain

Pain is temporary, but quitting lasts forever.

—Lance Armstrong

I often joke that the reason that I shave my head before a marathon is so that the hair follicles can't hurt because everything else will. I have heard about or seen many folks try to run through their injuries, who end up out of commission for weeks or months. I advise people all the time that if it hurts, stop doing it.

I did have to change that philosophy when I was training for the New York Marathon, which was my first. I was in pain most of the training period, but I attribute that to all the biking that I did. I found out two things: I don't like to be bent over for very long, and I don't like to be sitting on a narrow seat while doing it.

On July 19, 2000, I was going out for a simple thirty-minute bike ride. I had done this route many times and was going to go out to improve my time. That is the one thing I was really starting to like about endurance sports: you can go out by yourself, compete against yourself, and win—either by doing a distance you've never done before or in a time faster than you did before. You can even just set a time for the training event and see how close you can come to it. Or you can leave all the gadgets and watches behind and just run. Just you and the sound of your footsteps. You can leave the rest of the world behind. It will still be there when you get back.

I walked out of the house and looked at my helmet and thought, "It's only a thirty-minute bike ride, and there aren't many cars." I almost left it behind. The kids were with me, and we were looking forward to a weeklong houseboat trip the next day, so I grabbed it and put it on. I am still alive because of that decision.

I headed out for the ride, and everything was going as planned. It was a simple out and back, and during the back part, I lost control and came off the bike head first. In retrospect, as a car was coming from behind, I should have slowed down. However, I was out to improve my time, so that was not an option at the time. I remember thinking to myself as I went airborne that this was going to hurt. I landed on my head, right shoulder, and right hip.

I ended up breaking my collar bone in three pieces and breaking two ribs. The lady in the car that was behind me stopped and asked if I was okay, and I said no. She pulled off and left me on the side of the road. I picked myself up and started heading in the direction I was going. There wasn't much traffic on this road, but a car came toward me with two teenage kids in it and stopped.

They both got out and could tell I was in pretty bad shape. I was holding my collarbone with one hand and my ribs with the other. I got in the car, and when they asked where I lived, I was unable to give an address or directions. We kept going in the direction they were headed. I told them I was going in the opposite direction and asked them to turn around.

It would have been hard to do on that narrow road, so we went out on the major road and headed back toward my house. I assured them that something would look familiar—and eventually, it did. Back at the house, I walked in and noticed that the kids were home and that a bag was packed on my bed. I asked them why they were home and about the bag, and they reminded me of the boat trip the next day. I started to cry, not about my injuries but about not being able to take them on the vacation.

Someone took me to the hospital, and the doctor gave me two alternatives: I could have an operation on my collar bone so that it would heal properly, or I could take some pain pills and wear a brace to assist in the healing. I went with the pill option and went home and passed out—but not for long since the ribs really would not let me sleep for very long, no matter how many pain pills I took. One small problem was that you can't drive while taking pain pills, and we were taking the motor home to a nearby lake to pick up the boat. I got up the next day, stopped taking pills, and off we went for the boat trip. I got on the boat and back on pain pills, and the rest is history.

I learned a lot from that experience. The first thing was to follow your gut. Something told me to pick up the helmet, and throughout my life, I have used my gut to guide me through many situations. Some say "use your brains" or "follow your heart," but I believe your gut takes what you have learned over the years—your emotions and experiences—and gives the overall best decision.

I also learned that pain is temporary, but failure lasts a lifetime. I endured the pain so that I would not let my kids down. We all had a great time, and I racked it up as a life lesson. I didn't miss a day of work due to this injury, but because I didn't have the operation, I have a noticeable deformity of my collar bone. The two broken pieces healed on top of each other, so there's a protrusion big enough that you can notice it even when I have a shirt on.

About two weeks later, I was back at training for the marathon. I started out by walking a few miles a day. After a few days, I added riding a bike on a stand. One week later, I got back in the saddle and took a thirty-minute bike ride out on the road. It was not until five weeks after the accident that I was back to running ten miles on the road.

I was well on my way with my marathon training and, with a few months to go, was adding the required mileage at the same time. I was still busy running the kids to soccer practice and weekend games or tournaments, so some of these runs took place at odd times and venues. I continued with short bike rides, but swimming with a crippled wing was out of the question.

About a month before D day, I started the tapering for the marathon—just in time, because on just about every run, no matter the distance I was having knee pain of some sort.

On November 5, 2000, I lived out my dream and pinned on number 27925 to compete in the New York City Marathon. At that time, I was forty-five years old. I remember jumping over all the items that people started running with and then just took off in the first mile or so and left for people to trip over. We were packed like sardines, and it did not thin out much the whole way. Even if it did, it would bunch up again going over one of the five bridges. You couldn't stop, or you would be trampled by the masses behind you.

I flew the kids up to watch the race, and they were with my sister Gwen. I saw them right at about mile 20. It took everything I had to get that far. I was so excited to see them that it gave me an extra burst of energy, but it didn't last very long. Instead of me hitting the wall at mile 19, the wall hit me, and in a very big way. I didn't give up, but it took every shred of effort and mental power to finish.

You hear many stories about how much a mental game running a marathon is, and I have my own theories. It was so strange how hard it was to just keep moving. You always have a time in mind to finish, and now I am much better at it; but during my first, I noticed that as I was slowing down, it was harder and harder to calculate how long it was going to take me. It was as if I didn't have the brainpower to do simple math and keep running at the same time.

The joke I often tell is that near the end while I was trying to figure out when I would finish, I kept coming up with the answer, "Tuesday."

I just kept saying, "I think I can, I think I can," just like *The Little Engine That Could*. I have said a lot of different things over the past twenty years to keep me going, but that will always stick out.

Once I had achieved my goal, it was time to pay the piper. The pain of the stiff legs did not take long to take hold. It would take me forever to get up or to sit down, and no matter what I did or took, the pain was relentless. It brought back all the bad memories of running track in high school, all the pain trying to get home after practice and the days that followed. I remember having dreams as an adult trying to run and my legs not moving fast enough and everyone passing me by. I had the same dream the night after the race for the first time in years.

I now had bragging rights as a member of the small group of people who can say they have run a marathon. The very next thing that came to mind was wondering if I was going to be one of those folks who completes one marathon and checks it off their bucket list or one of those who continues on.

I didn't know it back then, but there were some other groups of people that take it to an extreme. Those who want to run a marathon in all fifty states. Those who find that 26.2 miles is not enough of a challenge. Those that want to run one on all seven continents. Then there is the last group of extreme folks who run fifty marathons a year. Marathons have completely taken over their lives. Turns out that I have flirted with each of those other groups except the last one.

I took a week off and was back at small distances, three to four miles a day just about every other day. On November 23, 2000, I ran Fast Freddie's Festive Five Mile Foot Feast. I dare you to say that five times fast. The day was very windy and cold, but I was able to pull off a 39:08 time with a 7:50 average per mile and a 7:41 best mile. A little over a week later, I drove the motor home to Indy and ran in the Jingle Bell 5K. In my seventh race for the year, I averaged 7:22 a mile. Not bad for my first year, especially since I didn't start until April and broke several bones along the way.

The next day I did a ten-mile training run over plenty of hills, and that pesky old right knee pain was back. It's kind of funny. Thinking back to those times, I don't remember the knee pain at all. It's kind of retrospective. It hurts at the time but doesn't leave a lasting memory.

There was so much about running that I truly enjoyed. It was my time to escape from the pressures of the world. To get lost by myself and at the same time do something positive that was good for me. So many people escape in detrimental ways, but that is not the case with running in particular or having a healthy exercise routine in general. Much has been written on how some have drifted off the edge with exercise and have gone to extremes that could be judged as unhealthy. Some might even say that I have approached that edge or even a time or two gone over that edge.

It has satisfied my competitive personality as a person who, in reality, is not very good at anything in particular. I would call myself a C+ person who works very hard to survive in an A+ world. These days I usually do about sixteen races a year. I guess you could say I'm hooked.

People often tell me that they no longer run because of their knees or other bothersome body parts, but the facts don't lie: those who run and stay active have fewer complaints than those who don't. Catherine and I try not to let the everyday aches and pain of daily life stop us from getting off the couch to breathe in heavy doses of fresh air, no matter where we are in the world.

We've both suffered pain, both mentally and physically. The only type of pain we've been spared, so far, is chronic pain. Catherine had a short bout with costochondritis, which is an inflammation of the cartilage that connects the ribs to the breastbone. She was told to take Advil twice a day, but that caused her blood pressure to rise. Luckily, the costochondritis was short-lived.

I still have vivid memories of pushing on the plunger to administer morphine right after my open-heart surgery. I did my best to quickly step down from all the hard-core drugs I was given to control the pain.

Neither of us, presently, has to take any pain medications on a regular basis. With that said, however, we both have had our share of routine pain. I mentioned to Catherine the other day, while out doing a four-mile run, that I really didn't want to run that day. It all started when I got out of bed and put my feet on the floor. My left ankle hurt, and my right knee was up to its old tricks again. I have written enough about my right knee and remembered my days as a young adult in college when I grew nine inches my freshman year and my knees couldn't keep up with the growth spurt so they both hurt all the time.

As we kept running, my knee and ankle pain subsided, and I mentioned how most people would have simply blown off the run. That's how it starts. Why bother trying to run through the pain? Why not simply take the day, week, month, or the rest of your life off?

Catherine and I are firm believers in "use it or lose it." Our lifestyle has helped Catherine by forcing her, on a daily basis, to continue to try to do the tasks that were once routine. It's the same way with our bodies: our muscles and joints actually feel much better when we stay active.

Yes, there are times when we've had to take time off, like when Catherine broke her ankle. But six weeks after it healed, she walked 13.1 miles in the very sandy Australian desert. Two weeks after that, in France, she was back to running.

Endorphins play a big role when it comes to pain. I always feel better after I run or go for a long walk. Endorphins also boost Catherine's mental health. As you exercise more, the likelihood of some form of injury—and thus, pain—increases. We try not to allow possible pain due to injury to persuade us not to continue our exercise routine.

Endurance athletes have their own relationship with pain. Your body uses pain to try to stop you from moving forward. Over the years, I've had many internal conversations with my body. As one part would subside, another one would raise its ugly head and scream at the top of its lungs for me to simply stop the madness.

# CHAPTER
# 10

## Running the Numbers

It's very hard in the beginning to understand that
the whole idea is not to beat the other runners.
Eventually you learn that the competition is against
the little voice inside you that wants you to quit.

—Dr. George Sheehan

Although Catherine and I didn't have a house, we weren't actually homeless. I liked to call us "nomads," and we did have a motor home at our disposal. We called it the Crib, and it was a 2005 38-foot Gulfstream Crescendo, Triple Slide-Out Diesel Pusher. Right before we sold our house, we loaded up with essentials and drove it to Atlanta, where we put it in storage.

After our trip back from Australia, we went to Louisville to get some yearly physical exams. My heart was still ticking, my blood looked good, and my dentist told me that my daily flossing seemed to be doing the trick; so the only question remaining was to find some local doctors and a dentist in Atlanta. We weren't sold on the place, so off we went looking for some place to take roots. The plan was to move the motorhome around to see if there was any place that tickled our fancy.

So far, we had traveled by planes, trains, and automobiles. Now it was time to take a two-week road trip in "The Crib." Our first stop was Greensboro, Georgia, where we enjoyed two very relaxing nights at a KOA campground adjacent to Lake Oconee. So nice to hear just the sound of nature while you fall to sleep. Then we were on to Athens, Georgia, to visit my daughter, Mariah, for a few days, then Augusta and Savannah, Georgia—which actually made it to the short list of possible places to live. We loved the friendly people, all the history, and the nightly tours of the ghosts that reside in the houses surrounded by moss-filled trees. The city came to life at night, with the sound of jazz coming out every corner of the downtown area. And the prices were right.

We found a UHAUL place that had outdoor storage, so we left "The Crib" there and flew back to Atlanta for a few days to get all our ducks in a row for the next thirty-day trip overseas, where the plan was for me to finish marathon number 60 in Bordeaux, France.

I had set the goal of running sixty marathons at the age of sixty. I love goals. I was still working on what to set my sights on for sixty-five. As a pilot, I always relied on numbers to do my job, and when I was in management in aviation, setting goals has always been very important, especially when it comes to motivating others. I'd given my next goal a good bit of thought: finishing a marathon in all fifty states plus fifteen half-marathons was a possibility.

Speaking of numbers, here are some to mull over. So far, we had been to seventy-six destinations, spending a little over 3.5 days per destination. We had visited thirteen countries and eleven states. We had run five marathons, one twenty-one-miler, and one half-marathon. The cash burn rate (our cost per day) was at $561.55.

Sometimes when you set a goal for yourself, it doesn't work out like you expected. When it came to me achieving the goal of running my sixtieth marathon at the age of sixty, the experience was perfection. I had planned this for several years.

The specific marathon was a major part of the plan. Le Marathon de Medoc in Bordeaux, France, is one of the most famous marathons in the world. It required extraordinary training since you run the 26.2 miles through fifty-nine vineyards which offered more than twenty wine-tasting stops—and all you could bear to eat oysters at mile 24. To add to the festivity, everyone dresses up in some outrageous costume.

The start of this trip did have one unexpected surprise. After our usual stop at the Atlanta Delta lounge, we made our way to the gate. I gave the agent my passport and ticket, and a red light and beep went off. The same happened for Catherine, and we were pulled to the side while another agent did some work on the computer. The only thing that came to mind was that we were being pulled from the flight for some reason.

The agent handed us our tickets and with a smile said, "You've been upgraded." It was like Christmas morning when I was a kid, and when we got on the plane, the first thing I did was stop the next flight attendant going by and ask for a Mimosa.

I wanted to stay awake the entire trip to savor all the amenities, but the seats were so comfortable that I slept five of the eight hours of the flight and arrived in Bordeaux ready to tackle the endless wine tasting for the next five days.

Our entire first day we went from one vineyard to the next, with each trying to prove that their wine was the best. After a few stops and lunch in a beautiful setting with different types of tapas spread throughout the expansive property, I was sure that I could actually tell the difference. As we drove along the roads from one vineyard to the next, there were ripe grapes as far as the eye could see. This was my first experience tasting actual grapes that were mere days away from being picked and would soon be wine. As I tasted each one, I tried to imagine what the wine would taste like when all done.

I was surprised to learn that almost all the grapes are hand-picked. It takes an all-hands-on-deck effort to pull it off in the two weeks allotted to get them all off the vines. A group of migrant workers move in and get a free room, board, and wine on top of their wages. After the grapes are picked, they move on. It was somewhat difficult for me to get my head around the fact that all those vineyards were going to get picked clean in two weeks.

On race day, Catherine got dressed in what I called Cat in the Hat ears, whiskers, and paws. I basically wore anything that I had previously worn for a race and put it all together with the thought of being as colorful as possible. The weather started out overcast, and right after the halfway mark, it rained cats and dogs. That turned the dirt and gravel roads into sheer mud puddles. It seemed as though most people sprinted from one wine stop to the next. They would pass me, and I would pass them back as they stopped to sample the different wines.

There was a six-and-a-half-hour cutoff, which I usually don't take into consideration, but in this case, I had to keep it in the back of my mind. My plan was simple: wear my costume the entire route, make it to the 37K wine stop within 5:30, and then drink my way to the finish.

I was told the best wine was there, so I figured why waste my time on anything but the best.

Along the way, there were times when it was impossible to do anything but walk or come to a complete stop while trying to maneuver around the mass of humanity that was drinking wine like there was no tomorrow. There were also teams of six to ten pushing or pulling various wagons and such, complete with stand-up bars to use at the different wine tastings. They were somewhat difficult to navigate around—in most cases they would run you right off the road.

I enjoyed a half-dozen oysters at mile 24 and came across the finish in a respectable six hours. That was probably the longest it had taken me to finish a marathon, but in this case, I figured I was going to get my money's worth, so why rush it.

If running through the vineyards wasn't enough, they had a ritual the next day called Balade. We all gathered at the selected vineyard for the year and then walked about five miles from one wine tasting to another. Each vineyard had music and endless wine. Instead of glasses, each of us got a tin sipping apparatus called a tastevin that was tied to a lanyard so we could wear it around our necks as we walked from stop to stop.

The last day in Bordeaux was topped off by a gala dinner inside the chateau of a famous vineyard, Saint-Seurin-de-Cadourne. The five-course meal included five different wines, each a little better than the last. The last one was poured out of a decanter instead of the bottle—I guess it really needed to breathe. It was served with the cheese. I didn't like the wine at all when I first tasted it, but for some strange reason, it really tasted good after a few bites of cheese.

We had an awards ceremony at the end of the night. There were awards for the best-dressed Couple, the fastest male and female in our group of ninety, and a new category, which was most colorful. I had to laugh since I was the only person of color in the group—of course, what they were really talking about was what I wore during the race. I would say if the shoe fits wear it. So my sixty-at-sixty experience ended with me winning the award and a very good 2011 bottle of wine. The wine was so good, in fact, that we drank it on the bus ride back to the hotel by pushing the cork into the bottle and passing it around the group.

After we left Bordeaux, we headed to Marseille for destination number 78, then on to Nice, France. Our apartment host, Michael, sent us directions to our apartment for the next ten days. It sounded like a good idea at the time: ten days to unwind on the French Rivera. But things were not going to work out exactly as planned.

When Michael opened the door for us, my jaw dropped. What I saw was exactly what I had seen in the pictures provided, but I hadn't realized how small the apartment was—or the fact that Michael was now showing us his two-bedroom apartment and that he was going to remain in the other room. Everything else, including the toilet and the shower, was to be shared. Lucky for us, he was going away for business the next day and he and his girlfriend were going to be gone for the next four days.

Don't get me wrong, they were perfect hosts and kept to themselves while we were there, but my college days are well behind me, and it just felt weird to have others in such close proximity to us. Everything really did work out: since we were on the French Rivera, we didn't spend much time in the apartment. We ran or walked along the strip adjacent to the beach every day, and I only got my feet wet while there. I didn't realize that the beach in Nice wasn't made of sand—big pebbles were more their style. Listening to the waves crash against them was mesmerizing but the thought of trying to wade out amongst them simply didn't appeal to me. Sitting outside at the many different cafes, bars, and restaurants watching the people go by also consumed a lot of our time.

The nights were filled with great meals at one of the literally thousands of restaurants there to choose from. World Cup rugby was in full swing, so many places had big-screen TVs set up outside for the fans. We were also able to find a few places that had live bands at night—one place even encouraged everyone to dance on the tables.

The change from a five-star hotel to this took a while to truly absorb. I wasn't quite sure why, when I was planning this portion of the trip, I didn't include a stop in Cannes on our way to Nice from Marseilles. This was a great opportunity to make a slight modification to our plans.

JW Marriott has a property right on the main street adjacent to the water, so with a withdrawal of a few thousand points, we made plans to take a few days in Cannes. The timing was perfect: As soon as our roomies got back, we left for Cannes.

The two nights at the JW were unimpressive, but the hourlong showers were delightful. The beach was made of sand, and the runs and walks were great, but it just seemed a bit too expensive for my taste. Gucci here and Prada there, but the usual guys on the street selling hats and selfie sticks brought balance to the experience. I love escargots, and having them in Cannes was a dream come true, but I now longed for the apartment back in Nice, smack dab in the middle of everything.

Before I knew it, we were back for another four college dorm nights in Nice—just in time for me to start trying to figure out how exactly how we were going to get from there to our next destination of Monaco, France. There I was expecting the lives of the rich and famous, and lo and behold, I wasn't disappointed.

I know my mouth was wide open the entire time we were there but I really didn't care. I had made it. I was now living amongst them in Monte Carlo, Monaco. We walked the first day, ran the second, and did the Big Red Bus the third, and I can tell you we saw it all. They actually have a casino so impressive that they charge you just to walk inside. There was also a path that ran from the hotel right along the water. Only separated by a small railing, rocks, and the splash of the water. I had now seen it all. (Or so I thought at the time.)

On what I commonly refer to as our "travel days," we don't accomplish much in the departure city or the destination. The goal is to arrive somewhere around the time on the schedule. Our next travel day was going to be somewhat complicated. We were trying to get from Monaco to Brussels, Belgium; and other planes, trains, and automobile events would be in order. Van to the train station, train back to Nice, extremely crowded bus to the airport, plane to Paris, then Air France flight 7185, which was actually a high-speed train to the main Brussels train station.

I thought a short walk would take us to the hotel. but I miscalculated exactly which train station we were arriving at, so the options were, bus, subway, or cab. You got it: twenty-five euros later we were in front of the Renaissance by Marriott.

Since we were going to be there for five nights, I opted for the Marriott extended stay apartments located right next door. We were here to take part in the Brussels Half Marathon. I have a love/like relationship with marathons and half-marathons. I love the sense of accomplishment when I finish a marathon, but I like running a half-marathon much better. I am sure I will be saying the same thing about 10K and 5K races when I turn eighty.

The weather was perfect. It was a mile walk to the packet pickup, a mile walk to the 10:30 a.m. race start, and another mile walk back to the hotel from the finish. Who could ask for a better half-marathon? Our finishing time was the best we had done in a while, and we got to run by all the sites Brussels had to offer. The day after the race we walked the streets and looked at all the old churches and buildings.

The next day we were on a quick nine-hour-and-fifty-two-minute flight back to Atlanta. Four movies later, we were back at our homestead of the Airport West, Marriott Courtyard, where everyone makes us feel like we are home. We did our superman impression: CVS, Target, Vitamin Shop, storage unit, UPS store, cleaners, a load of laundry, and even managed to get in a three-mile run. Forty-four hours later we were back on a Delta jet, this time headed to Kona, Hawaii.

In August 2011, we both became Iron Men in Louisville, and in Kona, we would live my dream of watching the true triathlon professionals compete in the World Championships Competition.

Kona was all that I had expected and more. We got to run along the same route the professionals would deal with in two days and were able to soak in the entire experience up close and personal. Even the hotel we chose was the same one the Iron Man used for their base of operations. The swim was right out back, the transition was right out back, and the after-party was—you guessed it—right out back.

We were there from beginning to end. We saw the last person out of the water, the first person on the bike, the last person off the bike. and the first male and female finishers. We even hung in (with some breaks to the pool) to see the final woman cross the finish a few seconds prior to the seventeen-hour cut-off at midnight. The thought of doing another Iron Man danced in my head, but I came up with the same answer I had before: "Sounds too much like work."

The trip ended with another example of getting exactly what you pay for. I had planned a year in advance and bought the tickets as soon as they went on sale for that time period, but somewhere I missed the fact that the Delta computer decided that instead of a roundtrip to Kona I would rather have two legs from Honolulu to Kona and no leg from Kona back to Honolulu. Cheap fare equals pay close attention to the details.

We finally made it back to Atlanta for about a week. It was a nice change of pace, and we even cooked a few meals. Our next flight was to Dublin, Ireland, destination number 87 in eleven months. The marathon there would be number 61 for me and number 74 for Catherine.

# CHAPTER
# 11

# Nothing or Nobody's Perfect

In my defense, I was left unsupervised.

—Lee St. John

Our fourth trip across the Atlantic could only be classified as "goofed up." I had no one to blame but myself since I did all the logistics. After twenty-seven years at UPS where logistics are Big Brown's forte, I figured I could handle it. Not on this trip.

This excursion was to last thirty days, but from the onset of the planning process, it was one misstep after another. One thing I have never wanted to happen was to show up at the airport and be told my flight left yesterday, but we came pretty damn close. I'm not sure if I was getting battle fatigue from all the planning or was just lackadaisical, but for whatever reason, my flights didn't match up with my hotels at all.

The mere fact that this trip was to take us from destination 87 through 95 can't be used as an excuse. The majority of the scheduling screw-ups were self-induced, but I did have some help from those folks that operate the airplanes. It started out with those friendly words at the gate when a friendly voice requested us to bring our boarding documents up to the gate agent. As we approached, she had a big smile, and then she uttered my six favorite words: "I have good news for you."

It turned out they had changed planes and needed our seats, and since they had a few extra up front, we got upgraded. That was the second time in four trips heading eastbound across the Atlantic that this had happened. So far, so good.

After a long flight over the ocean the last thing I wanted to do was try to navigate in a brand-new country, so took a taxi to our hotel in Dublin. It should have taken fifteen minutes but instead was over an hour. Watching the meter keep rolling as we sat in heavy traffic was excruciating. It turns out there was a train strike going on, so everyone was in their cars.

Prior to the marathon, they had a friendship breakfast run. It was a two-miler that ended up at the coliseum for breakfast. There they had everything from soup to nuts and plenty of Irish songs and clogging.

Dublin is the home of Guinness beer, so this was my first introduction to that fine liquid. There is a two-step process to pouring Guinness. First, you fill the glass until the head of the beer touches the top of the glass, and then wait for a minute. There is an interesting story as to why—you can Google it someday. Then you fill the glass. There is also a process of how to drink Guinness. Much like you would with my first love, Kilkenny, you take several swallows—not sips—to get all the flavor of the foam head. The long day before the marathon ended with a banquet-style meal at one of the oldest and highest, in elevation, pubs in Dublin called Earlsfort Terrace, where several groups of tap dancers performed for us.

The marathon was a bit cold and wet, but that didn't stop all the locals from coming out and cheering us on. We're back-of-the-pack runners who take walk breaks, but even in the hard rain, the Irish were still out in droves—even the "wee ones," as children are often called there.

The next day we were off by bus for our next destination of Galway. The most memorable spot on this trip was Ennis, where we stopped to see the Atlantic Ocean from Ireland at the Cliffs of Moher, which were carved out during the Ice Age.

It was at the Grand Hotel in Ennis that the screw-ups started. I had gotten an email a few months back letting me know that our trip from Dublin to Porto, Portugal, had a misconnect in Madrid. British Airways/Iberia decided to move the flight out of Madrid two hours earlier, so now we wouldn't make our flight, and the only alternative was a flight that had three stops.

I didn't notice that the date had also changed, so now we were going to be in Dublin for an extra night. The good folks at Marathon Tours didn't notice that when I sent them my flight information, so we had two alternatives: Change the flight back to the original day or stay a day longer in Dublin. I keep saying "Dublin," but actually, we were in Ennis, which is clearly on the other side of Ireland.

I sent my new flight information to Marathon Tours and they happily pointed out that our flights were from Dublin. I sent our Marathon Tour coordinator a quick email and asked her for the price of a private car transfer from Ennis back to Dublin. It was my lucky day, since four others had made the same mistake and had flights out of Dublin, so we could carpool together.

Our last meal in Ireland was at the Bunratty Castle, where Catherine and I were designated the King and Queen for the night. We sat at the head of the table in special chairs, each wearing a royal crown. We had mead to drink, and when some folks disobeyed my order, I ordered them to the dungeon. On a trip when so much went wrong, it was fun to be in complete control for a couple of hours.

After Ireland, we spent four very relaxing nights in Porto. Our hotel backed up to a huge mall with great restaurants and a movie theater. It has easy access to the metro and were across the street from the famous Porto soccer stadium, Estadio Do Dragao. We were even able to get in a seven-mile run along the bay in Porto out to the Atlantic Ocean and back. Porto definitely made my list of places I'd like to come back to. Everything was rather inexpensive there, and I'd love to see an actual game in Estadio Do Dragao.

Our trip from Porto to Lisbon was one of the best train rides I've ever had. We had assigned seats in the comfort car. We had internet, power chargers, someone to give out magazines and newspapers, and at-your-seat lunch and bar service—all for fifty-seven euros.

Good thing I rested up. In Lisbon (or Lisboa, as they call it), it was nonstop. We got in a great run near the water, and then it was walking either up or down to see the sites—and I mean straight up or down. I would never do a marathon here, even though there was one here a few weeks before we arrived.

You can't do or see it all, but we tried our best. We stayed at the very stylish Fontecruz Lisboa, Autograph Collection, which is a Marriott-brand hotel. When I say "stylish," it's more iconic. Big red wingback chairs met us in the lobby, and the whole hotel was moodily lit in darkened tones.

On the downside, there were plenty of opportunities for people to ask us for money, from the high-end Gucci stores down to trinket guys trying to sell us anything and everything, to folks roasting chestnuts, to the panhandlers walking or lying along the sidewalks. The secret there is to never make eye contact, which for me is easy since I could simply look straight ahead over their heads. There was even one guy who had two small dogs tied to a fire hydrant. He had one bowl of water, one filled with food, and a little straw hat for donations. He sat across the street, in the park, to keep an eye on the hat, I'm sure.

The food was great and not very expensive: a meal for two with a bottle of wine was around fifty bucks. A must-see in Lisbon is the São Jorge Castle. It was built back in the second century BC and, over the years, has been a royal palace, a military barracks, home of the Torre do Tombo National Archive, and a national monument and museum. For eight euros, you can take in the great views of the city below and get in a good workout walking up the stairs—but be careful if the stones are wet on the way down.

Portugal is noted for its tiles along the side of the houses and the mosaics that line the streets and sidewalks. It makes for a pretty dangerous run if you're not careful: (1) they're very slick if wet; (2) some stones are missing; and (3) it's always tempting to stop and take pictures of the intricate designs.

On Friday night, the thing to do in Lisbon is walk the streets in Bairro Alto. Once again it was a hike up the hills, but well worth it. The entire area isn't more than one square mile but it was always filled with people pouring in and out of the hundreds of bars and restaurants jammed into the area. They're famous for a drink called morangoska. It's basically crushed strawberries with vodka and brown sugar, and it's deadly.

Saturday turned into a rest day with breakfast just before it closed at eleven. I can't pass up an included meal. We did some people-watching while eating dinner near one of the many squares and were early to bed for our flight the next day to Madrid.

They do it right at the Lisbon airport. They toss a lot of folks at every step of the process. We didn't wait in line for anything. We boarded the flight almost an hour before departure, taxied out fifteen minutes early, and landed over twenty minutes before our scheduled arrival time. I wished all our travel days could be like that.

At the hotel, there was a note posted about how there were traffic problems due to the Madrid marathon that morning. I do remember deciding not to participate since we were just coming off the Dublin marathon three weeks prior and had another marathon in Istanbul the next week. We might have to come back to Madrid sometime in the future to run the marathon, but I doubt it since I've already done one in Spain and there are over 190 countries that have marathons. It's a big world, and there's so little time.

We did enjoy Madrid, though. Our hotel was near one of the biggest parks, Parquet Del Buen Retiro. It was so big you could easily hold a half-marathon inside its gates, and it was full of thousands of people running, biking, skateboarding, roller-skating, walking, and rowing small boats in the lake outside the Monumento al rey Alfonso XII. This is a monument you just have to see for yourself, with its statues and ponds and columns. There were entertainers in all shapes and sizes throughout the park. We were able to get in a nice four-mile run, the last one prior to the marathon in six days.

We didn't go inside the world-famous Museo del Prado, but we got some great pictures of the outside and the beautiful church next to it. With only three nights there, we were unable to see and do it all, but there's a very good chance we'll return, now that I think of it.

Madrid also has a very dense bar and restaurant district, Cortes, along with a huge square where there were thousands of people just milling around. No outstanding building, monument, or fountain to look at, just a lot of folks.

We spent the last full day in a very unusual way. As I have mentioned, due to my artificial heart aortic valve, I test my blood once a week to make sure it's thin enough to keep from causing blood clots around the valve, but not so thin that it causes excessive bleeding.

I drip a drop of blood on a test strip then put it in a handheld machine, and in a few minutes, I know how my blood is doing. Sometimes when my blood gets out of whack, I have to test more often. I left the States with plenty of strips—or so I thought. Lo and behold, my blood got out of whack, and I found myself running low on strips.

We were going to be in Lisbon for six days, so I had UPS send me the strips at the hotel. Big Brown made a wrong turn right off the bat when they sent the package back and forth to Philadelphia twice. I used to be responsible for all the pilots flying out of Philadelphia, so I knew that sometimes things did end up in the wrong place or on the wrong plane. No big deal, there was still plenty of time. The package finally left Philadelphia, headed to Cologne, Germany.

This is where it got interesting. Tracking showed that the package was in Portugal on Tuesday with delivery due on Wednesday. I wasn't leaving until Sunday, so I was now a happy man. The next day at 4:00 a.m., I woke up and checked the trusty UPS tracking site and my blood drained out of my head.

What the hell were my strips doing in Hong Kong? No more sleep for me. After phone calls and emails that day, I found out that my package never really made it to Portugal, but instead was missorted once again and sent on a big shiny 747-400 or MD11 to Hong Kong.

I didn't think they were going to make it to me by Sunday, so I needed to move on with how to test my blood. I had the machine so all I needed was some strips that I was sure could be bought anywhere. Not true. I called the company that makes the machine, and they said they'd only sell me strips if I could produce a prescription from my doctor. The bigger problem was that they don't send them out of the US.

On the desk, in our room, there was an info sheet that listed everything from where to eat to the closest hospital. The hospital was only 1.5 miles away. I figured I could get there in thirty minutes, spend a few hours there, and have another thirty-minute walk back. I would be able to kill two birds with one stone. What could go wrong?

Much had so far on this trip, so I crossed my fingers and laced up my shoes, and off we went. So far in Madrid, everything had been easy to figure out. Everyone spoke English and the city was really easy to get around. Things headed south quickly once we got to the hospital. The first lady we saw didn't speak English. The second lady didn't speak English, but I refused to give up. They found a young security guard who knew some English, and he directed me to where I needed to go.

After a few minutes, I was in the patient registration area. I only knew that because Google Translate has a feature where you can take a picture of words and it translates it for you.

Inside, however, I hit another roadblock: No English spoken here. The receptionist used her translation app on her computer, and I typed in my answer on my phone. After a few phone calls, the security guard and the first information lady were back to my rescue. After a lot of conversation, which I pretended I understood, I was now heading to the emergency room. As I entered and saw all the people sitting around, I knew this was going to take a lot longer than two hours.

The first nurse said I could use her machine, which we figured was for diabetics. She suggested that I take a number and, after paying 180 euros, I might get tested today but doubted it because of all the people ahead of me.

Then the strangest thing happened. The security guard said that he knew a great doctor who maybe could help, but I needed to keep it on the down low—my words, not his. Lo and behold, a doctor came out and directed me back to where they draw blood. In a minute they had their tube of blood and told me to sit quietly for an hour for the results. About ninety minutes later, he handed me what were, by my standards, perfect results. Two hours after we arrived, we were enjoying our brisk walk back to the hotel.

Lesson learned: take twice the number of test strips that I might need when I go out of the country and forget about getting anything from the states to me. That pretty much threw the idea of being an expat out the window.

This episode also made me reconsider the question I'm often asked by my daughter who is working on her PhD in linguistics: "Why don't you learn another language?"

I have two not-so-good answers. First, I'm somewhat dyslexic, which makes learning another language very difficult. Second, I travel to so many places, so which language should I choose? I try to learn how to say "thank you," but I mostly point myself around the world.

The next day we were off to Istanbul, Turkey, our ninety-second destination in 327 days, to meet up with our fine folks at Marathon Tours once again. Granted some of these places, like Atlanta, we have visited many times, but that is still unpacking our bags every 3.5 days.

At Istanbul airport, we waited for our three bags. One came down from the belt right away and then…nothing. After the belt stopped, that sinking feeling set in. Off we went to the lost bag office, and within a few minutes, the very nice lady indicated that two of our bags didn't get on the plane and would be on the same flight tomorrow. No big deal. I bought a T-shirt, a pair of underwear, and socks and was all set for tours the next day.

Our bags arrived before bed the next day, but I could only think: what else could go wrong on this trip now? I had to put all this in perspective when we woke up to multiple CNN reports of a string of terrorist attacks in Paris. It was so surreal to be in Istanbul, where the majority of folks are Muslims and hear about the fact that ISIS was taking credit for killing 131 people in Paris.

During our travels, we have visited places like Paris, Nice, Belgium, and Istanbul where some terrible events happened after we left. We just try to put those thoughts in the back of our minds but don't let them stop us from seeing the world. The first day of our walking tour consisted of the Basilica Cistern, an underground water system built over 1,500 years ago; the Hippodrome, where chariot races were held; and the Blue Mosque, which actually has a deep-blue glow off the tiles in sunlight; and the Ayasofya (Hagia Sophia), an incredible church built back in the AD sixth century, which is now a museum. It's listed as the fourth-largest building constructed as a church in the world, and I must say it was truly unbelievable to think how long ago it was built. We finished off the day with a visit to the Grand Bazar.

The second day consisted of a tour of the Topkapi Palace, which was home of the Ottoman Sultans who once ruled three continents. It's a museum today and home of the famous Harem. It took several hours to tour this massive complex. It had numerous buildings, most with intricate stained glass ceilings of different shapes and designs. At the end of the day, we stopped at the spice market, where I made my first major purchase of our trip: nuts, dried fruit, and tea. As I always say, "If we can't eat it or drink it, we don't buy it."

The day prior to the marathon was a rest day. We barely made it to the included breakfast prior to the 11:00 a.m. cutoff. I spent the entire day with my legs up, watching endless CNN on the Paris bombing on the TV. Every few hours we would hear chanting from the loudspeakers of the nearby mosque. During the nights in Istanbul, we passed Syrian refugees begging. All this unfolding in front of my eyes gave me much to think about while running the marathon.

For the race itself, we were bussed to the Asia side of Istanbul to run across the Bogaxic Bridge that spans the Bosphorus. So if you're trying to run a marathon on all seven continents, you can run this marathon and get either Asia or Europe checked off your list, but there's an unwritten rule among world-traveling marathoners that Istanbul can't count for two continents in one race.

The phrase "Nothing or nobody's perfect" came to mind once again while we were running the thirty-seventh Istanbul marathon. You would have thought it was their first time.

We had our own private charter bus to the start, but the roads were closed early that day so we had to leave at the crack of dawn for the 9:00 a.m. start. No complaints, since we took the extra time to go up into the hills of the Asia side to see the great views at sunrise.

There was a five-and-a-half-hour time limit for this marathon. This was less than the usual six hours, but our info packs gave us the impression that you could still finish if it took you longer—you just had to move to the sidewalks because they were going to open the streets back up. I wasn't taking any chances, so we did something out of character and moved up near the start as the race began.

All was going well, but then a rush of folks started to weave in and out of our group of marathoners. These really fast folks were running the 10K that had started ten minutes behind us. That didn't seem to make much sense, but I just tried not to have any of them run me over. The 10K finish came and went, and off we were for a short out and back, then the 15K split.

The 10K and 15K folks really looked like they were having more fun, but this was going to be Catherine and my fiftieth marathon together, so I put my head down and kept moving forward. This is where it got ugly really quickly.

It was beginning to get warm, the humidity was increasing, and we were faced with a mile-long hill. So far so good but the wheels were all coming off at the same time. Then I noticed that they had only water at all the stops—no Gatorade, Powerade, or off-brand equivalent. I was about out of what I had brought from the Dublin marathon and I was starting to worry. Here my mind played a dirty trick. I started to ration what I had, and without me knowing, dehydration started to set in.

I remembered back to the beginning of the marathon craze when people were dropping like flies due to drinking too much water and having their cells explode. So at the water stops, I was only pouring it over my head and rinsing out my mouth. I did bring one tablet to put in some water, so around 20K I split it with Catherine, but the damage was already done. The only saving grace for us was our new best friend, Elayne, who we could see off in the distance.

I like to keep an eye on the folks headed in our direction both when we are behind them or when we are ahead of them. I shout out encouragement to those I know and those that really look like they need it. I also try to pull strength from the faster ones and take it from those that no longer need it, because it's very clear they are simply waiting for the sag wagon to pick them up and take them back to the finish.

The term "our new best friend" is one I have coined during our trips. When people ask if we miss our friends back home, I always say, "Not really, since we'll have new best friends on this trip." We're very outgoing people and can strike up a conversation with anyone, even if English isn't their native language or they don't speak English at all. So out of our Marathon Tours group of thirty-five, we chose Sarah and Elayne as our new best friends for the next ten days. As an extra bonus, they both lived in Atlanta. As the kilometers came and went, we started to catch up with Elayne and could clearly see she was starting to slow down, since we weren't getting any faster.

As we caught up with Elayne, we offered some words of encouragement. Back then our marathon strategy was to run for five minutes and then walk for one minute. As we walked alongside Elayne during one of our walk breaks, I remembered telling her a few days before the marathon that if we caught up with her, we would help get her to the finish. We weren't going to renege on that statement. I mentioned what our plan was to make it to the finish before they pulled up the mats. Our buzzers went off, ending our walk break, and I asked her to join us. I guess she figured, what did she have to lose since it was clear we were getting near the back of the pack.

We would say when it was time to run and when it was time to walk, and it seemed to help all of us take our minds off the most boring part of this out and back. The cheering crowds had all gone home, and the folks at the water-only stops were busy texting away on their cell phones. We could see the empty boxes of bananas and power gels, and I was starting to have this sinking feeling that, with sixty-one marathons and hundreds of other races under my feet, this was going to be my first DNF: Did Not Finish.

My mind was playing one last devilish trick, that of doubt. Nothing or nobody's perfect, so this was when I did some calculation and issued the word of warning to Catherine and Elayne: "At this pace, we're not going to make it." I figured with a five-thirty cutoff and ten minutes to get everyone in the marathon off and running we had better get to the finish by five-forty gun time.

The plan was to walk faster during the walk breaks. We each took our last power gels, and off we went. The ladies were determined to make it to the finish, but I was getting into oxygen debt. I hadn't experienced that in several years, and panic started to set in. They kept looking over their shoulders, and to keep up I had to run longer, while they were still able to take their one-minute walk breaks.

I wanted to tell them to go ahead, but I knew that if that happened, I would never make it. The 35K marker was off in the distance, and I could see a crew jumping out of a truck to work on the mats. As we got closer it was clear they were rolling them up. I yelled for them to wait, and the man looked up and said in broken English. "It's over." The only thought that came to mind was HELL NO.

My plan was to beat him to the 40K marker and get back on track. I did some more mental calculations, told Catherine and Elayne what we needed to do, and off we went. I knew that the finish was in the old city, and we had two steep but not so long hills to climb, and that worried me, but my plan was to deal with that when we got there.

As we approached the 40K marker, there was that damn truck again. This time we were only ten seconds behind the man as he started rolling up the damn mat. Our walk buzzer went off, and we took a left turn into the park, with a steep hill ahead.

The buzzer once again went off and I said, "We are not running up this hill." There were no complaints. At the top, the buzzer went off again. I gave the command to run, and off we went through the now-crowded park. We had to dodge everyone as they shouted out and clapped, and it was downhill so we rode it for all it was worth. We had one last hill to go, and I knew running up it was out of the question.

You hear so many stories of people dropping dead at the finish, and that isn't how I wanted my life to end. As we turned the corner and looked straight up at crowds cheering on both sides, I simply said, "We will walk to the top." Everyone was telling us to run, and I just yelled back, pumping my fists. I realized that was using much-needed oxygen, but at that point, who cared?

We made it to the top, and there was a small group of Marathon Tour members yelling and clapping. The three of us grabbed hands as we made the turn to the finish. Little did I know there were two turns to the finish, so we dropped our hands, clapped to the crowds of diehards who had stayed to cheer on the final few. I only had one last thing to say to my teammates—that the clock was still counting and we could slow down.

With a few steps to go, we grabbed hands once again for what we thought was going to be a fantastic photo finish, but then the strangest thing happened. There was a guy on his knees rolling up one of the four mats at the finish, and he was directly in front of me. We were still holding hands and we were all looking for the photographers who were no longer there, and I found myself headed right for this guy.

He kept rolling up the mat, and I tripped over his leg. I tripped Catherine, who went down, but luckily Elayne was able to go around without a scratch. I got the worst cramp ever in my leg and could barely walk. Two guys carried Catherine off to the medical tent. I peeked in to see if Catherine was okay. I didn't see any blood, which I had seen in the past, so now my focus was on getting our medals. I couldn't find the usual line of folks that usually put them over your head, and after what we had gone through, we weren't going to leave without them.

I asked everyone I saw and was pointed to a guy standing behind the back of a truck.

I rushed to him and he handed me two medals from a bag. I rushed back to check on Catherine. They were finishing up taking her blood pressure, which was reading normal, and she kept trying to tell them that she hadn't fainted, she was tripped.

Nothing or nobody's perfect, but this was the worst marathon I had ever run. It was one of the most memorable, though, and after a few days I was glad I did it, but all the missteps on the organizers' part make it one that I do not recommend for marathoners like us who run from the back of the pack and try to enjoy themselves.

For me and Catherine, it didn't really matter if we got an official time by hitting the mat prior to the five-thirty cutoff. I heard the beep of at least one of the mats, and we had medals. I was told later that you had to cross every mat to get a finishing time, but when I went to check, our last recorded time was at 30K.

Getting a finishing time did matter for Elayne since this was her marathon in Asia as part of her plan to run one on all seven continents. For her sake, I hoped that what we had seen were the "live stats" times and that after a few days we would all get the official times.

That night our tour group met for dinner at the Han restaurant, where we sat on the floor for some great Turkish food. We licked our wounds and swapped great stories. There was a small group of ten or so who had done the Athens marathon the week prior, and they each had two medals around their necks.

We had run Athens back in 2010, which was the 2,500-year anniversary of when Pheidippides ran from Marathon to Athens back in 490 BC. There, as you may remember, he died. We also did back-to-back marathons in 2012 when Paris and London were a week apart. We even did two marathons a day apart back in 2005 while training for a fifty-miler. All of those races were easier than Istanbul, simply because they were more organized and had plenty of supplies for all the runners—even the ones in the back of the pack.

The next day, eight of us headed to Cappadocia. (It's actually spelled several different ways, but I won't go into them all now.) The tour guide, Ali, who we had had for the last few days, was going to lead us into that very magical part of Turkey.

It began when Ali asked if we wanted to do a morning balloon ride. I had done one in the past so it wasn't high on my list. It was close to being a budget-buster and it was early in the morning, which meant Catherine might not get her usual nine hours of sleep. So I said no at first, but on the ride to the airport, we found out that Sarah and Elayne had signed up. I really didn't want to hear about what I had missed, so we had Ali make a quick call and we were all set for a 5:20 a.m. van pick up the next morning.

In Cappadocia, as the facts and figures rolled off Ali's tongue in rapid-fire, I just listened and looked with my mouth wide open. We visited numerous churches in their elaborate system of caves. Some of them were still being used, but most were abandoned back in the '50s. There was also a jaw-dropping underground city which was eight levels, built five stories below ground. It dated back to 400 BC and had been home to over three thousand people, who could live underground for six months at a time. They had all the comforts of home, even one section where they made their wine.

There were traps with slabs and holes to drop spears on invaders throughout. To make it harder for enemies to even find them, instead of building chimneys to vent the smoke where they lived, they used tunnels to channel the smoke far away, so people trying to find them would go to where the smoke exited, which was nowhere near the settlement. Pure genius.

We checked into our new home for the next three nights at the Yunak Evleri Cave Hotel. That's correct; our hotel was made from a cave as many in the area are.

The hot-air balloon ride was the highlight of our trip, nothing like I had expected. I was thinking we'd take off, fly around for an hour, and land. Maybe we'd have a glass of Champagne and we'd freeze our buns off in the process.

Instead, we had a great breakfast while we waited for the red flags on the balloonists' maps to turn green to let us know that the weather was good for flight today. After we finished up our Turkish tea and olives, we were off for a short ride to the launch area for what turned out to be over fifty balloons taking flight. With the different wind directions at different altitudes, we were able to dip down and get up close and personal with all the different caves and mountains in the area. It was truly magical.

After a flawless touchdown and the usual Champagne toast, we got the added benefit of a medal put around our necks by the Captain, who was also the Chief Pilot of Royal Tours. I highly recommend it if you're ever in the area.

There was another couple in our group that we referred to as a much younger version of ourselves. They were in their midtwenties and had worked and saved for a few years after college. They had quit their jobs and were traveling the world for the next eighteen months, with a plan was to go back to work after that. They figured that this experience would be something extra to go on their resumes when it was time to reenter the job market.

It was hard to top the balloon ride, but Ali did his best. We had lunch at a local family restaurant where we were the only ones being served—there must have been six different courses. After that, we went for a leisurely ninety-minute hike through some more caves. One of which contained a huge wheel to grind up grain.

I was falling in love with the area. Most folks were very friendly and spoke very understandable English, and Ali's connections made us feel like family. We visited a workshop where they made rugs. They gave us a very informative demonstration of the entire process, which ended with some soft selling as they unrolled rug after rug. Since we don't have a home, it was easy for us to walk away.

The last day consisted of seeing more cave churches and dwellings. The mountain range off in the distance included the second tallest mountain in turkey, Uludoruk. We stopped off to see an Einstein look-alike at a pottery shop. He was the third generation, with over fifty years at the kick wheel. He had three daughters, so in a male-dominated profession he would pass the tradition on to them. He also selects ten women from around the world to come and be trained by him. The selection process is a bit odd: for the women to enter the lottery, they must send him a lock of their hair.

After that, we went to another family-run restaurant where here we had eight different courses. The first desert was number four: They felt that having something sweet halfway through the meal helped clean the palette. With full bellies, the only thing left for us to do was go for a strenuous hour-long hike.

That night we witnessed the Sema (otherwise known as the Whirling Dervish Ceremony), which represents the mystical journey of man's spiritual ascent through love, finding the truth, and becoming "Perfect." Once he has reached maturity and a greater perfection, a man's mission is to love and to be of service to all creatures without discriminating in regard to belief, class, or race.

After some of us met around the outdoor fire pit with Ali to reminisce about all that had occurred for the last ten days. Of course we did a quick check of the race stats before bed and saw that it was official: We had run our fiftieth marathon together, my DNF less streak was alive and well, and our new best friend Elayne didn't have to repeat Asia.

After a short flight back to Istanbul, we stayed the afternoon and evening before our predawn departure back to the States the next day. Of course, when I was planning this trip, I once again failed to notice exactly when and where we needed to be prior to heading back to Atlanta. The helpful folks at Marathon Tours pointed out that our flight was leaving nineteen hours after our arrival from Cappadocia, so thirty thousand points later, I booked us at the Renaissance hotel.

Upon check-in, the kind lady pointed out that we had, in her opinion, the best room in the hotel. It was on the top floor and a view to die for. I did see the presidential suite down the hall. I had no idea what it looked like, but I was pretty sure it wasn't perfect.

# CHAPTER
# 12

# Where It All Began, One Year Ago

> Don't call it a dream, call it a plan.
>
> —Calibe Thompson

A year into our voyage of running all over the world, we were in San Jose, Costa Rica, staying at the San Jose Marriott, Costa Rica. I had been there on a layover when I was a pilot, and I remember lying by the pool on a layover, thinking to myself that when I retired, I was going to come back and spend a week.

The first day was a travel day; so we only managed to eat breakfast in the executive lounge, lie by the pool, take a short walk, and graze once again in the executive lounge. There was plenty to do and see here, but as you might remember, we can't do and see it all.

We had done numerous tours over the last year, and I had decided I wasn't doing any risky behavior until I was around eighty, so whitewater rafting and zip-lining didn't make the cut. One hour and six hundred bucks later, we had the plan laid out for the next three days.

The first day of tours started with a two-hour drive to the Poàs Volcano. It was cloudy and raining, so after a fifteen-minute walk up to the site we were able to see absolutely nothing. After a forty-five-minute hike around the area, we arrived back at the volcano, and it was our lucky day: we were able to see the crater with steam coming out.

Next we moved on to the rainforest and the La Paz waterfall. It had been raining before, but it was really coming down in the rainforest. The views of the five different waterfalls were fabulous, and the outdoor zoo was an extra treat. My favorites were the butterflies and hummingbirds. I didn't know that hummingbirds didn't have a sense of smell and can fly up to 50 mph.

After lunch, we continued in the animal park with views of jaguars, chimps, and many varieties of birds, including toucans and macaws.

The second day was Catherine's favorite since she was on a horse for an hour ride. She was all smiles while I ended up with a saddle whose stirrups were too short. It didn't make for a very comfortable ride.

After that, we caught a cable car down to the nature walk that lasted over two hours. Our guide made us feel like we were back in school with his way of giving the information by first asking us a question about each tree, flower, or animal. The highlight here was us crushing the actual sugar cane the way they did it back in the day, with an oxen-drawn press. We even got to drink some of the fresh-squeezed nectar right on the spot.

Another thing I learned is that they only have two seasons in Costa Rica. The rainy season runs from May to November, and the dry season starts in December. It rained on and off the entire time we were there during the dry season, so I would hate to be here during the rainy season.

The last day of tours started with a van ride to the main Soccer stadium, Estadio Nacional. There we got on the VIP bus for their version of the big red bus. We got off several times for a walking tour that made it a good immersion in the way of life in Costa Rica. Everyone was very friendly and the prices for everything was very reasonable.

The San Jose airport is twenty miles from the capital of Costa Rica, San Jose. Traffic on the way back reminded me of trying to get from the airport to the hotel in Dublin. The reason was two-fold: First, everyone got their holiday bonus checks that day, so everyone was out shopping. Second, that Saturday was their annual holiday light festival, so they were putting grandstands and food stands up all around town, which closed down many lanes of traffic.

Our third voyage with the Windstar Cruises line took us back to where it all began one year ago. Turns out this seven-day cruise would end on December 19, the same day one year ago that we got on a Windstar cruise in St. Maarten to start this nomadic lifestyle.

I had a book I had been carrying around for a while and looked forward to replenishing the old vitamin D while sipping on a cold blended drink and watching the world slowly go by as I occasionally looked up from my book. It was an uneventful passage through the Panama Canal, and as always, we did meet a few of our "new best friends."

About a month prior to our trip, I got an email from Delta Cruise, where you get rebates, miles, and a personal agent to assist you. The email said that Windstar had upgrades for $500, so I jumped on the offer. On the ship, I learned from our new best friends Barbara and Bob from Naples that you can simply ask while on board, and if upgrades are available, you can get one for free. They had managed to do this since the ship was only three-quarters full.

As we were preparing to leave for dinner the second night, I noticed a stain on our bed cover. I did a quick clean-up job, and off we went for an incredible meal. Upon arrival back at our cabin after dinner, I noticed a typewritten letter on our bed apologizing for the water leak in our cabin. The stain was now much larger, and looking up, I could see the water dripping from the ceiling overhead.

We went to reception and asked for another cabin. We were given keys to one of the "owners' cabins," as they are called. Needless to say, it was huge. It was the perfect place to have a few of our new best friends over to watch the Canal crossing from our party balcony.

A few folks were a bit upset over the fact that due to the relatively small size of our yacht, as it was called, we had to go through the locks at night. The big ships go through during the day. It was all lit up, so it wasn't a problem for us. We hit the first lock right after dinner at 8:00 p.m. and the last on at two o'clock the next morning.

As we transitioned through the various locks, our yacht's big screen showed the Nova movie on how the Canal was built. We also had a lady on board who gave us a blow by blow of the process over the PA system. Watching the whole process in action, it was amazing to know that it was built over one hundred years ago, despite all the obstacles and lack of equipment they had to solve many of the engineering problems that had to be solved. This should be on everyone's bucket list. We call ours the "Life List."

The seven-day cruise took us from Port Puerto Caldera to Quepos, where we went for a run, then on to Bahia Drake, Puerto Jimenez, and Isla de Coiba. There we had the traditional private island barbecue. We stopped at Balboa/Fuerte Amador and then went through the Panama Canal. At the last stop, we ran along the causeway to the Biomuseo, a museum focused on the natural history of Panama, whose isthmus was formed very recently in geologic time. The structure of the building had some very dramatic geometrical shapes. I never did open up the book I had planned on reading.

The next morning, we departed the ship in Colon, which is on one side of Panama, and then got in a bus for a ninety-minute ride back to Panama City where we stayed at the Marriott Executive Apartments, right in the middle of downtown. The best description I can come up with is that Panama City is a tale of two cities: one for the "haves" and the other for the "have-nothings."

The tall skyscrapers looked illusive with the sun beaming off their windows, but at street level, it was an entirely different story. Large pockets of the city were up to their ankles in the garbage, cluttered with broken-down, rundown, and—in some cases—abandoned buildings. Quite a contrast to say the least, but the people, for the most part, seemed friendly and happy.

One part of town called, Casco Antiguo, had once been overrun by gangs, but the government had solicited their help to revitalize the area—with some success. A ten-block square area had all the shops, restaurants, and bars, but outside that area was still a mess. They did have one heavily used Metro line (with plans for three more), along with a slew of jazzed-up busses filled to the brim that crisscrossed the city.

What about those crazy buses blaring music? They're called the *diablos rojos* or red devils. If you want to sample a ride on one, you'd best be quick because they're being phased out. Each diablo rojo bus is owned individually. They are decorated to the taste of the owner/driver to attract passengers. They often travel with their door open to give occupants a cooling breeze.

Later that day, we drove to the airport to pick up Catherine's daughter Christie and her family, who were there to spend the week of Christmas with us. Driving in Panama is a cross between New York and Tahiti. In other words, anything goes, and this was the first time my iPhone app refused to give me directions. I had to use Google Maps, and since some streets didn't have street signs, stop signs, or lights, it was a challenge to not get run down or totally lost. It usually only takes me a few days to get somewhere without my phone in turn by turn in my lap, but in Panama City, it took me the entire week.

Horn-blowing was a common practice in Panama, but using turn signals was not—instead you blew your horn when you were making a left or right turn from the outside lane. You also blew your horn when you didn't want someone to do something with their car, like changing lanes as you approached them. Cabs, which made up 75 percent of the cars on the road, blew their horns when they thought pedestrians might want a ride. If we were waiting at a corner to cross, they would slow down, blow their horn, and ask, "Do you need a ride?" We kind of got used to it after a while.

Meanwhile, we had a fantastic time at the pool, the Meso rainforest, and seeing the dry land view of the Panama Canal and Old Panama. We enjoyed some authentic Panamanian dishes, and since Christie is fluent in Spanish, I was able to sit back and relax instead of me trying to figure out what people were trying to say to us. We were even able to get in one short run at sunrise along Panama Bay, and it was spectacular.

Christmas evening was very special. Seemingly everyone in Panama City made their way to the water. Not to get in, since Panama City water quality does not allow for actual beaches, but to be out by the water. We made our way to the area called Amador, where the cruise ship had docked; and even there, people were out on rental bikes, scooters, walking, running, or simply watching the Christmas evening full moon, which was beautiful.

They call Panama a "developing country," and my impression was that it still has a long way to go. The expats are rushing into the hills and high rises, but no one is paying attention to the details that might make this a great place to live. I had high hopes, having read so much about it in International Living Magazine and other publications, but I doubt if I'll ever be back. I felt the same way about Belize and Tahiti, so the quest for the perfect place to live continues.

Our next adventure was going to be a Caribbean Running Cruise out of Tampa with our buddies at Marathon Expeditions. Prior to the cruise, we were spending some time in the Crib in Orlando, Florida, when I got word that my ninety-four-year-old dad had passed away. So off to NY we went. There was a big storm headed for the northeast, so we were going from sun and fun to the eye of the storm.

His memorial service was the next day, so we resolved to give our best effort to be there. I was sure there would be many twists and turns, but our cruise ship left in eight days, and I figured one way or another we should make it back to Tampa by then. As I told someone the other day, "We don't have a home, so it really doesn't matter where we spend the day or night."

Our next stop was the Delta lounge at the Orlando airport for breakfast. Halfway between my decaf and oatmeal, I got a message on my phone that our flight has been canceled. The agent rebooked us on the delayed 2:30 p.m. flight, and I was back to my oatmeal. I was prepared for a long day, so all was still good.

Not so fast, as they say. The agent came by mid-swallow and gave us new boarding passes for our original flight. The reason given was that the computer was supposed to have canceled the same flight for tomorrow but was a day off. Just the thought of all that rebooking made me chuckle. On to my fresh fruit.

Of course the flight was delayed, and since the original estimate was forty-five minutes, they gave folks the option to get off the plane. That sounded like a reasonable idea, but something told me that someone was going to get left. No more than ten minutes later they announced that they were cleared to leave right away.

We arrived in New York ready for the snowstorm of the century, which was headed our way on the day of the memorial service for our dad. During his remarks, one of Dad's best friends chose to pick one word to describe him. That word was "stubborn." He didn't want a service, and the storm was his way to try to have the service canceled. As his kids, I guess you could say that trait was passed down to us. Even though cars were banned from the roads, we trudged through the knee-high drifts and crowded subways. We were so determined that we had decided to would walk the entire way back to our hotel, in fifty-mile-per-hour winds, if the subways were shut down. We all had a good chuckle on his behalf. As my sister Sarah put it during her remarks, "I'm sure he is sitting on his perch laughing his ass off."

Judson G. Parker, Sr. was born in Washington, DC, on March 25, 1921. His early years were spent in Tarboro and Durham, North Carolina. He received a BS from the Philadelphia College of Pharmacy and a Master's Degree in Social Work Administration from Columbia University. Before retiring in 1988 from the City of New York Human Resources Administration, he served as a top administrator under Mayor Ed Koch. Although he lived in many places and traveled the world, he was a New Yorker at heart.

That urge to travel the world was another trait he had passed down, and his funeral inspired me to continue running all over the world as long as I could.

Our New York odyssey finished up appropriately at a nice, quaint, restaurant/bar called the Drunken Monkey. There we met this energized waitress who was also a runner and had run the Denver Marathon, which we were scheduled to run on Catherine's birthday, May 1, 2016. We told her our story and that all we had was two suitcases and two backpacks. She said that some people "truly believe the world is their possessions," and I was happy to think that, with our lifestyle, our most precious possession was the world.

# CHAPTER
# 13

# How to Not Go Overboard on a Cruise Ship

To move, to breathe, to fly, to float/To roam the
roads of lands remote/To travel is to live.

—Hans Christian Anderson

Y ou hear it all the time: "I put on ten pounds while on the cruise ship, and now it will take me a month to get back into those jeans that I love."

The other misgiving people have about the typical cruise ship experience is the many hours of just sitting or lying around at the dinner table, during the many off Broadway-type shows, in the lounge chairs, at the casino, or being rocked to sleep in your two-by-four cabin. John "The Penguin" Bingham and Jenny "The Coach" Hadfield have the answer for you.

The idea that these two life coaches came up with ten years ago is to combine all the benefits of cruising and staying fit into a seven-to-eight-day adventure that you will write home about. We first met up with John and Jenny (otherwise known as "J and J") back in 2011.

The gist of the program is to bring a manageably sized group of like-minded runners/walkers to different regions to do a staged marathon or half-marathon over the course of the week. The great part is that you don't do it all at once, but when all is said and done, each

individual has completed either 26.2 or 13.1 miles. If you're the traditional competitor, this might not be for you. Each race has a first-
place winner for both males and females, and the winners get the
coveted yellow hat. (My understanding of the premise of the yellow
hat is to mimic the Tour De France's yellow jersey, with the exception
being that you get to keep the hat.)

What constitutes winning each day is actually calculated by
J and J. It might be the absolute fastest time among the men and
women or something as random as who gets the king of hearts out
of the deck of cards as they are handed out when you cross the finish
line.

The last race on the trip is the one we all look forward to. They
call it the Amazing Race. Groups of two to four crisscross the major
tourist attractions, from churches to fountains, with the goal of being
the first ones across the finish with a picture of the group in front of
each tourist attraction, in the proper order.

Both Catherine and I already have our autographed yellow hats,
so what brings us back is enjoying the company of like-minded individuals in the most picturesque of settings while keeping a reasonable
exercise routine going. That exercise surely comes in handy when
trying to counterbalance the endless opportunities to eat, lounge,
and sleep.

A very important quality each participant must possess is flex-
ibility. You are on and off a cruise ship for seven or eight days, so if
you're one of those who insists on the race starting at 8:00 a.m. sharp,
you might want to keep collecting states or continents. The most
memorable upside was another Caribbean excursion a few years back
where, not only were we the first ones off the ship in Aruba, but also
got a police escort to the race start where the roads were closed for
our 10K race along the coast. The local running group put the race
together for us, including an official clock at the beach finish with
coolers full of beer and soft drinks and barbecue to eat as we cooled
down our legs in the water.

If you're one of those types who calculates all your marathons
down to the penny, since you are doing thirty to fifty a year, you'll
need to take a chill pill before signing up. They say money can't buy

happiness, but this comes pretty darn close. We're planning our seventh trip with them since we've found it to be a very cost-effective way to enjoy the benefits of cruising and living an active lifestyle.

John and Jenny are the proverbial who's who when it comes to running. John has brought millions off their couches to the sport of running/walking, and Jenny coaches just as many to reach their goals from just completing their first marathon to qualifying for the prestigious Boston Marathon.

John is a featured columnist for Competitor Magazine and his popular column, "The Penguin Chronicles," ran for fourteen years in *Runner's World* magazine. Known by fans as the Penguin for his back-of-the-pack speed, John writes and speaks about his childhood dreams of athletic glory, sedentary years of unhealthy excess, and a life-changing transformation from couch potato to "adult-onset athlete." He has inspired many to get off the couch, put out the cigarettes or put down the bottle, and lace up your shoes. With his trademark sense of humor, he reminded us not to worry about where we came in during the race and to embrace the thought of getting healthy by simply showing up.

Jenny "The Coach" Hadfield is the coauthor of the best-selling Running for Mortals and Marathoning for Mortals book series as well as a columnist for *Women's Running* magazine and RunnersWorld. com. Jenny practices what she preaches and is an accomplished endurance athlete, having competed in over forty marathons all over the world including the Boston Marathon, the Antarctica Marathon, and three of Mark Burnett's Eco-Challenge Expeditions.

My personal take on this duo is that John is the inspiration and Jenny is the brains of the pair. Jenny often quizzed us over a beverage about where else in the world we could possibly go, and from those intense conversations blossomed our Florence, Danube, and (soon to be) Southern France adventures. John kept us inspired in between bouts of sheer laughter.

Our Caribbean running cruise had plenty of twists and turns to keep the dynamic duo on their toes. It started out very calm with the evening welcome event, where the Embassy Suites Hotel offered drinks and snacks to loosen up those of us who came in a day early.

The Gasparilla Pirate Festival was going on that weekend, so we got our fill of much-needed pirate outfit ideas.

The next morning, we were off to stretch out the old legs along the water on a slow two-mile run. The Vision of the Seas cruise ship, our home for the next seven days, was a short walk away. After the mandatory safety drill, all 142 of us met in our new meeting spot, Some Enchanted Evening Lounge. There we got an overview of the upcoming week's events and races.

In Key West, Florida, we were met by the local running club and ran either a 5K or 10K, with the winner being the fastest male and female in each race. We chose the 5K to give us more time to view the buoy making the southernmost spot in the US—and to visit my namesake, Captain Tony's Saloon.

After all that we were back on board for a day at sea and a 5K race on the deck. The boat was pitching, but we had felt worse during the Alaska cruise. This was a "predicted time" race, so some might say the winner was somewhat random, but it was a lot of fun and there was cheering from everyone.

The next day we were back in Belize City. We had been here back in April last year, and it was nice to see the area from a different perspective. I wasn't impressed the first time, but seeing it through the lens of a cruiser was something of a contrast. They know where the money is, so they made sure we all had a great experience.

It turns out we made history by being the first to ever hold a race of any type at the Mayan Ruins of Altun Ha. It was a four-mile relay race, so Catherine and I did two miles each, a half-mile at a time. It was a bit hot, but after the race, the folks there gave us a tour of the largest temple-pyramids, the largest of which is the fifty-two-foot-high Temple of the Masonry Altars, which was quite a hike after a run.

On our last visit, we were not allowed to enter the cruise terminal, and it was a vast difference to the area just one mile away. Money talks and nobody walks. There were a couple of watering holes with music to choose from, and anything and everything you could ever want to buy on hand. My favorite phrase was, "I have all the junk you don't need at half the price."

Back on the ship, we learned that you can order two of each appetizer, entree, and dessert. I even saw someone order three deserts. As runners, we can eat anything we want. The folks in our group were not the types who try to win each race.

The next day the seas won and we were unable to make land at Costa Maya or, as we called it, Costa Maybe. This was a first for J and J, but they called an audible and put on a couple of deck events. The ship supplied champagne, and we all racewalked a few laps around the top deck on the ship while drinking a glass of champagne in between laps. I made it to the final round but Harry, the professional racewalker, beat me out. I did come back with a team victory for the spoon egg carry.

Some might have noticed by now that the mileage, so far, is not near where you would think it would be for either a marathon or half-marathon. Turns out that J and J had decided that it wasn't feasible to have people out running or walking that many miles in the Caribbean heat and humidity. No complaints here, but for those who need to accomplish more mileage in a week, do as some of us did and just keep running or walking. Others in the group simply found a nearby race when we got back on land at the end of the cruise.

Our final race of the week was the Amazing Race in Cozumel. We didn't really get all dressed up, but some of the folks on this trip went all-out with their pirate costumes. I even saw a few stuffed birds on their shoulders. At the start, everyone took off in one direction each clutching their maps and clues, while we went in the opposite direction to get in a good two-mile run. We all finished up at Margaritaville, and some took an extra stop at Senior Frogs at the cruise terminal.

Only about half of us made it to dinner that evening. We were now back at sea for the trek back to Tampa, and the boat rocked and rolled the whole way back. It did make for an interesting awards ceremony in the Majestic Theater at the front of the ship.

Besides the overall winner presentation, J and J also select their Inspiration, Dedication, and Perspiration awards. It was a very pleasant surprise for Catherine and me to be awarded the Inspiration award for our cutting-edge approach to running all over the world. I sometimes have to tell her and remind myself that if it was easy, anyone would be able to do it.

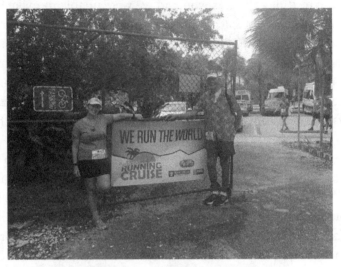

I could not say it better myself.

# CHAPTER
# 14

# Does Running Slow Down Alzheimer's?

> What is good for the heart is also good for the brain.
> —Robert Roca

As we were running all over the world, dealing with physical, logistical, and financial issues, sometimes I couldn't help asking myself, "Is this really helping Catherine?"

Before I answer that question, here's some context. According to the Alzheimer's Association, an estimated 5.8 million Americans have the disease. Alzheimer's doesn't just cause dementia: It kills more Americans than breast cancer and prostate cancer combined. Since 2000, deaths from the biggest killer, heart disease, have gone down 7.8 percent while deaths from Alzheimer's have gone up 146 percent.

Many people think of Alzheimer's as genetic bad luck, but scientists have also been studying associations between Alzheimer's and a variety of lifestyle choices. In the report, "Dementia and Risk Reduction: An Analysis of Protective and Modifiable Factors," Alzheimer's Disease International identified four categories of risk factors: developmental, psychological, lifestyle, and cardiovascular—all of which have been repeatedly linked to Alzheimer's.

Most doctors and nurses who treat Alzheimer's patients now believe that common-sense lifestyle adjustments can help people avoid the disease or slow its progression. As Robert Roca, vice president of medical affairs at Baltimore's Sheppard Pratt Health System said in an interview with the Woman's Brain Health Initiative, "The good news is that if you take simple steps that are beneficial for your overall health, you can reduce your risk."

We've all seen the PSAs about quitting smoking and the ads telling us to eat this or that "heart-healthy" food, but partly because we know less about it, there has been less public education about Alzheimer's. As it turns out, some of the same choices and habits that protect against heart disease (including regular exercise) also protect against Alzheimer's. "What is good for heart," Roca said, "is also good for the brain."

Ann McKee, the associate director of Boston University Alzheimer's Disease Center, agreed. "The brain and the heart actually have a lot in common. Both organs are responsive to what is going on in the rest of the body—and to our life experiences."

When it comes to treating the symptoms of Alzheimer's, there are five FDA-approved drugs. Unfortunately, according to Robert Stern, director of the clinical core at Boston University's Alzheimer Center, "Medications can bring about some improvement for some people some of the time, but they don't modify the course of the disease."

In fact, according to David Bennett, director of the Alzheimer's Disease Center at the Rush University Medical School, "The best current tool involves not taking medication but building up resilience."

Bennett said that people who got more education early in life have a greater amount of "cognitive reserve"—a technical term for a variety of cognitive skills—which can help them compensate for the damage to their brains. And no matter how educated someone is, they can improve their resilience by learning new skills. In an article for Scientific American Mind called "Banking Against Alzheimer's," Bennett wrote steps that we can all take to age-proof our brains to make them more resistant to dementia: remaining socially and intellectually active, achieving goals that we set for ourselves, and even helping others. I would say that our nomadic lifestyle forces us to do all those things.

It's hard to say exactly how much benefit Catherine got from our constant flow of new experiences, but Yaakov Stern, a professor of neuropsychology at Columbia University's Taub Institute for Research on Alzheimer's Disease and the Aging Brain who has published several papers on cognitive reserve, has said that "...experiences acquired over a lifetime can stave off dementia—often for several years."

What's easier to say is the benefit she got from regular cardiovascular exercise. Aerobic exercise protects against Alzheimer's through its impact on the heart, but it can also slow down the deterioration of the brain. In a neuroimaging study published in the Annals of the New York Academy of Sciences in 2007, Bonita L. Marks, a professor in the department of exercise and sport science at the University of North Carolina at Chapel Hill, showed that greater aerobic fitness was associated with more white matter integrity in several regions of the brain. A 2016 paper published in Alzheimer's Dementia, by Dane Cook (not the comedian but a professor of kinesiology at the University of Wisconsin at Madison) showed that regular physical activity can protect against temporal lobe atrophy.

What does "regular physical activity" mean? One book I read called Cured has an entire section on Alzheimer's and exercise. It turns out that merely exercising several times a week is not enough. It's great to get your ten thousand steps a day, but to reap the true benefits, you need to participate in intensive exercise for at least thirty minutes at least four times a week. Other articles I read recommended an hour day at least six days a week.

The science behind the need for this much exercise is complicated, but the bottom line is that you need to get your heart rate up, you need to sweat, and you need to be worn out when you're finished. They say that it reduces the inflammation in the brain, which they feel is the root of the problem. As time goes on, I have read more and more about inflammation, and I have adjusted Catherine's supplements to help with that issue. Since I'm not doing a clinical trial, I can't give a scientific answer as to whether running helps, but it certainly doesn't hurt.

Our travels, coupled with our exercise routine, have given us the ability to run marathons and other various race distances so far. It will give us the ability to continue this lifestyle as long as feasible.

I have found that it satisfies Catherine's desire to regularly exercise, compete in races, and see new sites. It definitely wears her out so she can get plenty of sleep, which is highly recommended for people with Alzheimer's.

# CHAPTER
# 15

## We're Supposed to Be Here

> Permanence, perseverance and persistence in spite of all
> obstacles, discouragements, and impossibilities: It is this, that
> in all things distinguishes the strong soul from the weak.
>
> —Thomas Carlyle

I took the phrase "we're supposed to be here" to heart during our next two adventures. In retrospect, this was what we were supposed to be doing. With all that was and is going on in the world, you really can't put things off until tomorrow anymore. I recently heard of the passing of two UPS pilots that were both my age. They put up a good fight with cancer, but neither of them won. I'm sure they both had big plans for their retirements.

Life is entirely too short, so we were doing our best to do as much as we could in the undetermined time we have left. We both really enjoyed our visits to Brussels and Istanbul last year, but we would never return. We were supposed to be there when we were there.

All that being said, why would anyone go to Tel Aviv to run a half-marathon?

A few answers came to mind, in no particular order:

- Because I can.
- It sounded like a good idea at the time.

- Because it was on the calendar of Marathonguide.com, the road racer's bible.
- We had a tough race schedule of eight marathons, three half-marathons, and one very hilly twenty-one-miler last year, so we wanted to start off easy.
- Because I had some miles and points to use.
- Because we don't have a home and have to be somewhere.

The trip to Tel Aviv was like an endurance race itself. I figured it would be about twenty-seven hours from the time we checked out of the hotel in Atlanta to when we checked back into another Marriott hotel. A mere 6,420 miles apart. We departed at 8:40 p.m. from Atlanta to Paris's Charles De Gaulle. This is my least favorite airport. I never schedule less than two hours to make it through that maze.

The world has changed a lot since I was a kid. A trip overseas was a piece of cake then, but now it's a totally different story. Each airport has its own way to combat terrorism, and as I have often said, "I really don't care what they make me do, just as long as the plane doesn't blow up." You hear folks complain all the time, but I like the fact that they keep us passengers guessing. Better safe than sorry is my motto.

Terrorists want us to stay home and fear the world, but I refused to stop doing what I loved to do, and going to Israel was another example for my list. Not only that, they were the ones that invented airport security. It would be interesting to see it up close and personal.

At customs and immigration in Tel Aviv, we chose the slowest line and the one where the officer gave everyone the tenth degree. "Why are you here? Where are you staying? For how long? Let me see your return ticket." The other folks were only getting stamps and smiles in their lines. When the officer asked me "Why are you here?" I was prepared with a quick answer: "To run the half-marathon on Friday." I think she was impressed.

Our Renaissance Hotel was on the beach of the Mediterranean Sea and smack-dab in the middle of Tel Aviv. I was highly anticipating plenty of runs along the sea. A very healthy breakfast buffet was included, with a state-of-the-art fitness center and an Olympic-sized pool to keep the calories in check. The Tel-O-Fun Bike rental system station right down the street made it effortless to get around town easily.

The next day, we were off for a full-day tour of Jerusalem. It was an hour drive to our panoramic view of Jerusalem from the Mount of Olives. We also had a great view of the Mount of Mariah, where Jesus was crucified. From there, we stopped at Mount Zion to visit King David's tomb, the room where the Last Supper took place, and the Dormition Abbey. After another short ride, the walking tour continued with a visit to the Old City and a walk through the Armenian and Jewish Quarters to the recently excavated and restored Cardo, the Roman Road.

We went on to see the Western Wall, otherwise known as the Wailing Wall, where we left notes praying for Catherine and her Alzheimer's. In the Christian Quarter, we walked along the Via Dolorosa and visited the Church of the Holy Sepulcher. After the Old City, we went for a nice, leisurely self-guided tour of Yad Vashem, the memorial to the Holocaust. A number that will forever stick in my mind was that 1.5 million children had perished one way or another.

We had a quick twenty minutes for lunch in an area that reminded me of the Grand Bazar in Turkey. I didn't much like the thirty-minute stop at the tour guide's designated souvenir store. This is typical for all tours, so you kind of get used to it. More than half the people in our group bought something, so I guess it was worth the stop—for them, at least.

Getting to the start of the half-marathon, which was four miles from the hotel, was going to be a bit tricky. Since all the roads to the start were closed, a taxi would only get us so close. The train stop was near the start and finish, but the nearest station was more than two miles away. Walking the four miles was also an option, but the Tel-O-Fun bike rental system seemed to be the best bet.

There was a station on the way to the start, so with a swipe of a credit card, we were on our way. They charge a daily access fee and then start charging for usage after thirty minutes. So if you get it to the next station by then, you are only charged a small fee for that day. They had a large holding pen set up at the start, we were able to check our bikes in and then check out another bike for the ride back to the hotel.

That was simple enough and was a good four-mile warm-up before the race. The race itself was one of the best I've ever done. I was really starting to prefer half-marathons over full marathons. No real issues with the body, and recovery was a snap.

We decided to start at the very back of the pack for several reasons. I figured if anything strange was to happen that would have already occurred before we had even arrived. I felt very safe, but with all that is going on in the world, better safe than sorry. Also our very good friend and running coach, John "The Penguin" Bingham, has always talked about starting at the very back of a race. We had plenty of time to complete the half, so I figured this would be a good race to do so.

At the back of the pack, you get to see all those who might be making their first attempt at such a distance, and you're able to give them much-needed encouragement. There was plenty of organizational support, and our course took us right by our hotel twice, with several miles along the road adjacent to the beach. There was not a lot of fan support, but I figured with all the races they had going on that day, everyone must have been running or walking in one. The race is held on a Friday simply because road closures on Saturday and Sunday were out of the question. Sunday is actually the start of their workweek, with Friday and Saturday being their weekends.

They are big into their pubs in Tel Aviv. Something else that was a stand-out for me was their cocktail bars, where they take pride in mixing some one-of-a-kind drinks. At a place called Moonshine, all their drinks were based on the moonshine concept. It was happy hour, so we were able to sample four different drinks, and they all seemed to come in different, unique glasses.

This usually does not happen, but I must say, seven nights was just not long enough in Tel Aviv. The people are incredibly friendly. It was kind of odd: They seem to be in their own world, speaking Hebrew, but when asked a question they spoke some of the best English and went out of their way to help you. There were too many examples to list here, but it was a pleasant surprise to be on the other side of the world but, in many respects, to be that welcomed.

Our journey back to Atlanta started with a 3:30 a.m. local wake-up and a sad face by Catherine as we got in the cab to the airport. We gave ourselves plenty of time, but leaving Tel Aviv was a quick process. Other than a checkpoint where an armed guard peeked inside every car, it was nothing much out of the ordinary.

Hindsight being twenty-twenty, I have come up with the answer to the question "Why would anyone go to Tel Aviv to run a half-marathon?" It's a great city with outstanding people and an incredible race.

When we got back to Atlanta, we decided to modify our goals moving forward. I would do the Boston Marathon in April, which would mean we both will have completed the six world major marathons. Catherine was only five states away from completing a marathon in all fifty states (I was seven states behind her), so on May 1, we would go to Colorado, since both of us need that state, but we would only do the half. Our goal now was to complete either a full or half-marathon in all fifty states. Then we would do a full marathon in Prague, only because they don't have a half distance.

I don't usually modify my goals, but as I have learned in life, especially as time moves on, you have to remain flexible. We would still do five to eight half-marathons a year. Tel Aviv taught both of us that half-marathons are much more fun and you can have much more fun afterward. We would probably do at least three more full marathons in the next five years since I'm a numbers person, and the goal of sixty-five marathons at the age of sixty-five sounded good.

After ten days in "The Crib" in various parts of Florida, we were off to Mexico City to run another half-marathon but this time it didn't start until 6:30 p.m. I was very apprehensive about this race. Mexico City is 7,500 feet above sea level. They are not noted for their air quality, and you throw in some humidity and that makes for a bad combination. This was a "Rock and Roll Series" race. They usually put on great races, but this was their first time doing Mexico City. I heard the first time they did Las Vegas at night it was a mess. People actually got lost on the course. We arrived three days before the race to help acclimate ourselves to the altitude.

The first night I woke up gasping for air. Two days before the race, we took a tour of the Teotihuacan Pyramids, which required a lot of steps to get to the top of the Sun Pyramid. We were on our feet all day and had no altitude problems, so I felt like we were ready for the Sunday night run.

The hotel was across the street from the city's major concert venue, and the night before the race we noticed the place was set up for a red-carpet event. We went to see what was going on, and it turned out they were having a premiere of the Superman vs. Batman movie. Ben Affleck and the rest of the cast got out of their limos to cheers from the crowd and walked the red carpet to the viewing area. Next door to it was a military complex that had the largest flag I had ever seen. Some estimates were that the pole itself was five hundred feet tall.

I was watching the weather very closely, but it turned to be near perfect conditions. It could have been five degrees warmer, but I was dressed appropriately and I'd rather be a bit cold than hot.

They did a perfect job routing the race. We were mostly on wide well-lit streets and went by some of the most spectacular monuments and fountains. The downtown skyscrapers were all lit up, and we got to see the majestic JW Marriott Hotel competing for views with the full moon.

We started and finished at their horse-racing track where the infield was set up for a concert for the locals and the racers. Since this was a rock and roll race, they also had bands out on the course. It was strange to see fans out on the course paying more attention to the bands than to us going by. They even had food trucks/carts by the bands along the course—in case the fans got hungry.

Once again, we started near the back of the pack, and it came in handy for the last four miles of the race. That part was on closed sections of the highway, and by then people were walking up and down the long ramps. We were able to pass one after the other and got a great sense of motivation from each of them. Two miles out, we could see and hear the band off in the distance, and the infield was packed.

We worked our way closer and closer, bit by bit, and near the end, we ran between a band and its fans. They were screaming and singing to the music and gave us a great lift for the last one-half mile. We ran the backstretch of the racetrack on packed dirt and were able to have a very strong finish. When all was said and done, it was about the same time we typically do a half-marathon in but I was amazed that I never got into oxygen debt or got any cramps.

When we got back to the hotel, the staff had a table set up with fruit, water, Gatorade, and a sign saying "Mission Accomplished." That was an extra special sight after running the race. There is so much to see in Mexico City, so we will have to come back. And when we do, we will be sure to stay at the JW Marriott. The staff at the hotel made us feel like family. Once while we were sitting in the lobby for a few minutes, the manager on duty came up and asked if we needed anything. He gave us his card and told us if we ever needed anything to let him know. We got that same warm feeling from everyone we came in contact with at the hotel.

This was another one of those times when we really were not ready to leave. Like in Tel Aviv, the people here were so very friendly and actually went out of their way to help. When we left with our bags, every staff member at the hotel stopped what they were doing to say goodbye.

Mexico City is not perfect. I was glad we hadn't experienced a smog alert, when they only allow vehicles with odd or even last number on their tags into the city, depending on the day of the week. Also, I had never seen so many food carts on the side of the road, next to buildings, and even being pushed or pedaled down the street. It was a bit depressing to see ladies on the side of the road with their kid or kids alone with a cup in their hands. We had seen this before in our travels and had found it helpful to keep a pocket full of change to hand out as we passed them. It seemed to help me mentally to feel that I was helping out.

One unusual aspect of Mexico City was its taxis and buses. None of the taxis had meters, so they seemed to invent the fare out of thin air. I didn't feel that I was overcharged: in fact, the price we paid from the airport was a lot less than the hotel had listed as the usual fare. When we checked out, the hotel got us a taxi that I could pay a fixed fare. That was great since we always try to use up all the local currency before we leave a country. Also there was a discount for cash.

Traffic can be bad in Mexico City, but what they did for the buses, I had never seen before. They had bus-only lanes and cars couldn't get into those lanes due to barricades. So while the traffic was moving at a snail's pace, the buses were using the middle lanes in either direction and moving at normal speed.

As we walked the terminal for our gate, I was thinking how we were supposed to be in Tel Aviv on a peaceful day, and how we were supposed to be in Mexico City when the air was clear and the bands were playing their hearts out as we ran around the racetrack.

I was driven to travel to all these places by wanderlust, which I get honestly. My parents divorced when I was around eighteen, but I watched them closely in their sixties to eighties as they both traveled the world. Our mother would pack her bags for a few months of travel and would go from child to child, with stops to check on her condo in New York. She would often go on cruises and safaris with the grandkids. Our dad was known as a world traveler and would tell stories of his adventures in vivid detail. It's in my blood, and I was so fortunate that I found the right career, as a pilot, to live out those deep desires.

Sitting at the gate, I asked Catherine if she was tired of all this travel, and she simply replied no. It's in her blood as well. When she grew up, her parents were always taking the five kids on camping trips, and that made her an adult who was closing in on getting a marathon or half-marathon in all fifty states. Her mother, at eighty-one, informed us that she had just bought a mini motorhome and was off to Alaska to start a trip down to California.

We're destined to travel—or, better yet, to wander.

# CHAPTER

# 16

## The Boston Experience

The past is really almost as much a work
of the imagination as the future.

—Jessamyn West

Our next stop was Playa Del Carmen, which I nicknamed PDC. In my flying days, that stood for "Pre-Departure Clearance," the automated message you would get on your onboard computer for your route of flight that day. This was only fitting since we would be taking a close look at PDC as a place for us to settle down at some point in time. Not permanently, but maybe for a month or two at a time.

One plus was the fact that the first class was not in high demand on this route. We got an upgrade pretty easily, and there were plenty of empty seats on the two-and-a-half-hour nonstop flight from Atlanta. Catherine wanted to be near a beach, and our Airbnb was only five blocks away, so that was another plus.

The condo included not only a welcome basket with a bottle of bubbly but a fully equipped kitchen, so if we were to stay longer, we could save on the cash burn rate by cooking. At the rooftop pool, the lounges were in a few inches of water and a few steps away from the five-foot pool, which was not quite long enough for laps but easy to cool off in.

We ran or walked numerous miles while we were there. There were also plenty of sights to see nearby, but we decided to make this a tour-free trip because we only had a few days to rest before we left for Boston where I could achieve one more goal, I had set for myself.

Catherine qualified for the Boston Marathon back in 2002 and ran it a year later. She has held that fact over my head ever since. In 2007 I came within twelve minutes of qualifying with a time of 3:57, but I hated the entire race with me watching my watch the whole time. At about mile 19, I knew it was not going to happen and I slowed down the rest of the race. On the fly I set another goal to break four hours, so all was good—or so I thought.

I figured I would continue my training and as I got older and the qualifying time got longer, I would eventually qualify for Boston. About a year later, as I continued to slow down as opposed to getting faster, I realized that I would have to be around eighty-five to ever make the cut-off. I thought my slowing down was simply old age, but I learned in the spring of 2012 that I had a heart murmur, and you know the rest.

So how was I actually going to run the Boston Marathon? A simple answer would be that money does buy happiness in some cases. For those who want to run but don't have a qualifying time, there's a second way to get into Boston: to raise funds for one of their charities.

I was willing to go that route with a minimum fundraising amount of $5,000, but it turned out that, as long-time sponsors of the event, our friends at Boston-based Marathon Tours and Travel also get a few slots each year. I was selected for one of those coveted slots due to the amount of business we had done with them over the last five years and the fact that I was able to come back from open-heart surgery two years prior to be in a position to finish consistently under the six-hour time limit set up for the Boston Marathon. It would be my eleventh marathon since my operation. Only time would tell if I'd actually complete the course under that time limit, but I felt good about the possibility.

I could kill two birds with one stone by finally running the marathon itself with all its history, and also finish my sixth World Major Marathon. Catherine got her sixth last year, so now we would be on equal footing—sort of. Of course she'll always say that she actually qualified for Boston and that her fastest time in a marathon is eight minutes faster than my time. Who says we're not competitive?

I had another goal during the actual marathon, and that was to smile and enjoy the entire 26.2 miles. I planned on giving plenty of high fives and staying in the moment since I didn't plan on doing this again. I heard the fan support is outrageous.

My brother Garrett and his son Coleman and my sister Gwen were coming to cheer me along, and I hoped to run into a few racing buddies while there. Gwen was there for my first marathon in New York, so it would be a very special experience for me to have her here again.

We were planning dinner after the finish, so all I had to do was get there in time. I was a bit anxious, which was new to me. You would think, this being my sixty-third marathon, that this would be old hat for me. I came to the conclusion that the fact that I only had one chance at this made it truly a one-of-a-kind experience. I decided to handle it just like I did during my open-heart surgery. I was prepared, I was in great health, and I would just enjoy the ride.

The expo was like no other. We usually just go get our numbers and leave, but we had to take in the whole (crowded) experience. We stopped at the Marathon Tours and Travel booth to say thanks for the bib number and hug some of my favorite tour guides. And we had to buy some official Boston Marathon gear: a T-shirt and mug for me and a jacket for Catherine. I had bought my jacket a month ago and couldn't wait to wear it after the race.

After that, we were able to catch up with Mariellen, who lives in the area and was with us back in Dublin last year, during another Marathon Tours trip. We will meet up again in June at Easter Island. Her local running group was working the water stop at mile 12.

The day before consisted of getting one last look at the finish area from the perspective of a spectator. Next we were off to the pasta dinner hosted by Marathon Tours and Travel where, as usual, we ran into some runners from other adventures over the years. We swapped stories and had the pleasure to listen to two icons in the running community, Roger Robinson and Kathrine Switzer.

They gave away a few books and had some great stories to tell. Roger ran for England and New Zealand at the world level, set an overfifty record (2:28:01) at New York, and is the author of the acclaimed *When Running Made History*. Kathrine was the first woman to officially run the Boston Marathon fifty years ago, when she was twenty. She was now in training to do it one more time next year. We sat across the table from a lady who had qualified for the race for the third time at age seventy-five.

The race itself was an out-of-body experience. The bus to the start was at 7:30 a.m. to the parking area. On the way to the athletic village for security screening, the temperature was up to seventy-two in the Hopkinson area. It was ten degrees cooler back in Boston, so I just needed to get near there before I overheated.

My wave started at eleven-fifteen after a one-mile walk from the village. I was very surprised how much trash was left by the runners. They were going to run 26.2 miles but were too lazy to pick up their own trash. It took me another five or so minutes to get to the actual start and it was all downhill from there.

The first few miles are mostly downhill. I tried my best to stay on my 12:30 per mile pace, but just like everyone else got caught up in the downhill and screaming crowds, so the first five miles were just a bit faster than I had hoped.

I learned a trick from Mariellen, which was to reset your watch every five miles. It forces you to concentrate on the race five miles at a time, which helps mentally. The second five miles was more like rolling hills, and once again I was a bit ahead of my predicted pace. I figured I was going to need it later since the Heartbreak Hill of the course runs from mile 15 through 21. I ran into Mariellen at mile 12, where she was working the water stop for her local running team. The hug came in handy. I could hear the girls from Wellesley College, who were still about a mile away.

Up to then, I had given out many a high five and even a hug to a stranger at mile 5. The ladies at Wellesley required me to use both hands to give high fives to as many of them as possible. I was starting to slow down a bit, but all was good since I was still smiling and the crowds kept me going.

My family was waiting for me halfway up one hill just past mile 16, and after a few minutes of hugs and pictures, I was on my way again. I then had something happen to me that had never happened during a marathon before. Each of my leg muscle groups decided that they really did not want to go any further. I had been talking about how much I liked running half-marathons rather than marathons after our great experiences in Tel Aviv and Mexico City, so my legs started to rebel.

I still had five more miles of hills to go, so I put my head down and started to worry if I was going to be able to finish. None of my cramps forced me to stop, but each would give out that warning clampdown at random times. It didn't matter if I was running or walking, so I just kept going. At each water stop, I grabbed two cups of Gatorade and took all the electrolytes I had with me.

I made it up the actual Heartbreak Hill but must admit I had to walk it. I was now doing thirteen- and fourteen-minute miles, and the time I had in the bank looked pretty good right about now. It was pretty much all downhill into downtown Boston. The temperature had cooled off, but that wasn't a problem since I had some arm sleeves and my Paris headscarf to keep me warm.

I was now on pace to finish with a 5:30 total time, half an hour prior to the cutoff. My muscles started to cooperate, so it was back to giving the deserving crowds their much-needed high fives. There was another section where two hands were necessary, but my legs disagreed with that idea. It required me to run sort of sideways, and they clearly pointed out that was not part of the agreement.

I had a flashback to the bike portion of the Ironman competition, where I had to have a long talk with them to get to the transition area. The agreement back then was that they were going to work during the uphill, but I was to coast downhill. I felt so good near the end that I started pedaling downhill, and both calves screamed out for me to stop that. Once I complied with their request, we coasted into the transition area, and off we went on the run portion.

I was right before mile 25, which I was happy to realize was not 24 again. Math becomes increasingly hard during this phase of my marathons. One more hill to conquer and there was a long line of yelling and screaming fans along the right side, so I decided to take one more detour to give them what they wanted.

As I approached, I started yelling, "Get me up this hill!" over and over. My hand was out and everyone responded in kind with not only hits to my hand but also my back, and they got me up that hill. You could see the high-rise buildings in the distance and there were now police everywhere.

Right before the last turn onto Boylston Street, I heard my name and looked to the left. There was the gang from Marathon Tours and Travel! I ran over to give them all a hug. I was wearing my Marathon Tours and Travel T-shirt which they gave me years ago, so it was a great photo op.

I turned the corner, and there was the finish—but in this case, it seemed like two miles away. In reality, it was only about a half-mile since I did see the twenty-six-mile post off to the left about a quarter-mile away. The street was very wide and the barricades kept the spectators up on the curbs, but you could hear people yelling out various names on either side. By now there were not many of us running in, so I turned from side to side to see if there was anyone else that I knew.

Shortly, I heard a lot of people calling out my name, and when I turned to the right, I could see a large group chanting, "Tony, Tony, Tony." At first, I didn't recognize any of them, but in a second, I recognized Gwen and Catherine. I ran over and gave them hugs. Turns out the people near them asked what my name was so they joined in yelling out my name to be sure I didn't run by without noticing. I didn't expect them to be there, so it was a great surprise.

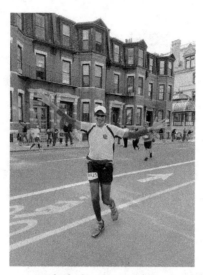

*Right before I turned final*

That lifted me to the finish, where I heard my name announced as I approached. It was a nice touch for them to add that I'm presently running all over the world. I remembered the days when I was a consistent midpacker, but finishing the Boston Marathon was nothing to sneeze at. More than 10 percent of registrants didn't start and another 3 percent didn't finish, and I was overjoyed I was not one of them.

Afterward, my brother, sister, and another running buddy, Lori, who works in the area met us for dinner which was quite a feat, since my legs were still trying their best not to cooperate. We cheered my success, and Catherine gave me a nod, knowing that her fastest marathon time was still intact.

# CHAPTER
# 17

## Running All Over the World Is Not for the Faint of Heart

Life begins at the end of your comfort zone.
—Neale Donald Walsch

You can look at this in two different ways: (1) It does take a pretty strong heart to do all the running that we do in a year, and (2) the world is not as safe as it once was. With the internet, there seems to be a heightened awareness of all the turmoil around the world. During our travels, we heard of bombings in places that we had just visited or were about to visit.

While we were recovering in Acapulco, Mexico, after the Boston Marathon, I got a message from one of our running buddies about a shootout that took place on the Sunday of our stay. It turns out that some drug lords were not happy with the recent arrest of one of their kingpins so they decided to take the vengeance to the streets.

Boston was one of the hardest marathons I had run to date. The course was tough and the late start and heat made it particularly hard for me. Running in the heat puts a strain on me in particular, and trying to get some running in during our time in Acapulco wasn't easy. We did manage to get in two runs, one on the beach and one on the road. Running in eighty-five degrees on loose sand was probably not the best of ideas, but as they say, what doesn't kill you makes you stronger.

Since my operation, I have a pretty good sense of how I feel, and I must say I did push my limits. For some reason, I don't sweat as much as the typical person, and the humidity didn't help. The good thing was that we did have a very nice pool to cool off in afterward, and I was even able to get in some laps on the days we did not run.

After Acapulco and eighteen hours in Atlanta, it was off to Fort Collins, CO, to check Colorado off Catherine's list of states where has completed a race. Her original goal was to complete a marathon in all fifty states, but we've decided that after one more marathon in Prague, we're going to cut back to only doing half-marathons for the next four years.

We were so glad we made the switch since when we got to Fort Collins the temperature had dropped from the sixties to the thirties. The race start was at 6:30 a.m. but the bus departed at five, so we stood out in the cold for an hour in light snow. I was so freezing that I broke down and put on someone else's discarded warm-up bottoms.

Catherine was layered, but for some reason, she really did not adjust to the cold weather. The folks that did the full marathon started at the same time we did but 13.1 miles further up the mountain, so I can only imagine what the cold must have been like. During the race, we kept telling each other how glad we were that we were not doing the full.

The race ended in the town square with beer and some entertainment, so I was happy, but since Catherine was still shivering, we caught the hotel shuttle back for the much-needed hot showers.

After twenty-seven hours on the ground in Atlanta, we were off to Prague, Czech Republic, for our final marathon for four years. Prague would be number 64 for me, and I decided to wait until I was sixty-five to do marathon number 65.

We connected through Paris Charles De Gaulle airport, my least favorite, and after a two-hour layover on to Prague, where we once again met up with our Marathon Tours and Travel folks. With a welcome reception that evening at the hotel, we decided to push through and stay up during the few hours between our arrival and the reception. With only a few hours of sleep on the plane, we usually crash out for a few more hours of sleep as soon as we get to the hotel.

It worked well. We both slept like babies that night and transitioned our body clocks to being six hours off better than ever before. The next day was a walking tour of the city where we were able to take in all the nearby sites. We were able to see Old Town, New Town, Lesser Quarter, and the Castle Town. We got to walk across the famous Charles Bridge and go up the 250 steps to get to Prague Castle and Saint Vitus' Cathedral. We didn't get to go inside since the lines wrapped around the building. and I could not stop thinking about all the cobblestones we were going to have to tackle the next day. The marathon start was in Old Town Square, and we ran back across the Charles Bridge early on in the race.

The race itself was very memorable. A 9:00 a.m. start and seven hours to finish made for a relaxing day. The start/finish was only one-fourth mile away from the hotel, so it was easy peasy as far as logistics went. Since we're so slow, we were in corral L, which was another one-half mile from the start. Our plan was to start at the very back, so we just waited near the start line, and when everyone had gone by, we jumped right in and we were the very last to cross the start line. The added advantage was that we were able to watch the seventy-nine elite runners take off. This was one of the last qualifying marathons for the Rio Olympics.

I'm not sure why, but for this race, I decided not to wear a watch. I guess I wanted to try something different for my last marathon for a while, and with the seven-hour time limit, I thought it would be a good idea. I didn't realize how strange it was going to be. To make matters more interesting, they didn't even have a clock anywhere on the course. I broke down at the halfway mark and pulled out my cell phone to get the time so I could figure how slowly we were going. At that point, we were pretty much on pace for our usual 5:30 to 5:45 marathon time. Shortly after that, the wheels came off of Catherine's wagon. It did not help matters that she was still fighting the cold she got while in Fort Collins.

The second half was not pretty, but we got it done and were able to finish once again, holding hands and all smiles. The race reminded me of Rome, which I did not much like. People everywhere going from major tourist site to the next and only a few that were actually cheering you on. Also, like Rome, there were cobblestones every-where. Catherine almost went down when she tripped on one sec-tion, but she somehow managed to stay on her feet.

I tried to stay motivated by giving out high and low fives as often as possible, but the decision to hang this up for a while was looking better and better. During our limited discussions during the race, Catherine pointed out that actually she wants to do two more marathons. One for my sixty-five and one for her to have eighty marathons.

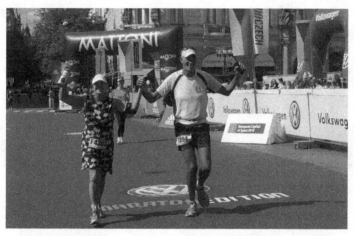

*Holding hands at the finish, marathon number 51, together*

After the race, eighteen of us with Marathon Tours and Travel toured Vienna for three nights and Budapest for three nights. I never thought I would ever do this, but a couple on the tour with us found a local chapter of the Hash House Harriers group who were having a run a few hours after we arrived. The Hash House Harriers (abbre-viated to HHH or H3) is an international group of noncompetitive running social clubs. An event organized by a club is known as a hash or hash run, with participants calling themselves hashers or hares and hounds.

At a hash, one or more members ("hares") lay a trail, which is then followed by the remainder of the group (the "pack" or "hounds"). Sawdust, flour, chalk, and toilet paper are used to mark the trail. The trail periodically ends at a "check" and the pack must find where it begins again; often the trail includes false trails, shortcuts, dead ends, back-checks, and splits.

These features are designed to keep the pack together despite differences in fitness level or running speed, as front-runners are forced to slow down to find the "true" trail, allowing stragglers to catch up. Members often describe their group as "a drinking club with a running problem," indicating that the social element of an event is as important, if not more so, than any athleticism involved. Beer remains an integral part of a hash, though the balance between running and drinking differs between chapters, with some groups placing more focus on socializing and others on running.

Generally, hash events are open to the public and require no reservation or membership, but most require a small fee, referred to as "hash cash," to cover food, drink, or other costs. The end of a trail is an opportunity to socialize, have a drink, and observe any traditions of the individual chapter. When the hash officially ends, many members may continue socializing at an "on-after," "on-down," "on-on-on," "apres," or "hash bash," an event held at a nearby house, pub, or restaurant.

Our hash was an easy four-mile run through some trails and the traditional "circle up" provided for some great entertainment. These folks did have some strict rules: You can only point with your elbow. You must have a cup or can of beer held over your head when you want to speak. You can't have a hat on while you're inside the circle.

Since we were visiting, they did give us plenty of opportunities to chug a few cups of beer while we were in the circle itself. Hashers love their somewhat lewd singalongs, and we finished up with a group picture. We joined them for an on-after at a nearby pizza joint and laughed all the way back to the hotel reliving the adventure.

The next day we took a city tour, and our guide pointed out that the ring road that started near our hotel basically went around in a circle for four miles that went by some very impressive statues, museums, and churches. It had very nice walking/running and bike lanes. We were a bit too busy to partake in a run, but it would be good to do when we come back in the future.

During the tour, we learned that Vienna had been voted the healthiest city in the world for numerous years. They also have the best quality water in the world. We got to tour St. Stephen's Cathedral, the Homburg, Imperial Apartments, and the Sisi Museum. We had been there before on a running cruise in 2013. Even though we had seen many of these timeless structures before, it was like seeing them for the first time.

We ate at one restaurant whose name was so long that they just called it 12A, which is the number of the building. When we arrived, we weren't sure we were in the right place, since it was completely empty. We enjoyed a typical Austrian meal consisting of beef goulash, boiled beef, and one of the best Champagnes I have had. It was so good that we bought an extra bottle for our boat trip to Bratislava the next day.

A high-speed catamaran goes there several times a day, and within seventy-five minutes we were in the country of Slovakia. We took a one-hour little red bus tour of the city and got some great views from Bratislava Castle. There were plenty of shops in the Old Town area, but since we usually don't buy anything unless we can eat or drink it, after a few hours we were ready for our boat ride back down the Danube to Vienna.

During our three-day visit, we were only able to scratch the surface of Vienna. The price of food was a bit high in both Prague and Vienna, but they are also both very clean cities, and the people seem friendly enough.

Keeping our average of 3.5 days per destination intact, we took a bus to Budapest. The location of our hotel, Novotel Budapest City, was not the best, but unlike everyone else I really didn't mind—we were across the street from a nice mall with a few great restaurants and grocery stores. We went for a five-mile run in the rain up to the Royal Castle area, and the next day, we went on a guided bus tour of the St. Stephen's Basilica, where I was, once again, mesmerized by the intricate stained glass domes. We saw Hero's Square and Kodaly Circle then finished off back in the Royal Castle area, where we had great views of the Danube River and the surrounding residential area.

The next day was our travel day to Helsinki. Since our flight didn't leave until 9:00 p.m., the hotel gave us a very reasonable half-day rate of $25. We were able to get a run-in at the gym and still have time for dinner across the street at the mall.

After the late-night flight to Helsinki and the time change where we lost another hour, we made it to bed around 2:00 a.m. local time. The sun was up at 5:00 a.m. and the blackout blinds did a fair job, especially since it rose right outside our window. Sunset was not until 10:00 p.m., so we got plenty of sunshine while we were there.

We were able to get in two six-mile runs and really enjoyed the mild temperatures (in the fifties). We had great views from our room and the executive lounge. Since we kind of went over budget for the first part of this trip, we ate all our meals in the lounge. We didn't have to sacrifice since they had delicious meals each day.

We were also able to enjoy the sauna in the hotel. Helsinki is noted for its saunas. They have more of them per capita than any other city. Saunas can be found in college dorms and just about every apartment has one. There's a nearby island that is full of them.

Some words of wisdom that I have received so far on this trip.

- If you think you can, you're right.
- If you think you can't, you're also right.
- Happy hour only lasts an hour.
- That beer is not going to drink itself.
- Trust but verify.
- Love is traveling the world together.

Our overall impression of Helsinki was very positive. The people speak perfect English and are very helpful. The Hilton did a great job of making us feel right at home. The temperature was perfect for running, but a tad colder than I would like. I bet this place is great in the summertime.

On our travel day to Amsterdam, we woke up to another example of how running all over the world is not for the faint of heart: Egyptair's flight from Paris to Cairo was missing. We were on a similar route from Paris to Tel Aviv back in February. I remember the fact that when we entered Egyptian airspace, we had to all remain seated for some unknown reason. I don't really think about aircraft crashes as we run all over the world, but stuff does happen.

Our hotel in Amsterdam, the Renaissance was an easy walk to anything you might want or need in Amsterdam. The only thing we couldn't find was the police. We walked around all the happening spots of Amsterdam for two days and only saw one on a bike and one in a car. I guess they figure who needs them if you make everything legal.

We found a very nice park about a mile from the hotel, and for some reason, I refused to learn my lesson that you can't go back a different way and not expect to get lost in Amsterdam. So many canals and so many streets going off on angles, making it impossible to just use your sense of direction to get you back to where you can come from.

I felt bad that we were only eating at the hotel's lounge again, but we're on a budget, even if it does sound a bit crazy when you all add it up. This limitation did help in another way: there were so many places to eat, so it saved us from making the difficult decision of where to eat.

Amsterdam is unlike anywhere else, for some obvious reasons and others not so obvious. The one that boggled my mind was the amount of money being spent there. There were people shopping everywhere and for everything, both for things that are legal everywhere and also for those things you can only buy here. It's not because the prices were that good, either. The shops were full, and so were the streets outside of them. Even in the rain, the place is packed, even on Sunday.

We have been places where the sales staff is out on the street trying to get people to come in to shop. Not in Amsterdam, where so many people were in each store that the sales staff was busy ringing up the sales. The only downside is that it was a rather dirty city. We have been places where you could eat off the sidewalks, whereas I would hate to even touch these sidewalks.

After five nights in Amsterdam, we were back in Atlanta for three days, then off to Charleston, South Carolina, for my middle child Shawn's wedding to his college sweetheart Cassie. All the family was flying in, so it would be good to see everyone together once again.

I often told Catherine that if running all over the world was easy, anyone could do it. We haven't run into anyone else doing this, and no one that we talk to seems interested in doing it themselves. They all comment on how they like the idea but don't see it fitting into their lifestyle.

Another way that our lifestyle was not for the faint of heart is the fact that we both seemed to catch a cold every two to three months. This time around I'm sure it didn't help to go from Mexico to Boston, back to Mexico, and then to Colorado and on to various parts of Europe. Once we started wiping down our seats on the airplane and the surfaces in our hotel rooms with a sanitizer, we stopped catching colds. We still use sanitizer on our hands all the time, hoping that will help. Our continual exercise routine keeps us in good shape, both in body and mind.

# CHAPTER
# 18

# The MINDSET Trial

We can't choose where we come from, but we
can choose where we go from there.
                                        —Stephen Chbosky

Since Catherine's Alzheimer's diagnosis, we had tried to get in various drug trials but hadn't met their criteria. They don't actually tell you why; they just say yes or no. A few months back, on a conference call put on by ALZ.org, we had learned about MINDSET, a Phase III clinical research program evaluating an investigational medication, RVT-101, for mild-to-moderate Alzheimer's disease.

Researchers were investigating how effective RVT-101, in combination with Donepezil (which Catherine was already taking), would be in helping with patients' cognition and ability to perform daily living activities, as compared with Donepezil alone.

Donepezil, the most widely used medicine to treat Alzheimer's, increases the level of acetylcholine, a vital chemical in the brain that helps with cognition and performing daily activities. It does this indirectly by preventing acetylcholine from being cleared from the brain, similar to blocking a drain. According to the MINDSET literature, "RVT-101 increases the release of acetylcholine directly, similar to turning up a faucet" so that in combination, RVT-101 and Donepezil should work together to increase acetylcholine by both turning up the faucet and blocking the drain.

The screening process for this study was extensive. It took three visits to complete all the verbal and written tests to confirm Catherine's level of cognitive impairment. She took a blood test, had an MRI, and underwent various neurological tests. They even had many questions for me to answer.

RVT-101 was an investigational medication that was available only through this clinical research program, so we were excited to be accepted into the trial. We did have to adjust our travel schedule, though, since the study included nine visits to the Atlanta Research Clinic over thirty-three weeks, the first four of which had to be exactly three weeks apart.

The first six months were a "double-blind" study, meaning Catherine would have a 50 percent chance of receiving RVT-101 and a 50 percent chance of receiving a placebo. After six months, all study participants had the opportunity to participate in a twelve-month "open-label" extension study in which everyone would receive RVT-101. The belief was that after that period of time, the drug would be approved and on the market.

When we finally got approval to enter the program, we were given a bottle that was simply listed as RVT-101 or Placebo. The questions they asked me about Catherine gave me a good idea of where she was in terms of cognition. They stated that previous studies had shown significant benefits, so we should see some improvements quickly or not.

The staff was skilled and understanding, and we both actually got paid: $80 per visit for Catherine and $60 per visit for me. We also felt good about taking an active role in finding a cure for this disease.

We believed that our nomad lifestyle was a benefit to her. I had noticed that Catherine hadn't really gotten worse in the eighteen months since we started running all over the world, so if we had to wait another six months before she will definitely get the new drug, it would be well worth it. I doubted her health would decline during that period of time.

After we made it through the first phase, we were approved for the second phase, which was getting the actual drug RVT-101. We had an entire day of testing, and I could say that she hadn't gotten much better, but she also hadn't gotten any worse.

Her short-term memory hadn't improved, but I must admit her cognitive skills had gotten better. It was interesting to watch the difference. There had been things she just figured she could no longer do, and I would have to take up the slack, but now I saw her trying to do those things. She has become more independent and self-assured.

As an example, she was trying to figure out where we were going in the future. She used to just rely on me but now wanted that information so she could refer to it on a calendar and not have to ask me several times a day. It wasn't easy for her, and from time to time there was frustration, but I applauded her for the effort. I truly believed that over time it would get easier.

After Catherine had been taking RVT-101 for a month now, in addition to her desire for independence, which was great, I also noticed that, instead of just taking things as they were, she now felt free to ask for things the ways she actually wanted them. At first, it was an adjustment for me because I would try to accommodate her requests, but then I figured out to allow her to make her own adjustments to her desires. In other words, if she wants something done a certain way, I now ask her to do it herself.

Her independence manifests itself in her desire to go for walks by herself. It's nothing major, but seeing her walk around the campground or hotel complex and return with a big grin on her face is something I came to cherish. I really looked forward to the one hundred or so questions they asked me at the MINDSET appointments because they gave me a great gauge of where we were and where we might be going in the future.

I truly believe they will find a cure in Catherine's lifetime, and as the doctor who came up with RVT-101 said, "Within the next five years, people like her will live a good life and will die from something else, just like everyone else." Until that time we will continue to enjoy each day that is provided to us.

The drug did, in fact, improve her cognitive skills, so after our last visit for the clinical trial, I tried my best to have Catherine continue in the program but was unsuccessful. To get into the program, we had to cut her dosage of Donepezil in half, so our first step after the trial was to increase that dosage again.

There was another clinical trial being done by a physician in the Atlanta area, but that would require RVT-101 to be entirely out of her system, which would take several months.

I also got a message from a friend that mentioned another study that sounded promising. Australian researchers had come up with a noninvasive ultrasound technology that clears the brain of neurotoxic beta-amyloid plaques, structures that are responsible for memory loss and a decline in cognitive function in Alzheimer's patients.

By oscillating super-fast, these sound waves gently open up the blood-brain barrier, which protects the brain against bacteria and stimulates the brain's microglial cells to activate. Microglial cells are basically waste-removal cells, so they're able to clear out the toxic beta-amyloid clumps that are responsible for the worst symptoms of Alzheimer's.

The team reported fully restoring the memory function of 75 percent of the mice they tested it on, with zero damage to the surrounding brain tissue. They found that the treated mice displayed improved performance in three memory tasks: a maze, a test to get them to recognize new objects, and one to get them to remember the places they should avoid.

They were hoping to get human trials underway in Australia at about the time Catherine would have to come off RVT-101, and I wouldn't mind if we had to live in Australia for a while. We were planning a half-marathon in nearby New Zealand in November anyway.

In the meantime, we decided to try a recode protocol developed by Dale E. Bredesen, MD, in his book *The End of Alzheimer's*. The premise is that the amyloid-beta plaques and tau tangles that develop in the brains of Alzheimer's patients are a perfectly normal response to an attack on the brain, so his protocol involves finding the underlying cause of those attacks.

Once the harmful identities are determined, a doctor develops a diet and prescribes appropriate vitamins and minerals. It sounded like we might have to go back on a gluten-free diet, coupled with stress reduction, adequate sleep, and exercise. We already had the last three covered.

Bredesen's book had gotten mixed reviews, but I was rapidly coming to the conclusion that this disease would not be defeated with a single pill. It would require a change in lifestyle, and we were more than willing to make those changes.

# CHAPTER
# 19

# There's a First Time for Everything

Every journey begins with the first step.

—Lao Tzu

Running all over the world thing is full of "first times," but our latest trip had more firsts than usual.

The twenty-day jaunt started with the wedding of Shawn to Cassie. I knew this day would come the first day I met her. I believe everyone had the same impression of the two of them. Gwen officiated at the wedding and used one-word "delight" to describe them.

Tropical storm Bonnie had plans to disrupt the outdoor wedding in Charleston, SC, but she was no match for the Parker clan. We left up the tent used by another wedding the day before, the clouds parted just prior to the ceremony, and the rain didn't begin again until we were all back at the hotel after the reception.

The next day, we were off to Santiago, Chile. After a nine-hour flight, which we both slept seven hours of, we safely arrived. For the first time in our experience of flying all over the world, we were in the same time zone after nine hours in the air.

After a hair-raising taxi ride where I had to give the driver directions, we arrived a day late for the events Marathon Tours and Travel had planned. We missed a day and a half of tours in Santiago, but after all the late-night festivities of the destination wedding weekend, we really needed the day to rest up.

There was a great mall nearby, and we actually did some shopping for things we couldn't eat or drink—another first. We didn't buy tourist trinkets—it was more like hair care products and cosmetics. As time went on, sometimes we weren't able to bring everything that would last the entire time we were away from Atlanta. Nothing was cheap in Santiago and very few people spoke English, but my pointing skills continued to serve me well.

The next morning, we all met in the lobby at 5:30 a.m. for our 8:30 flight to Easter Island. Running the half-marathon there was the real reason for us to come to Santiago, but it was strange to arrive and depart a major city without touring it or all least running its streets.

Due to time zone changes, our flight arrived two hours before it left. Our modified goal was to run a race of some sort in as many countries as we could, and Easter Island would make continent number 5 and country number 21.

We spent a day and a half touring the island. The tours included a visit to Orango, where we learned the history of Birdman. There were three periods in Easter Island history, and the time of the Birdman Cult was the second one. Each year, they would have a competition to decide who would lead the Rapa Nui. The competitors would dive down dangerous cliffs of Orongo and swim to the small inlet named Moto Nui, wait for the first bird egg of the season, and then swim all the way back to Orongo with the egg.

We stood on the edge of the cliff and could see the inlet off in the distance. At Anakena, a white coral sandy beach along the otherwise rocky coastline, we got to see one of the many Moais located throughout the Island. The Moais are human figures carved by the people of Easter Island between AD 1250 and 1500. The production and transportation of more than nine hundred statues is considered a remarkable creative and physical feat. The tallest is thirty feet high and weighs eighty-two tons.

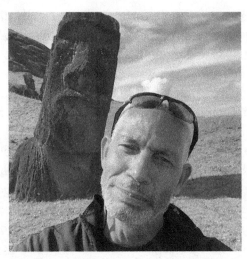

Most of the statue is underground

The arrangement of races connected to the Rapa Nui Marathon was unusual: They had the typical marathon and half-marathon on Sunday, but also a trail bike race the day before, either 35 or 70K. The day before that, there was a triathlon, either sprint or half Ironman distance. Each race had a limit of 250 participants. I'm sure there were some who did all three, but we stuck with the plan to run the half-marathon.

We went horseback riding to the highest point on the island on one of our free days. When we got to the top, we could see the entire island, but it was hard to even stand up since the wind was blowing at over 50 mph. The horses didn't seem to mind. The one I was riding on was rather short, and my feet almost dragged on the ground.

The hotel we stayed at the Hanga Roa Hotel was more of a resort, and another first was the fact that this hotel didn't have TVs in any of their rooms. There were some interesting restaurants nearby, including one that didn't have any electricity the day we ate there—so we dined by candlelight and flashlights.

Race day began with an outdoor opening ceremony where they blessed all the participants with an offering of meat and vegetables cooked in a ground pit. It was a great race, and once again, I didn't wear a watch and was able to take a lot of pictures of fellow runners since it was a mostly "out and back" type race. Catherine and I got third place in our respective age groups. We were both very happy that we didn't do the full marathon, since everyone who did said it was very challenging, and right now in life, we were preferring enjoyment over the challenge.

The next day we flew back to Santiago for a true touch and go. We were at the Holiday Inn at the airport for exactly six hours, followed by a 4:00 a.m. wake-up for a flight to Lima, Peru, connecting through someplace I had never even heard of before: Cusco, Peru. I had sweaty palms during the mountainous approach to the airport.

We spent one night there at the Aranwa Cusco Boutique Hotel. We were above eleven thousand feet elevation, so they pumped oxygen into the rooms and even provided portable oxygen bottles for anyone who needed them. They recommended chewing coca leaves and drinking coca tea, but my preference was the coca beer. I didn't have any ill effects from the altitude but did find myself catching my breath from time to time.

The restaurant we ate at that night served guinea pigs. I did partake, which was another first. The pig was tasty, but there was not a lot of meat on the bone, and I wished it had come with an apple in its mouth. In yet another first, I even had a piece of alpaca, which was a bit chewy.

They say that Cusco is the oldest city in South America, at over three thousand years old. We did a half-day tour of the city and got to visit the Inca fortress of Sacsayhuaman, Sexy Woman. Looking at the huge stone walls that surrounded the area, I found myself wondering once again, "How did they do that?" I think someone should come up with a contest to award a prize to the first group of folks who can move similar-size boulders from the mountains 40K away with only the tools that were available back then. We also got the opportunity to walk through a tunnel that was completely dark, and which our guide told us had cleansing properties. As always when we entered a church or a setting like this, we thought of Catherine's Alzheimer's, even though we're not very religious and more spiritual.

We took a very bumpy and curvy two-hour bus ride to the train station and then a ninety-minute train ride to Aguas Calientes, where we would start our tour of Machu Picchu. "Wow" is the only word I can think of to describe the train ride. We were basically following the Urubamba River all the way, with mountains on either side. We crossed the starting point of the Inca trail and saw a few folks taking the four-day trek on foot.

The train stop was within walking distance of our hotel, El Mapi by Inkaterra, which was smack dab in the middle of everything. As I always do, I turned on CNN; this time I learned of a terrorist attack in Tel Aviv. We had just been talking about how great our trip was when we were there in February, and how we wanted to go back next year. Not so much now.

The next morning, we were once again up at the crack of dawn to wait about forty-five minutes for the scariest thirty-minute bus ride known to man. A total of twenty-seven busses run the mostly one-way, switchback dirt road up to Machu Picchu. It is a dance they all do as they go up and down. The fact that they don't run into each other or off the road is a miracle itself.

You might think that, being so remote, the area would be somewhat behind the times, but I guess the constant flow of money to see one of the Seven Wonders of the World has brought all the technological devices to track everything you could ever want to see. All the folks on the trains and busses and at the venues were dressed in fashionable suits and ties or scarves.

The Seven Wonders of the World have changed over the years. The original Seven Wonders included the following:

- The Colossus of Rhodes
- The Great Pyramid of Giza
- The Hanging Gardens of Babylon
- The Lighthouse of Alexandria
- The Mausoleum at Halicarnassus
- The Statue of Zeus at Olympia
- The Temple of Artemis at Ephesus

The Seven Wonders of Modern World, according to the American Society of Civil Engineers, are:

- The Channel Tunnel
- The CNN Tower
- The Empire State Building
- The Golden Gate Bridge
- The Itaipu Dam
- The Netherlands North Sea Protection Works
- The Panama Canal

We had seen six of these, and if we made it to the border between Brazil and Paraguay, we could finish the list by visiting the Itaipu Dam.

On July 7, 2007 (7-7-07), an organization called New Seven Wonders announced a "new" Seven Wonders of the World based on online voting from around the world:

- Chichen Itza, Mexico
- Statue of the Christ Redeemer, Brazil
- The Great Wall, China
- Machu Picchu, Peru
- The Ancient City of Petra, Jordan
- The Roman Colosseum, Italy
- The Taj Mahal, India

We had been to a number of these but were still looking forward to someday seeing Chichen Itza, Petra, and the Taj Mahal.

On the first day in Machu Picchu, we did a tour of the main structure and then walked into the clouds of Sun Gate. We got some great views, but I must say that the hike up is not for the weary. At the top, where the Inca Trail ends, we saw a lot of people coming down to catch the bus back down to Aguas Calientes.

On the second day, we were once again in line at 6:00 a.m. for the terrifying ride up the mountain. This time we took the most difficult hike I have ever done up to Machu Picchu Mountain, which is also called the APU Hike. The planes I used to fly had APUs (auxiliary power units) and wished I had one for the hike. You actually had to sign a book as you entered and sign out when you get back down. I'm not quite sure which was the scariest since some of it was extremely steep and some of it was on very narrow, cliff-face trails. I had to face one of my demons, a very rare condition called the high-place phenomenon, where you want to jump off bridges or cliffs. You don't have suicidal tendencies, and they say no one with the condition has followed through, but I'm not sure how they actually know that.

I huffed and puffed like a freight train all the way up, which took over ninety minutes. In some cases, I was on all fours and tried not to look down the cliff face. On the way down I got a headache from concentrating so intensely. The last time I had concentrated that hard was back in my days as a pilot in training when you had to take off in the simulator in mountainside terrain, fully loaded, with one lost engine and the other on fire.

The train ride back to Cusco was very scenic, but this time they threw in a dancing devil routine and full fashion show. Back in Cusco, we pretty much stayed in bed right up to dinner. We found an Irish pub and were able to have another first since it was the highest Irish pub on the planet.

The next day was another travel day, but first we had to see the festivities. All of Cusco had been celebrating the competition among different dance schools all month, and over the weekend they took the celebration to the streets. With the bright costumes and impressive dance routines, it was like Macy's Thanksgiving Day parade—minus the floats and with judges and winners.

It is a really big deal to them and was a lot of fun to watch. We were also able to take a tour of the nearby church called, Basilica Cathedral. Unfortunately you are not allowed to take pictures inside, but I highly recommend the audio tour, which gives you the complete history of the first Christian church to be built in Cusco, which is also a major repository of Cusco's colonial art and archeological artifacts.

That afternoon we headed back to Lima, Peru, for one night en route to Rio de Janeiro. In Lima, we stayed in the Miraflores section, which is supposed to be a safe part of town, and I was glad we did. When we arrived and departed there were people everywhere. I thought leaving at 6:00 a.m. we would be fine, but traffic jams had already started with buses and cars filled to the brim.

Two flights later, we were in Rio, and we made sure we made full use of the twenty-four hours we were there. The next morning, we were up and went for a run along Ipanema beach. Catherine loves the song by Frank Sinatra, and it started to play as part of her playlist while we were there.

We didn't want to leave, so by the time we got to the gate, they were already boarding our flight. I thought the gate agent's head was going to explode trying to understand our lifestyle. It was fun to watch.

Mohammed Ali passed away during our trip. One of his many memorable quotes is "Don't count the days, make the days count." This seemed appropriate, as it had been two years since I had my faulty aortic valve replaced. A lot had transpired and changed in my life since then.

Health-wise, I felt great and very satisfied with my decision to have my valve replaced with a mechanical one. The daily dose of Warfarin and the weekly testing of my blood had become pretty routine for me. I use Cardiac Remote Services to help monitor my international normalized ratio (INR) and had only had one mishap where I ran out of testing strips while in Europe. I really didn't think about that part of my life since I was much too busy living life to the fullest.

The only thing I have noticed is that I do bruise easily since I'll be on Warfarin for the rest of my life. I can bump into something one day and see the bruise the next. So far, it hadn't been a big deal since all my bruises heal rather quickly.

Looking back on two years of adventures, I was very grateful for the great work of the team at the Cleveland Clinic in general and my surgeon, Dr. Gosta Pettersson, MD, PhD, in particular. The heart-valve-surgery.com website was also a great benefit. Adam Pick, a former heart patient, put together this blogging site where fellow patients could share stories with others who were also having open-heart operations. Writing down my thoughts before and after the surgery had been very therapeutic, and reading the writings of my heart brothers and sisters on the subject was extremely helpful. I learned a great deal from the experience, but I definitely hoped that my first heart surgery would also be my last.

# CHAPTER
# 20

## We're Not on Vacation,
## This Is Our Lifestyle

It's better to look back and say, "I can't believe I did
that," then to look back and say, "I wish I did that."
—Richard Branson

I say, "We're not on vacation, this our lifestyle," over and over to
people we meet. What it means to me is that, unlike others who
have saved up for a trip or adventure and want to see it all, we have
to budget and can't do and see it all in each particular place we visit.
For the money to last until I'm being pushed around in a wheelchair,
we can't spend like there is no tomorrow. Also, we need to take a day
every now and then to just kick our feet up and relax. If it was easy
anyone could do this.

So far, we were on destination number 176, and day number
593 of running all over the world. That averaged out to 3.37 days per
destination. In other words, every three or so days, we were packing
up our bags and heading somewhere else. Originally the plan was to
do this for five to seven years, but now I can't imagine living out my
retirement days any other way, and I'm sure Catherine would agree.

After a quick stop in Atlanta, we were off to Africa, where I was
determined to overcome another fear of mine: wild animals. I was
once actually afraid to fly, but I managed to fly planes as my career. I

dug deep into what got me over that fear and applied the same principles when it came to the Africa trip.

Catherine wasn't looking forward to Antarctica next March, so as a trade-off I was going to Africa. She was afraid she would get seasick on the ten-day cruise there and back. She has been on many cruise ships and has done fine, but people who have done it before have said that the ship making that journey really rocks and rolls.

Our first night was in Nairobi, and we did a day tour where we got up close and personal with some orphaned, baby elephants and visited a giraffe-petting park. Some fed them by putting the food pellets between their lips, but I just gave them a few the old-fashioned way—with my hand. Baby steps, I always say.

Our second night we stayed at the ARK, which got that name honestly. It looked like one, and plenty of animals came up to the nearby watering hole at all times of the day and night. They have an elaborate notification system depending on what is going on outside the ARK: one chime in your room for elephants, two for rhinos, three for hyenas, and four if there was some action going on. We heard there was some action the week before we arrived, but there were no kills during our overnight stay.

After the ARK we went to the Silo ranch, where we saw plenty of rhinos, giraffes, and various other animals in the wild—but no lions. We did see some of their leftovers, but since all the other animals seemed so relaxed, we guessed the lions were enjoying their recent kills under the tall bush.

At Aberdare Country Club, plenty of somewhat domesticated wild animals roamed around during the day—but at night it was a different story. All we could hear was screaming from all the nearby animals. I'm not sure exactly what was going on, but I took a Sleep Ease tablet and got 8 great hours of sleep.

Our next destination was Sweetwater's Tented Camp. I was not looking forward to the whole tent idea. I spent my high school summers at Boy Scout Camp, but as an adult, I enjoy the finer things in life like actual walls and a roof, especially since it was going to get down to the midfifties at night and I didn't have much adipose tissue.

Large sections of the roads were dirt and or gravel, with speed bumps everywhere for no apparent reason. A few were so extreme we had to go over at one mile an hour to keep from severely damaging the van. Every now and then we'd see a shakedown point along the major highway system. A few cops along the side of the road would pull over vehicles because they were speeding—so they would say. The driver would then have to negotiate and pay in cash to continue on. Our van got stopped once and the driver was able to get the price down to twenty bucks. We all anted up a dollar each to reimburse him.

It turned out that tented life was not so bad, especially since they provided plenty of covers and a hot water bottle to snuggle up to at night. On the game drive the next morning we saw a few lions and a lioness cooling out in the shade of a huge tree. Plenty of baboons were hanging out in the tree since they didn't want to be a lion's meal. We even saw both white and black rhinos on this trip. To be honest, they're both grey in color, but the white are grazers with a wide mouth and black eat off tree branches and have a narrow mouth.

A small setback took place when Catherine stepped on a spiny, needlelike object that fell off a yellow fever tree. It went right through her shoe and into her foot. It was the same material that was used for Jesus's crown of thorns, and Catherine said it hurt like hell. The name really scared us, but the nurse said it wasn't poisonous.

We were planning to run a half-marathon in three days, and I was sure this wouldn't stop her. She walked a half-marathon in a boot six weeks after breaking her foot in three places and just two weeks ago ran a half-marathon after bruising her little toe when she hit the foot of the bed. She's very competitive, so the thought of me completing a race without her was out of the question.

After one more cold night, we were off to a place called the Sanctuary at Ol-Lentille. The road trip was a true adventure. We actually got lost but did get a preview of the racecourse we were going to run.

The mastermind behind the Ol-Lentille development, Gill, gave us an intriguing talk on his vision. After his career, he wanted to give back and decided that Africa would be a perfect place for that vision to become a reality. After a year of research, he decided to take this side of the mountain that had been abandoned by another developer and create a place that would marry conservation, tourist development, education, and health care. With his plans in hand, he convinced the local elders to let him finish the development that can only house sixteen folks at a time.

He bought all the land and paid for the building, then donated it back to the community and has been managing it with his wife since 2006. The project had a total staff of two hundred, including those onsite and the ones who patrolled the area for poachers and ranchers who wanted to use the land for grazing—there was no fencing anywhere in the area.

With guests year-round, Gill and his wife stayed at a nearby house they also built, and I could only imagine what that might look like since the Sanctuary was truly something out of a dream.

Listening to Gill speak about how he was able to see their vision come to reality, I could truly relate since I was seeing my vision of traveling the world also come to reality.

The four separate but semi-connected buildings can house from two to six people at a time. We got the Eyrie unit. When we first approached there was an enclosed area set up like a dining area with windows all around. Adjacent to that was the kitchen area where someone was standing by to prepare our breakfast and afternoon tea and do our laundry.

The living room area, where we relaxed and enjoyed our favorite beverage by the fireplace, had the same circular design facing the east. There was also an outdoor sitting area featured a tub overlooking the valley below, and last but not least, we slept on a circular bed with ten-foot windows and two doors halfway around.

Lunch and dinner were outstanding, and we had them both in the library since there was rain in the area. That was very unusual for this time of year, but nobody was complaining. After dinner, we were escorted back to our unit and told that someone would be in the living area all night if we needed anything and/or to protect us from whatever wild animals were in the area.

It was like nothing I had ever seen or experienced before.

Others in our group were staying in tents where the "long pits" were being dug. I had never heard that term before, but basically, it means holes in the ground for temporary latrines. I was glad we had paid for the upgrade. This wasn't going to be the most expensive trip we had been on so far, but it was pretty darn close. The jury was still out if it was worth it, but it was Africa, after all.

Included in that upgrade were nature walks and ATV drives. Catherine was a bit nervous about the ATV drive at first but was able to think back to her motorcycle days when she drove by herself to the west coast and back. Her true worry was that she was going to further injure herself prior to the race.

The next day we had the opportunity to visit the nearby village at a price: The elders there asked for fifty bucks per person, and it was worth every cent. They put on quite a show for us, and even let us go inside their dung and mud huts. Before we left, they laid out their wares for us to buy. It was very strange to see some of them checking their cell phones.

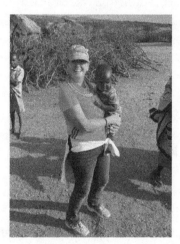

*Catherine was in heaven*

Race day was like no other. Since the creation of the Amazing Maasai race, they have raised over $150,000 for the girls in the area. That increases the GDP by 3 percent, which considerably increases their chance of breaking the cycle of staying at home and having, on average, seven children. (The mother we met back in the village had twelve children.) So far, proceeds from the race have helped 10 percent of the girls to finish high school.

Those who went on to the Tented Camp also had a tour of Daraja Academy, where the girls went to school, where their motto was "Mimi ni Daraja," meaning "I'm the bridge." All the 2014 graduates received national exam scores qualifying them to attend college.

All the girls from the Daraja academy ran the 10K race, and many of the young men in the area either ran the half or full marathon. Four Kenyans did lap us as we were passing 15K for us. The terrain was tough, and Catherine managed to stay on her feet even though there were a few close calls. The race started at an altitude of six thousand feet and at least half a dozen runners came in with cuts and bruises. The views were spectacular.

Every now and then, kids would run alongside us. All the different villages had folks out to cheer us along. Watching them herd their livestock for one grazing area to the next, all that I could think is that we take hot showers for granted. Catherine was clearly in heaven as she ran with many of them hand in hand. We were told that the only animals we had to worry about were elephants, but we didn't see any during our race.

Since we only did the half, we were able to go back to our accommodations to shower and have lunch. We returned in time to see others cross the finish line of the marathon. Luckily the clouds cooperated and stayed in the area, so once again we had a bit of rain and the temperature didn't get out of hand. A few people got lost. I wasn't sure exactly how, since I thought the route was well-marked with orange rocks. I guess if you zone out while running, anything is possible. The same is true for those that fell. Catherine's close call with terra firm-a was while she was giving high fives to some of the kids.

I had totally gotten over my fear of wild animals. I learned that they try to coexist with everything and everybody in their ecosystem. Yes, they can be dangerous to humans, but mostly because we as humans are just downright stupid. As they look as us drive by, they understand that the vehicle is not on their diet. It's only when you get out that they say to themselves, "Now that is a meal."

During the race we saw just about everything out there, and none of them had humans on their menu. It was great to run by them and see them just look up from their grazing routine—if that— then just continue what they were doing. Most of the time there was someone heading up the herd of whatever, and they would wave and say, "Jambo," which means "hello."

The day after the race, our private charter took off from a nearby dirt strip, headed Governors Camp in Masai Mara. For took the hour-long flight in a twelve-passenger Cessna Caravan, which really took me back to my early flying days. I sat right behind the co-pilot and had my poker face on so no one would worry. I usually don't like to see how the sausage is being made, but I just couldn't resist in this case.

Governors Camp is famous for its location close by the migration path of the wildebeest as they travel from Tanzania to Masai. The 1.5 million of them that make the three-month trek are not the smartest animals on the planet. The males lead the way, and the scent in their hoofmarks guide the rest, sometimes across streams and rivers.

This is where you really see the food chain in action. As they cross the water, many alligators and lions lie in wait for their daily meals. We were able to see many crossings of several thousands in large herds, and some would even go back and forth in confusion. We were glad that we didn't actually see a kill, but many in our group did.

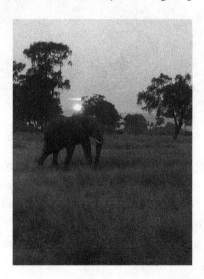

Like Ol-Lentille, the place had no fencing around it, so they had 24-7 guards protecting the guests, and no one could go any-where at night without an escort. All that wildlife came to pay a visit at night, and they sure did make a racket. I learned that it was best to take a sleep aid so that when all the screaming, yelling, and roaring woke me up, I could easily roll over and fall back to sleep. This was also a tented camp, so and if they really wanted to come visit or lunch on us, I'm sure they could have.

We did have an incredible experience of seeing a crossing of the Mara river during the last breakfast here. The first and near the last wildebeest were alligator bait, but I was enjoying my omelet during that time. Someone in our group was able to take a photo of a dead wildebeest hanging from a tree. A leopard, who can carry 1.5 times its weight, did the heavy lifting, and would come back and snack on its prize throughout the day and night.

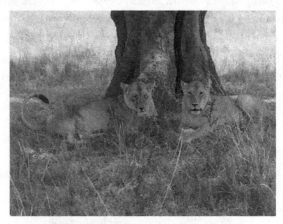

*Sister Sister*

It is going to be a very long day on the way home. I figured somewhere around thirty-six hours from checkout to check-in at the hotel back in Atlanta. There was, I thought, a strict thirty-three-pound weight limit per person for the flight in and out of Masai Marra, so we left a bag at the Nairobi hotel. We normally carry 140 pounds excluding our backpacks, so getting down to sixty-six pounds was quite a feat.

Something I hadn't seen before occurred as we were about one mile from the airport. The driver said that we had to get out, and he would meet us on the other side of an elaborate security system. We had to go through metal detectors, and the van pulled forward and was searched. After the gate and the tire puncher spikes were raised and lowered, we got back in the van and proceeded to the airport. Right at the door of the terminal we had to go through security once again.

Many of the people we met in Africa were talking about the adjustments they would have to make being back home. I made the comment that we don't have a home, and I was reminded that the entire world was our home because we're not on vacation, this is our lifestyle.

A few times when I have told people about our nomadic lifestyle, their response has been that I must have won the lottery. In some ways that's true. I was in the right place at the right time to have a very rewarding career in aviation. It wasn't because I was a better Pilot/Manager than anyone else, but more that good fortune has come my way time and time again. Along the way, I've worked hard and have always treated others as I have wanted to be treated. In retirement, I was trying to treat myself as I treated others.

On our last adventure to Africa, we met two guys who brought this thought home to me. James, was a Detective with the Chicago Police Department and recently retired. His plan was that when his daughter went off to college, he would retire. He knew that it would be an early retirement and he would have to deal with the financial consequences. That didn't matter to him because as he saw all the violence going on around him, and early retirement was worth the expense. His long-time friend, Alfred, was also on the trip and was counting down two more years until he could retire with his health care expenses covered.

I hear these types of rationales all the time. "If I stay X more years or months, I can make Y more or not have to pay for Z." What none of us know is how long we will be on this earth. We all have bucket lists or, as I call ours, "life list." We all have things we would like to do or see before we die, but most cannot be done while tied to a desk a cockpit or squad car.

I see others continuing to work or refusing to do any of the things on their bucket list because they're saving for their kids and or grandkids. That's a noble gesture, but since my parents and grand-parents didn't provide for me in that way, I have a hard time wrapping my head around that thought process.

Catherine and I were able to provide a college education for each of our children, so in my mind, that's all they can ask for. I was always been there for them in their formative years, and I'm glad to say they're all doing well for themselves.

Another rationale people use is that they really enjoy their job. I had a great job, but can honestly say that in the cycle of life, retirement is the best phase. I tell people all the time not to work a day longer than they have to. We all think we have time, but none of us know how much time there actually is.

You hear all the time about people who literally work themselves to death. By the time they finally hang up the keys to the office, they only have a few months or even days to enjoy the fruits of their labor. Some fear they wouldn't know what to do with themselves if they didn't work. To them I say, "Find and follow your passion."

I joke often about how I didn't let any of my kids move back into the house as adults. I'm not saying that any of them wanted to because, in their minds, they were ready to spread their wings when they went off to college. My goal now is not to have to move back in with any of them when I get old. I figure I'll take up risky behaviors if that ever becomes a possibility.

Over the last twenty months, we'd seen and done things that I could only have imagined many years ago, always with a healthy dose of activity, whether running, biking, or swimming. We'd done either a marathon or half-marathon in twenty-five different countries. There is something like 196 countries that have at least a half-marathon, and my goal was to complete as many as I could.

Our next stop was Chicago for the Organization of Black Aerospace Professionals (OBAP) convention. This annual event always seems to put things into perspective for me. I started in aviation in the late '70s, and back then the percentage of Black pilots was less than 1 percent. Some forty years later, the numbers haven't changed. It's inspiring to be there to meet and greet those who have that sparkle in their eyes as they aspire to be a major airline Captain.

I still remember the day they gave me my plaque for achieving that status—I even shook Colin Powell's hand during that ceremony. Now I'll go up during the Gala event and shake the hands of those who have been promoted to Captain over the last year. I get goose-bumps each and every time.

The Convention was a huge success, and we were able to get some exercise in with a great six-mile walk of the area one day and a rain-soaked run the next morning.

The next day we went to Swallow Cliffs, where folks can run or walk a large and steep set of stairs. It also meets up with an elaborate trail system at the top. We did the stairs three times and another half hour of trails.

As we ran, I recalled another not-so-original thought about time that was quoted by a friend from our African adventure.

"Time is nature's way to keep everything from happening all at once."—Albert Einstein

I remembered how time played a crucial role leading up to and during my recovery from heart surgery. On one end of the spectrum was the period right before and after the surgery. I saw the gas mask as it headed for my nose and mouth and was told to take a deep breath—then in the next second, in my mind, I heard Catherine and the nurse's voice in each ear, asking me to wake up.

I actually thought I was dead because when I opened my eyes, I couldn't see anything and really didn't feel anything. I guess some could say I was dead for about four hours as I was hooked up to all those machines, since they had to stop my heart to replace the valve.

During recovery I had to become a patient patient. That thought process was entirely new to me. I was used to going places at five hundred miles an hour, so having to wait patiently for hours for a blood draw was quite an adjustment.

We often try to wait for the perfect time to do such-and-such, but we might just run out of time waiting for that perfect situation to arise. As a dedicated nomad, I'm not waiting for that perfect situation to arise. Yes, it might be a bit complicated or downright distasteful, but the rewards are (most of the time) worth it.

After another touch and go in Atlanta, we were off to Kauai, Hawaii, to run the half-marathon there. They call it the Garden Island, and it rains on and off each day to stay so lush and green. The varieties of plants were outstanding, and most pictures I took didn't do the picturesque landscape justice. We rented a very nice condo for two weeks at the Kiahuna Plantation Resort Kauai by Outrigger.

The race itself was over-the-top. The start was right outside our condo building, and even though we had to climb the hills for 3.5 miles starting at mile four, the rest of it was back down to a great finish area with some of the coldest beer possible.

They even had chips, iced coffee, and turkey wraps. The ice bags at the finish were a great way to cool down. Since we only did the half, we were able to shower and return to the finish to cheer on the final few marathoners who braved the 85 degree plus weather.

I probably said ten times a day that I've found our new home if we decided to settle down one day. We loved this island so much that, even though we were actually on a budget and usually didn't splurge, I made an exception on Kauai.

I actually wanted to be a helicopter pilot when I started my flight training, but decided I didn't like the "drop like a rock" aspect of helicopters and the amount of maintenance needed to keep them up in the air. You would think after thirty-seven years of flying airplanes a helicopter tour of the island would be simple enough.

This was not the case, but Mauna Loa Helicopter Tours gave us the thrill and tour of a lifetime. For whatever reason, I thought we would be touring the island from thousands of feet over the ridges, mountains, and waterfalls. In truth, I felt I could have reached out and touched the leaves as we passed by. And of course, I opted for the "doors off" and extended version of the tour.

Once I got over the idea that this was how I was going to die, I truly enjoyed the experience. Catherine grinned from ear to ear the entire time. The cost was a bit steep, but it was worth every penny.

We were also able to get in some great runs around the different areas of the island. There are numerous hiking trails throughout the island, but we didn't do much of that. I'm more of an open-road type of guy. I don't like having to look down constantly to see where I need to place my foot so I don't trip and fall, twist my ankle, or get bitten by something hiding under a rock. Not to mention having to duck under all the branches that have been cleared by everyone much shorter than me.

We couldn't leave the island without taking one of the most popular tours, the infamous sunset cruise. We went with the recommended Captain Andy's Catamaran sailing adventure. We went with the sixty-five-foot boat option, where the dinner was actually cooked onboard. Even though the clouds hid the actual setting of the sun, the views of the inaccessible portions of the island and the colors of the sky just after the setting of the sun were breathtaking.

Back on land, we couldn't experience Kauai without experiencing the chickens and roosters. Simply put, they were everywhere. I'm not sure they actually served a purpose, but the reason they were so plentiful was because of their previous purpose. Cock fighting was big on the island, and due to a huge hurricane some time back, they were all freed by the high winds. Once they got out, they did what they do best and populated the island.

The locals don't like them since they're a nuisance, but for me as a light sleeper, it just meant that I was an early riser. Early to bed and early to rise was our agenda each day and night, which was no big deal since the first few days we were adjusting to the six-hour time change. Catherine thought the chickens were cute, so she took numerous pictures of them—and I couldn't resist taking a few myself.

We were now off to Europe for a month, starting with an eight-day Windstar cruise from Venice to Rome. My daughter Mariah visited Casablanca during her yearlong European tour after college, so we were going pay a visit ourselves before heading to Amsterdam for a half-marathon.

They say, "Time flies when you're having fun," but it also speeds up when you get older. For a two-year-old, one year is half their life, but for me it's $1/61^{st}$ of my life. We were starting day 649 of being nomads, but it only felt like day 2.

# CHAPTER
# 21

## Why Do We Travel?

Travel is rebellion in its purest form
We follow our heart
We free ourselves of labels
We lose control willingly
We trade a role for reality
We love the unfamiliar
We trust strangers
We own only what we can carry
We search for better questions
Not answers
We truly graduate
We, sometimes, choose to never come back

—Anonymous

Most people will conclude that Catherine and I have taken travel to an extreme. We've met a number of people who have retired and gone on the road but all, so far, actually have a home. There are folks who have sold their home, bought an RV, and have been full-timing in their rig ever since.

We only live in our motor home only a few times a year. We usually spend around a week each time and have been moving it around over the last several years.

Travel has been in my blood my entire adult life, but it goes deeper than that. As we took self-guided tours of Venice, I realized, that certain things about travel intrigued me. I'm a planner and manager by heart. I have spent most of my adult life managing assets and find that to be a better fit for me than actually flying airplanes from point A to B safely. I really enjoy the planning part of travel and then putting those plans into action. The points of interest are nice to look at, but figuring out how to get around on my own is where the real thrill exists.

Venice was a real challenge with all its narrow streets, more than four-hundred-foot bridges and numerous canals with few signs, makes it almost impossible to get around without getting lost. It was like the largest corn maze in the world. I tried my best not to double back and was proud that I only pulled out my map a few times and my phone once.

The challenge kept me going. Over three days, we walked twenty-two miles but did take time out for the (rather expensive) thirty-minute gondola ride. The fare is regulated by the government and you can tell they're pushing the envelope on what people will pay. It was worth it, but only for the tourist factor and limited learning experience.

After a while, I did start to wonder why there were thousands of little shops selling stuff we didn't want or need. There were great-looking churches, and it was fascinating watching the water transportation system. The other part of travel that I love is seeing how people all over the world go about their daily lives dealing with the same thing all of us have to deal with: sleeping, eating, entertainment, getting rid of garbage. In most places I try to use mass transportation as much as possible because the different ways that is handled vary greatly.

We were staying at the Venice Airport, Marriott. From there it was easy as pie to get to Central Venice by bus. The bus stop was right across the street from the hotel. In twenty minutes, we would be in the middle of it all, and from there it would be a tram ride to the cruise terminal we were leaving from—or so I thought.

It turned out that our yacht, as they like to call it, wasn't large enough for the actual cruise terminal, so we had to drag our bags, along with another misguided couple, to where it was actually docked. The Windsurf could carry 330 people. We only had 260 folks on our trip, with a crew of 190, so you do the math. To put it simply, if you dropped your napkin, three people would be right there to pick it up. There were five crew members we knew from previous cruises, and we ran into one gentleman who had done ninety-two cruises with them.

During the planning phase of this trip, I was looking for somewhere to go prior to Amsterdam, and for some strange reason I picked Casablanca.

Here are a few random reasons why we went there:

1. Because we had never been there before.
2. Because my daughter has.
3. Because we have no home and have to sleep somewhere.
4. Because it is not on our way to our next stop, Amsterdam.
5. Because we really liked the movie.
6. And the most important one being: Because Catherine didn't say we couldn't.

Don't waste your time. The Sofitel was in the middle of it all and was imaginative, but the city itself was basically a hole in a wall. They did have the Hassan II Mosque, which was jaw-dropping, but everything else was very dirty and not appealing to the eye. The hotel had a great lounge with an outstanding jazz singer, and two great restaurants. One night we had a sampler meal of all the Moroccan dishes known to man

Another reason why we travel is that you just have to see things for yourself. You can hear stories from others or look at pictures in books or on the internet, but the expression "seeing is believing" really comes to life when you travel. I guess I also travel for the stories you can tell. I'll say Casablanca made for a great story.

The train station was right across the street from the hotel, so the trip back to the airport should have been easy. The problems getting out of the country started the moment we stepped off the train. The train was packed, we were at the end of it, and they had security screening before you could leave the station. Only one guy was checking to make sure everyone had a plane ticket. Then there was one belt for everyone to put their bags on, and one guy to check you through the metal detector.

I usually plan to arrive at the airport three hours before the flight, and the first hour went by just trying to get off the train and on airport property. The ticket counter was just as bad. They had no record of me paying for my third bag, and they wanted twice the price at the airport. We went back and forth for another hour, and after a manager's intervention we were on our way to customs and immigration.

As we turned the corner, I could hear yelling from a sea of people trying to be processed by four agents. It became crystal clear we were going to miss our flight, so I took the opportunity to cut the line. Staying another night in Casablanca was not an option. The agent was not happy, but I held my ground and Catherine flashed her smile and baby blues, and we were on our way.

Security screening was a joke, with a cop with a gun standing in the metal detector and basically frisking everyone, since it was obvious the machine itself did not work. We made it to the gate with a few minutes to spare, and were happy for an on-time departure for Madrid and our connecting flight to Amsterdam.

I thought the worst was behind us, since our flight was on time and we had almost two hours to go through customs in Madrid. They had twice the number of agents for EU folks as for the rest of us, so we slowly made our way to a point where you had to pick a particular agent to stand in line for. Just like at the grocery store, I picked the wrong one. First our agent went to lunch and the new agent took a while to settle in. She was busy talking to her friend between each passenger, so her process rate was nothing to write home about. She was also not happy with a few folks, so that also took a while.

We now had forty-five minutes before departure and the signs indicated it would take thirty minutes to get to our gate. First we went several levels down to the underground train, and after a long ride to the terminal, back up we went. They can give your seats away within fifteen minutes of departure time, so when we saw the departure board saying final call, we started a slow jog to our gate.

They hadn't given our seats away, but it was close. Our reward for all that trouble was an easy ninety-minute flight to Amsterdam. This was our third trip there. We had decided that whenever we went to Europe, we would stop there for a few days each way. After an easy train ride to Central Station and a short bag drag to the Renaissance by Marriott hotel, we were in the Executive Lounge having dinner.

We were there for the half-marathon, which was the best race I had run in recent memory. They encouraged everyone to catch the Metro to the start, and even though the trains were packed, the 1:50 p.m. start for our corral made it easy as pie.

It was a Sunday race, so with the afternoon start, we were still able to enjoy the night life of Amsterdam before and after the race. The weather was perfect, and the people along the course were not plentiful but very friendly. The views were great, but I understood some of the marathon course did go through a very industrial part of town, so I was again glad we were doing the half. The real reason this was one of our favorite races was simply because it was in Amsterdam. What is there not to love about the place?

After a few more days, we were on our way to Marseilles to meet up with our running cruise group for another trip. It started with three nights in Marseilles, followed by a seven-night cruise up the Rhone river from Arles to Lyon. We had been to Marseilles the previous year, but we did get to see more of the city on a couple of bus tours. In one outdoor area there was a mirrored canopy overhead, and I couldn't resist taking a picture of ourselves below.

We also did a morning run along the Mediterranean which was simply gorgeous, with the turnaround point being the Square du Lieutenant Danjume. It was nice to experience more of Marseilles this time. We did something we had never done before during our adventures: eating at the same restaurant three nights in a row. The Le Petit Pernod was worth it, and each time more and more people joined the group.

A private bus charter took us to Arles to meet up with our new home, Amadagio. This was actually one of the oldest ships AMA Waterways had, but you really could not tell it. It holds 120 and had two groups on board for this sailing: ninety-four runners and walkers with Marathon Expeditions, and twenty from Expedia. During our trip we went through twelve locks, and there were mere inches on either side through most of them.

To say the least, this was a very active cruise. I came to believe that John and Jenny could get this group of lemmings to do anything. I'm not saying that in a bad way, but we all did the fifteen-mile bike ride in pouring rain. Our group covered the distance in about an hour, so it was not a leisurely ride by any stretch of the imagination. We rode along the famous ViaRhôna, a bike route between the Swiss Alps and France's Mediterranean Coast.

I noticed this group seemed to be a bit more cohesive than usual on these cruises, probably because only a few folks had not been on a trip with Marathon Expeditions before. This was our eighth trip with them.

During this trip I have been asking random people why they travel, and here are some answers that I have been given:

- It's something I have always done
- For the excitement
- To meet new and different people
- To see it for yourself
- Because my father didn't
- Because my parents did
- Because we can
- For the adventure
- It makes for a good story to tell others
- You only live once
- To get a better perspective of the world

As we get older, we have to deal with health issues from time to time, and sometimes thoughts about how we're doing get in the way of being able to enjoy what is going on around us. A turned ankle here, a slip and fall there, and we're thinking about how much longer we'll have here on earth.

An eighty-year-old fellow runner/walker, Nancy, gave me these words of wisdom: "Stay active as long as you can, and don't let your age dictate your brain." I translate that to mean to keep up with the running in spite of the continual fact you're slowing down or can't run as far. Also don't dwell on your current age or how much longer you might have. Living each day to the fullest seems to help, and travel is probably the best way to achieve that.

For our next race, everyone had to run either 5K or 10K without a watch and predict their time. We chose the 10K—some said it turned out to be about seven miles. The rolling hills through the various vineyards always seemed to make the distance enjoyable. After that, we went to the top of the vineyards in the area for a fantastic lunch, final awards ceremony, and wine tasting.

One day we went for a seven-mile guided hike through the Alpilles Region from Les Baux through the Lumieres Quarry to the Van Gogh Asylum, with a tour there. After a short bus ride to St. Remy de Provence, we had an over-the-top outdoor buffet lunch of the specialities of Provence at the Manade Caillan, a farm with black bulls of Camarque. These bulls are trained to race against men. The winning man is the one who has gotten the most scarves off their horns, and the winning bull is the one that still has his scarf on his horns.

We had a red wine and chocolate pairing tour in a castle, Château-musée de Tournon-sur-Rhône, which was off the charts. They selected three wines for us to taste and gave the information to a master chocolate maker in the area. After tasting each wine, he made enough chocolate balls for those of us in the tour based on the wine. We basically were taught everything you ever wanted to know about how to make chocolate in general and why he came up with those ingredients for each individual chocolate. It was mind-blowing and I planned on going out to buy some fine chocolate the next time I bought a bottle of wine.

We always have a variation of the Amazing Race on these trips, but they changed the format for this particular race. The winning team of three to four had to get back to ship after going to as many checkpoints as possible in sixty minutes. Some checkpoints were worth more than others, and if you were a second late you were disqualified. We went for a leisurely 4.5 mile run of the area and ended up at the start of a marathon in historic Avignon. The roads were all closed in the area so it was perfect for us.

The fun and activities didn't let up once we got to Paris for the three-day pos-cruise package. The fifty or so of us who stayed on met up that evening for a night-time, four-hour bike tour of Paris with Fat Tire. This was not for the faint of heart, but it was worth the risk.

We took several stops to see the famous sights of Paris, along with a stop for ice cream or an Irish Coffee. Another stop near the end was for a thirty-minute river cruise where we cut the chill with some wine as we admired the lights of the city.

It was a good thing we took some afternoons off, because the next day we were back at it with a Hash House Harrier run through the Bois de Boulogne, largest park in Paris. It's three times bigger than Central Park, and our hound made sure we got to see all the great sites. This was by far the best hash we had done, featuring plenty of food and refreshments at the finish.

The next day we took a twelve-passenger Mercedes van to the Reims/Champagne region for two Champagne tastings. Our first stop was a small vineyard, Ployez-Jacquemart, and the other was the famous Moet & Chandon, which was established in 1743.

The contrast between the vistas and valleys was awe-inspiring, with vineyards as far as the eye could see. I learned more than I ever expected about how Champagne is made, so I now have a greater appreciation of the price per bottle. Unlike other wine tours, they did not teach us how to drink it. I was disappointed since we found out on our way to the vineyards that there were bisques you can buy to dip in your champagne. I didn't buy any, thinking we could get some later. Moet sold everything else, but no bisques.

This particular thirty-four-day trip taught me a couple of things. The first has to do with preconceived notions about places. By traveling and seeing them yourself, you can either confirm these thoughts or not, as we did in Casablanca. I was also reminded that there are places in the world, like Paris, which are diverse, and other places that are not so much if you take tourists out of the mix. I still didn't see many middle-aged African American males like me during our travels.

Another reason to travel is to learn. As we age, our brains don't do as well as when we were younger. Seeing new and exciting things keeps those synapses fired up, especially for folks like Catherine with younger-onset Alzheimer's. I have noticed the difference for myself too. These memories will stay with me for a lifetime, as opposed to who said what to who on the latest TV show.

When we touched down back in Atlanta, it would be destination number 196, not including the many ports of call on six different cruises. On day number 683, we were still averaging around 3.5 days per destination. Given that, there was one last thing I was trying to figure out as we went from place to place and noticed the people around us: Were we two peas in a pod or two nuts in a shell?

# CHAPTER
# 22

## A Time Warp, Then Time to Reflect

Not all those who wander are lost.

—J. R. R. Tolkien

After a week in Atlanta, we flew to Miami to meet up with our Marathon Tours and Travel team for a tour of Havana, Cuba. The group of more than ninety of us was split into three groups at two hotels. We stayed in the old Havana area at the Saratoga Hotel. The other two groups were at the Melia Cohiba Hotel, which was located along the race route and the famous Malecón.

Officially the Avenida de Maceo, this broad esplanade, roadway, and seawall which stretches for 8 km (5 miles) along the coast, from the mouth of Havana Harbor in Old Havana, along the north side of the Centro Habana neighborhood, ending in the Vedado neighborhood. New businesses were appearing on the esplanade due to economic reforms that allow Cubans to own private businesses.

There's so much to say about our trip to Cuba. Havana was somewhat like many places we have visited during our travels, but more like all of them rolled into one. There were parts that remind me of Casablanca, Morocco, with dirt and filth were everywhere, and then there were areas that reminded me of upscale Mexico City.

I kept asking people who we were traveling with what surprised them the most about what they saw. Their answers were varied, but one we could all agree on was that none of us expected to see as many old cars as we did. They were everywhere. Some were broken down on the side of the road, but most were set up for people to take pictures of or to serve as taxi cabs.

We were also very surprised to see all the buildings in disrepair. You could still see the artistic details from Cuba's rich and checkered past, but some had scaffolds in place and many more looked like they would fall over any minute. Apparently the capitol building has had its scaffolding up for several years.

They did have local busses running throughout the city, but beyond that anything was up for grabs. Lines for what looked like a rideshare system were everywhere. They also had people-powered bikes for hire including the driver and the strangest of them all was the motorbike-type taxicabs.

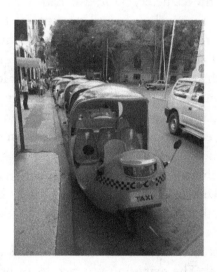

The first-day tour went by in a blur since I hadn't gotten much sleep the night prior and the seats on the bus were very comfortable. I enjoyed lunch at La Guarida (the location of the Oscar-nominated movie Strawberry & Chocolate), and I do remember our visit to a cigar factory. I was amazed to learn that over ninety different brands of cigar come from exactly the same leaf. The workers, mostly women, seemed happy enough, but I couldn't imagine rolling cigars day after day.

The next morning, we heard a presentation on US and Cuban relations. This was a high-level opportunity to discuss the social and political future of Cuba and the challenges awaiting the Cuban economy. Afterward, we paid a visit to an Art School called Instituto Superior de Artes (ISA). Before the revolution, ISA was the Havana Country Club. In 1961, it was converted by President Fidel Castro into an arts complex and was the subject of the film Unfinished Spaces.

The next day we visited the Colon Cemetery, founded in 1876 in the Vedado neighborhood of Havana on top of Espada Cemetery. Named for Christopher Columbus, the 140-acre cemetery was noted for more than five hundred elaborately sculpted mausoleums, chapels, and family vaults.

Following the cemetery visit, we had a panoramic tour of Modern Havana that included the University of Havana, Catalina Lasa's home (a mansion called the most beautiful house in all of Havana), and the Institute of Superior Art, to name a few. We stopped for lunch at El Divino, a private restaurant located at a beautiful organic farm. Following lunch, we visited Ernest Hemingway's home, Finca Vigia, where we saw his thirty-eight-foot wooden boat.

Something else the group was able to agree on was that we were pleasantly surprised at the quality of the meals. Yes, they had beans and rice for lunch and dinner, but the fish, pork, and chicken were also well-prepared. During the meals arranged by Marathon Tours, the welcome drink was usually the famous Mojito, which I still haven't acquired the taste for.

Sunday was race day and the start/finish was right outside the door of our hotel. The marathon was two loops of the course, and with the heat, hills, smog, and traffic, we were very happy to know that we were only doing the half.

After the race, about thirty of us continued with a day trip to Las Terraza, a sustainable community in the countryside of Pinar del Rio. We visited local artists and learned about rural life on the island. It was nice to get away from the hustle and bustle of the city for a while, and we got to see how they used to process coffee way back in the day.

It was funny to find out that the reason there were so few signs on the highway was because local farmers figured out the metal was good for building barns. We also got to see some low-tech forms of transportation, including horse-drawn carts and even oxen plowing a field.

The last day was jam-packed. After an outing to the Museum of Fine Arts, we visited the studio of Esterio Segura who was one of the most controversial artists in Cuba. His work was collected in museums around the world, including MOMA.

That evening, fourteen of us went to one of the locals clubs, Buena Vista Social Club, to see Legendarios del Cuajirito, also known as the "Afro-Cuban All Stars" in action. The ninety-minute high-paced flamenco show included three drinks for around $35 each. It was a great show and we were glad we went, but it meant another short night prior to our flight back to Miami the next morning.

Overall, we had a great experience of Cuba. It was a good history lesson, but it seemed to me they were stuck in a time warp. It was somewhat depressing to see all the folks who obviously didn't have enough to merely survive, even in some of the most touristy areas. I'd like to go back in five to ten years to see how they have progressed. A few days after we left, Fidel Castro died. Things do seem to happen after we leave a place.

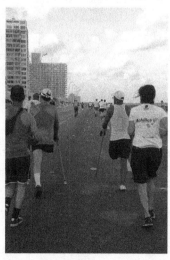

*What is your excuse?*

We made it safely back to the States, and after a good night's sleep at the Marriott, we picked up the Crib to enjoy six nights of relaxation at the Hollywood KOA. It's sometimes good to sit back, relax, and do absolutely nothing.

During the lull in the trip, I took a moment to reflect on the last two years of traveling to more than seventy different destinations in 713 days. When people asked how much longer we will be nomads, our most common response was that we were on the SKI program: Spend our Kids' Inheritance. Other times I gave the simple answer of seven to ten years or "until Catherine or I can no longer drag our bags."

I had done the calculations, and it simply didn't make sense for us to settle down and either rent or buy a place to live. I did an unscientific survey and decided that Catherine was the one who gets ants in her pants and wants to dance before me. In other words, she gets bored from lack of new stimulation way before I do.

Seven days was entirely too much time to spend in Atlanta. It was cold and cloudy most of the time, and without the vitamin D we both got somewhat depressed. I decided to try an Airbnb and the place was great, but with the lack of stimulation and endorphin fix, Catherine didn't do well.

The place had an incredible exercise facility, but it wasn't the same as breathing in fresh air out on the road. We did do a six-mile walk to, around, and from Piedmont Park. I love that park.

We were able to meet up with some Marathon Tours and Travel friends who we went to Istanbul and Africa. Sarah and Elayne had just gotten back from running a half-marathon in Lisbon, one of my favorite places.

We did take advantage of the time to have some doctor's appointments at the Emery Hospital Midtown. The doctors were fantastic, and if we showed up fifteen minutes early for our appointment, we could be out the door at the time of our appointment, feeling like everyone cared about our well-being. They even had a Starbucks inside.

At the same time, at the age of sixty-one, I felt like I was playing medical whack-a-mole. As soon as I hit one concern over the head, another one popped up. We found that travel and running helped us to keep our mind off the day-to-day aches and pains and upcoming exams, but I would rather know what was happening rather than being surprised to find myself in an emergency room one day.

By the seventh day in Atlanta, we were both ready to go to our next stop, San Juan, where we boarded a Windstar Cruises. The best excursion ever came in St. Maarten, where we experience America's cup sailboat racing firsthand. About thirty of us were split into two teams, and each had our own crew and ship. We all had our own job to do, and took instructions from either the captain or a crew member.

It was over-the-top thrilling, and our team even won. We got to watch another race that went out earlier, which the Canadian ship won. We brought the cup home by beating the Canadian ship by a full minute in the final race. We don't normally buy pictures but this was one of those once-in-a-lifetime experiences.

During the cruise, we had dinner with the ship's doctor. I had always thought about doing an ocean crossing with them, but the doctor pointed out that after a day, not even a helicopter could come rescue us if something happened on board, I decided maybe not.

After the cruise we flew back to Atlanta for twenty-four hours, then on to San Diego for the holidays. My eldest, Aaron, celebrated his thirtieth birthday three days after Christmas, and we were able to squeeze in a concert at the Observatory North Park. It was a flashback to my college days: George Clinton and Parliament Funkadelic were in town. The guy was seventy-five years old and still going strong— although he did have a swivel chair to relax in occasionally during the three-hour performance. I was amazed and pleasantly surprised to be able relive my youth with my kids.

As we approached the end of the year 2016, I looked back at some numbers. Over the last two years, we have run:

- ten marathons
- eleven half-marathons
- one 21-miler
- And numerous other races of various distances.

Over sixteen years of my running, biking, and swimming I have almost gone completely around the world: I've covered twenty-two thousand miles, and a circumnavigation of the globe is about twenty-four thousand miles.

I like having a New Year's resolution, and I came up with a pretty good one for 2017: to get either ten thousand steps walking and/or running, five miles, on a bike (actual or stationary), a half-mile swim, or a combination of all three every day.

We all have the tendency to dwell on the negative and not cherish all the positive things around ourselves. I'll use a general statistic as an example. I have often read that people who worry about having a heart attack are more likely to have one. Instead, we should all stop worrying about that possibility and just do positive things to prevent them.

# CHAPTER
# 23

## This Does Not Suck

Life is either a daring adventure or nothing at all.

—Helen Keller

The title of this chapter comes from a friend of ours, Jaime, who we met on a Marathon Tours and Travel trip for the Napa to Sonoma half-marathon. She used this term when talking about how things aren't perfect, but at the same time they could be a whole lot worse. Looked at the other way, things are pretty damn good.

This sums up our life as nomads. It's not perfect, and there are things that come up—health issues, the loss of loved ones and acquaintances, and all that was going on around the world—but we have to look at life in a positive light.

On the other hand, I was watching CNN in-flight and saw there was a shooting at the Ft. Lauderdale Airport. Once again, this was somewhere we had recently been, and this time five lives were lost. We usually don't worry as we travel, but as Catherine often says, you can get hit by a car crossing a street. As we traveled all over the world, my head was on a constant swivel. I used to tell my kids as they were growing up that if something happens around them, they need to move away as opposed to standing around watching. These days you see people all the time taking out their cell phones and taking pictures but for me, "head down and run away" was my plan.

Something you can't run away from, though. In January 2017, I found out that I had an aneurism and dissection of my right common iliac artery. I was going to have a CT scan of my groin area when I was back in Atlanta to see the extent of the aneurism and discuss the best course of action moving forward.

This news got me thinking about heredity's role in life expectancy. It's a double-edged sword: Both of our parents lived into their late '80s and early '90s, but they also both had a history of aneurysms.

To keep my blood pressure down and avoid the impact of running, I decided to stop running.

We had a few open time slots in the early part of this year so I would be able to schedule surgery, if necessary, and keep up with our nomadic lifestyle. This was a great example of "this does not suck." It was inconvenient and imperfect, but I had great insurance and a great team on top of the situation.

The CT scan showed that it might not be a simple procedure through the groin so I would have to find someone else to assess the problem and probable solution. I was hoping to hold off another surgery altogether, so I decided to get two opinions. Our first stop would be a great group of Surgeons at Harbourview Vascular Medical Clinic in Seattle Washington. After that, we would have two weeks in the Caribbean, followed by a trip back to the Cleveland Clinic for their assessment of my aneurysm.

I was still waiting for a call for an appointment, though, and there was no better place to wait for a phone call than Key West, Florida.

At first, I wasn't looking forward to the Key West half-marathon since I had decided to walk the entire 13.1 miles for the first time, but after a few miles I was able to get into the swing of things. We started at the very back and at first were able to go by slower walkers. As time went on, I picked up the pace and was doing about fourteen minutes a mile. I had planned on fifteen minutes a mile, so I was presently surprised.

Walking at that pace was hurting Catherine's shins so she decided to jog alongside me. To keep my mind occupied, I made a game of it. I would see someone one-fourth mile ahead and would try to catch them. One by one I would go by. I figured out I actually had two speeds: with my arms up, I was able to clip off a mile in thirteen minutes.

The last three to four miles were the best, since by then a lot of runners were struggling and walking slowly, so I was going by them like they were standing still. The original plan was to finish in about three-and-a-half hours, but I actually got it done in around 2:56. I was very proud of my sub-three-hour walk of a half-marathon. You could say it was a personal record, since I had never done that before. The next day some of my muscle groups that usually weren't used in that way weren't very happy with me, but no big deal.

I did have a bit of a problem near the end. I saw a woman grab her husband's hand. He was clearly struggling, but she made him start running so they could finish under three hours. You could tell he was not very happy with the idea, and as I went by, I mentioned that this was how people die at the finish, trying to accomplish something their heart had not signed up for. She yelled back, "You don't know my husband!"

I threw up my hands and said, "You're right, but please be careful." He took that to heart. He walked the last one-fourth mile and still finished under three hours. I congratulated them at the finish.

The appointment in Seattle went well. There was a lot of information to take in, but basically, I was two different people. On the outside and listening to me, you would say I was very healthy, but on the inside, I had some strange things going on. They weren't sure why I was having these aneurysm issues, especially at such a young age. One idea was that this current one was from an injury or a collagen problem. They also find these problems in smokers. I did smoke over forty years ago for a very short period of time, but they didn't think that was the problem.

Studies on long-distance bike riders have found that they were more prone to aneurysm in this area of the body. I did a lot of bike riding while training for the Iron Man back in 2011, so that might be the cause. Another possibility was the fact that they had to go through my groin for the cauterization during my heart operation, and maybe that pressure might have caused the problem.

They were tracking down my records from my previous doctors and working on a game plan, but the bottom line was that they did recommend surgery. The good news was that it wasn't something that needed to be done right away—but probably within the next three months. I was told to continue doing what I love, but not try anything new right now. Also to keep the strain off my midsection and not pick up anything heavy. We would have to devise a new way to move our two fifty-pounds bags around.

The surgeon, Elina Quiroga, gave me her card with all her personal contact information and told me to keep it on me in case there was a rupture before it could be repaired. She also said that she belonged to a world-wide vascular group and could recommend where I should go if there was a problem during my travels. I was pretty sure I would have the surgery done in Seattle. I felt extremely comfortable with the entire experience there, so I decided to cancel my appointment I had scheduled with the Cleveland Clinic.

It's easy to focus on the negative, but I would rather look at situations like this as minor inconveniences in the big picture. Since we wouldn't be going to the Cleveland Clinic, I went to marathonguide.com and found another half-marathon in Mesa, Arizona, on the date of the appointment.

I did get some great news about our quest to be recognized for having completed the six major marathons around the world. Since we did New York and Chicago before Abbott World Major Marathons had designated these marathons as part of the group, they wouldn't give us credit for them. Our good friends at Marathon Tours went to bat for us and others, though, and we were finally included in the esteemed group of runners who had finished all the majors.

On that positive note, we headed off to Gulf Shores, Alabama, for the half-marathon. A cold front arrived just as we did, so the temperatures dropped from the seventies to the high fifties, but I reminded myself that this does not suck.

At the same time, the weather was great for the race, which took us mostly through the trail system. The last four miles were along the major road along the coast, and the strong wind was in our face, but I put my head down and accomplished another PR, shaving one minute off my previous walking half-marathon time.

The Mesa half-marathon was our last training race for running on our seventh continent, Antarctica. The idea was to take it easy and cross the finish in around three hours. Sometimes things actually work out better than planned. It was rather chilly at the start, thirty-five degrees, so to warm up I started off the race with a vengeance. After about three miles I realized I was way ahead of my predicted pace, so we decided to keep the pace going.

This race was one that many runners used to get their Boston qualifying times, and I can see why, with the nice temps and the downhill slope all the way from the start to the finish. I was able to PR for the fourth straight time, nine minutes faster than my last half-marathon. I thought I might not ever run again. I was thinking seriously about tackling a marathon walking. That way I could get another PR for sure, since I have never walked one before.

It was funny to hear runners complaining about my long legs as I walked by them. When I run a marathon, I kind of shuffle, but while racewalking, I took nice long strides. Near the end, the runners were breaking down and I just kept passing them, since my pace remained the same the whole way.

Mesa was very nice, but as I commented to Catherine, with all the places I want to go to in my lifetime, we will never be back. I used to have what I called a "life list" of things I wanted to do, but now that we had been on the road for over two years it was more of a schedule based on what races we wanted to do and where and where the sun was shining the brightest.

After Mesa we were headed to Buenos Aires, stop number 218, for two days, then a short flight to Ushuaia, then across the Drake Passage through the South Shetland Islands to the Antarctic Peninsula. As I mentioned, Catherine doesn't like the cold. I pretty much cleared out our storage unit with cold-weather gear and was told to bring it all ashore in case we needed it during the race. I looked at being cold as a temporary inconvenience, just like the pain you feel during the marathon itself.

I was also praying for a smooth voyage across the Drake Passage. It's three days, and it can be rough as all get out. I tried to get anti-nausea patches for Catherine, but there was a moderate interaction with another medication she was taking. She brought her wrist bands that apply pressure to a vein, which have worked on cruises in the past. I did buy some Dramamine just in case.

Everyone kept telling me that the experience of Antarctica would be life-changing, but I had a theory about that. I hoped it wasn't one of those things people say when something really sucks, but they spent a lot of money so they don't want to admit to it. At more than $1,000 a day, I certainly hoped not.

They say no news was good news, but I'm not so sure when it comes to hearing back from my doctor. I was hoping to have the plan of action to repair my aneurism, but that didn't seem possible before we got on the airplane to Buenos Aires, after which we would be out of contact for ten days as we made our way to Antarctica and back.

On our first night in Buenos Aires, Marathon Tours had their typical reception and dinner—except this time, the president, Jeff, and the founder of Marathon Tours, Thom, surprised Catherine and me with our six Marathon majors medals.

We had gotten the certificates the week before and figured we would get the medals in the mail, but Jeff contacted them and had the medals sent to him so he could do the presentation in front of the two hundred folks headed to Antarctica. The surprise brought tears to Catherine's eyes.

In the morning, we went for an eight-mile walk at a very leisurely pace. Not really knowing where I was going, I headed in the direction of their famous park called Reserv Ecologica Costanera Sur. This was a popular area along the canal. Since we had plenty of time we managed to walk just about the entire park.

For dinner we ate at El Establo, which was famous for its steaks. I was one happy man. I went for the big boy steak, and Catherine got the smaller one. We also got some type of chips and they had a great salsa type sauce to go with them.

As we walked the streets near the hotel there were over a hundred folks calling out "cambio, cambio," alerting you that they were willing to exchange your money into pesos right there for a fee. I wasn't sure how any of them made any money since I never saw any transactions actually taking place, and some were literally standing next to each other.

The next day we rushed through breakfast prior to the 7:00 a.m. bus ride back to the airport for our domestic flight to Ushuaia. There are two ships used for this adventure, and since no more one hundred people can be on King George Island at a time, they split each boat up into two different flights each day.

We were on the second flight on the second ship, so would only have about an hour to tour Ushuaia. During the bus ride to the ship we were told that since we were running late, we wouldn't have any free time. Many of us were very bummed out, so the Captain ended up submitting to pressure and allowing us an hour to tour the town. Basically, this meant getting a picture in front of the Ushuaia sign and getting stamps and certificates for being in the southernmost part of the civilized world.

Accommodations on the ship were nice. Since we only planned on doing this once, we went for the Shackleton suite, named after the famous explorer, Ernest Shackleton, who was one of the first to this area some two hundred years ago. We had a good-sized sitting room with a desk and refrigerator. The bedroom had a queen bed with a normal cruise ship-sized bathroom.

The ship itself looked like someone had put some containers on top and made it look nice. It was a Russian research vessel out-fitted for tours with a mostly Russian crew operating the ship. The staff for tours and presentations were from all over the world. Since I upgraded to a suite, they had a bottle of wine waiting and an email address set up for us. It took me awhile to get used to having no key to the room (for safety reasons) and the constant broadcast through-out the day saying things like, "Whales off the starboard side of the ship at four o'clock." One lady who worked on the ship, was also a nomad, and had been at it for ten years.

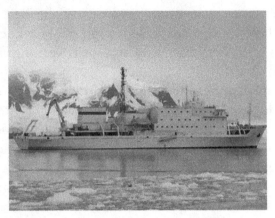

Our home for the next ten days

There was no TV or internet, but we could buy phone usage just in case someone needed to call home. We got outfitted for our foul weather gear, which was required when we go ashore for our expeditions. Catherine was feeling somewhat better after being on the verge of being sick. I felt great, and from what I heard the ride so far was not bad at all. One crew member said that on the last trip, even he got sick.

During our briefing on the Antarctic explorations from 1819 to 1922, our instructor tried his best to make it exciting. I didn't fall asleep, which was saying a lot. The takeaway was that even the Japanese came down here to explore back then. Few actually knew what they were doing and were lucky if they didn't kill themselves getting here or back home.

The food was actually pretty good on the ship, and there was plenty of it. They say you can judge how the people are handling the rocking back and forth by the number of people at each meal, and the dining room had been full. Crew members were actually calling the Drake Passage the "Drake Lake" for this crossing. Some said that if the ride was smooth one way, be prepared for the return. So maybe we would get the Drake Shake on the way back.

"Humps and Bumps" was a presentation of all you wanted to know about whales and seals but were afraid to ask. I snoozed a bit, but did wake up in time for the video showing the whales teaming up to kick a seal off a floating piece of ice so they could have a meal.

Only about 50 percent of whales survive the first year after birth, and females live about fifty years longer than males. The reason why was intriguing: Females are full of toxins that they pass on to their offspring, and a high percentage can't handle it. Since the mothers are getting the toxins out of their system as they nurse their young, they get to live longer. Since males have no way to rid their bodies of the toxins, they don't live as long.

We started our preparation for landing by signing a three-page release and making a detailed list of ailments and medications. If you don't sign, you don't get to leave the ship. Next we had to bring down all our outerwear that was going off the ship so it could be cleaned and sanitized so that we didn't bring anything foreign to Antarctica.

Finally we had to go to a presentation on how to get on and off the Zodiacs and everything we shouldn't do while on land. Once again, we had to sign that we were going to do all that they told us to do. I'll not say it was overkill, just something that has to be done by everyone who plans on commingling with this pristine part of the world.

Needless to say, Catherine was getting a bit stir-crazy, but all was well with me as we rock along toward King Charles Island. The ship ahead was already there and setting up the course for their race tomorrow. One more thing I choose not to do on this trip was kayaking. After seeing the whales team up on a seal in one of the videos, I decided the best way to stay dry was to avoid the kayak experience.

The afternoon presentation was on penguins, and our instructor did the whole thing in a penguin outfit. It was very informative about the three types of penguins in this neck of the woods: The chinstraps were the cutest, but some other breeds were more plentiful. The different breeds don't interbreed because they speak a different language.

Our first experience of Antarctica firsthand was on Aitcho Island. It was a bit chilly, but we had plenty of layers on to handle the cold and slight wind. The penguins were cute and curious, and the stench was not as bad as I heard it might be.

We also got to see two fur seals come out of the water right where we were standing and pay us a visit. We had to move a bit since they seemed to want to test the official distance between us and them, fifteen feet. It was fun to watch some trying out their swimming techniques for the first time. Many were molting, so we had to give them even wider berth, since that process was exhausting and we didn't want to give them a reason to exert themselves.

About an hour was all I could take before we got back in the Zodiacs to the ship. I thought that we would have enough layers for the race the next day but would test it out when we went back ashore on Robert Point.

On Robert Point, there were several types of penguins everywhere. We even got to see some elephant seals enjoying the sun on the rocky beach. Some of the leopard seals where a bit aggressive, so having a walking pole close at hand was recommended.

They call this part of this world pristine but there were remnants of penguin poop and various carcasses littered throughout the island, and the smell was a bit stronger that on Aitcho Island.

Race day was much better than I had expected. It was better to be over-prepared than under-prepared. Good thing I had worked for the largest logistics company in the world for twenty-seven years because it was a handful to figure it all out:

1. Dress in outwear for the Zodiac ride to the start line near the Russian base.
2. Once there, take the outerwear off and change out of your boots and into your running shoes.
3. Add any layers you think you might need for the run.
4. Put all the outerwear in a watertight bag along with your boots.
5. Start the race.

I had timed it so we were the last Zodiac going ashore, and once there we had fifteen minutes to get ready for the start. The hilly terrain had rocks, boulders, pebbles, and mud. They even threw in some snow showers along with the wind and cold at no extra charge.

We had to run out and back three times, and that was a plenty. The marathon was six times out and back, and I know I would have turned my ankles at mile 23 in the rockiest portion of the course near the Chinese base. Catherine and I both managed to stay on our feet.

We came in once again hand in hand, right on my predicted time. We were a bit slower than our last few half-marathons, but we did run/walk the entire time. When we started to heat up or there was a uphill, we would walk, and when we would start to cool off or there was a downhill, we would run.

We were so thankful that we chose the half, since the folks doing the marathon looked rather miserable. After the race, we took the Zodiac ride back to the ship in sweat-soaked clothes. It took some doing to get the mud cleaned off our shoes. I was very glad that our quest to conquer the Antarctica Half Marathon was over. We had officially completed either a marathon or half-marathon on all seven continents.

They say that less than 1 percent of the population has completed a marathon in their lifetime. Couple that with the fact that we have done all six major marathons and at least a half-marathon on every continent, and my computer can't do the calculations.

We had a bottle of champagne chilling in the fridge in our room back on the ship, so after the hot shower and the chili for lunch, all was now right with the world. Tomorrow we would have the awards ceremony to see who were the fastest male and female from both ships, along with age-group winners.

Overnight we made it to Mikkelsen Harbor and were able to go ashore and view many more penguins and seals. On Mikkelsen Island there were some cool whale bones strewn amongst the pieces of ice that had also come ashore. Small icebergs were plentiful, and the glaciers all around were magnificent with their dark blue color in the cracks due to all the oxygen being compressed out of the ice.

It was much colder and windier than where we ran the race the day before. I was very glad we didn't attempt a run this far south. They do have a race in the north polar region of the world, but I think this adventure will cap off my cold weather runs.

I never thought I would say that I enjoyed the awards ceremony and barbecue on the back deck of the ship in thirty-degree weather while a seal floated by on a small iceberg.

The cooks threw everything they had in their freezer, including the kitchen sink, at the barbecue. I hadn't had warm wine in a while, and the apple strudel was a fine finish to the meal.

Turns out I came in fourth in my age group and we were halfway down the list for those who did the half-marathon. It had been a while since I had been a midpacker in a race and doing so way out here felt like a real accomplishment. I was starting to see why some people say that this was a life-changing experience.

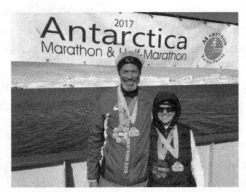

*With both our Antarctica and six major medals*

We pulled up anchor after saying goodbye to the folks from the other ship, who were going to start their trip back north. We kept heading south and some brave souls went on a Zodiac cruise or kayaking a few hours before sunset. I, on the other hand, enjoyed watching the floating landscape go by.

We did see a few whales from the ship, and during dinner everyone who cruised around in the Zodiacs was talking about the amazing time they had on the water amongst the humpback whales. Two even went under one Zodiac and came back up on the other side. I had visions of them teaming up and causing a wave to knock a few humans into the water for dinner.

I had to keep telling myself, like I did in Africa, that wild animals don't eat Jeeps—or in this case, Zodiacs—and if you stay in them, you'll be okay. We ended up going out for a morning cruise in Wilhelmina Bay, and we did see two whales doing their thing.

They would come up to the surface, then lead us to another spot where they would go under for a while and pop up somewhere new. We tried to get the perfect shot of the kayakers in the foreground and the whales in the background, but they were not cooperating.

Things didn't always go as planned especially here in Antarctica. We were going to do another landing to see the largest population of Gentoo penguins, but the whales and Mother Nature changed the plan. As we were heading to the landing, we could see a storm in the distance. While we stopped to come up with plan B, a hundred or so whales decided to put on a spectacular show for us.

They breached, slapped their tail, and even threw in a few fin waves. A few tried out a new trick of going back and forth under our ship. That was the only way I wanted to see them do that trick—not with a Zodiac like they had the day before. It was funny watching everyone going back and forth from one side of the boat to the other so as not to miss a moment of their entertainment.

After the show was over, we turned away from the storm just before it started to precipitate on us. We then headed for another bay and had our first landing on the actual Antarctica Peninsula. There were plenty of penguins there, and we even got see some come in from the water and feed their young after filling their bellies.

The one with the food would call out, and then the chase was on with the youngster trying to catch their parents for the food. It was definitely survival of the fittest. The fastest got fed, while the others had to wait for the next time around.

For our last day on the Antarctic Peninsula, we made a nice, steep climb up to the top to get a great view of Paradise Harbor. This was where the Argentine Research Station sits after it was rebuilt. It had to be rebuilt because there was a doctor who was not pleased that after he had spent a year there, the relief crew forgot to bring a replacement doctor with them. After his buddies left and he saw that he was looking at another year, he set fire to the station in hopes that the ship would see and return. They kept sailing, and by the time they heard of the fire, the station was mostly burnt to the ground. You could still see charred areas, but we were here for fun and the polar bear plunge.

Everyone made the climb to the top and then slid down on our rears. Most even stripped down to their bathing suits so they could say they did the polar plunge off the Antarctic Peninsula. We watched and took pictures, and made sure we were on the first Zodiac back to the ship, where we were greeted with warm rum cider.

The Drake Passage was forecast to be rough, so we started our trip back earlier than planned, since we would have to take the rough part slowly. We pitched our way through the Antarctic Charity Auction and dinner. As a group we did manage to raise $7,000 for the Oceanites Charity. They are billed as "those who count the penguins so we don't have to." Most us were in bed by 9:00 p.m., and we rocked and rolled all night long. We were able to come within three miles of Cape Horn and saw a presentation on what it was like back then to navigate these unforgiving waters back in the day.

We had two more full days of up and down and side to side. which gave me some time to reflect on whether this trip was truly a life-changing experience. I wasn't so sure about that. I have done and seen a lot in my lifetime, and this was interesting but not life-changing by a long shot. Having open-heart surgery was life-changing. Pulling back on the yoke of a five-hundred-thousand-pound plane and taking it seven miles in the air at over 500 mph and landing some five thousand miles away was life-changing. I could go on and on, but this didn't rate in that category.

It didn't suck, but there were times I wished I was somewhere else. Mostly somewhere warm and connected to the outside world. They say it's great to disconnect every now and then, but doing it for this long wasn't my cup of tea. I did find a book to read on my computer, but with the constant pitching and rolling that was not always a great idea.

I was glad I came to see for myself, but can't see myself doing it ever again. There are too many other things to see. I've visited sixty of the 195 different countries in my lifetime, so I still had some work to do.

I took another unscientific survey (by asking a few people) and the overwhelming opinion was that this was a life-changing experience for them. There were quick to give that answer, but I also noticed that most of them were under fifty. It seemed like they were used to roughing it and had saved up for this trip. Many of them were on their own personal quest to see as much of the world as possible, some in very unconventional ways: hiking or biking for months at a time or climbing the tallest mountain they could find. Money didn't seem to be a concern for them.

Some described lifelong friendships that had made. As a whole we did come together as a team so as to better experience all that Antarctica had to offer. I think that over time I have been somewhat desensitized by our extensive travel. This trip does rate right up there, but for me experiencing the wilds and people of Africa was a life-changing experience.

The running community helps me to understand just how small the world is in certain ways. The youngest runner, was eleven years old and was on a quest to run a half-marathon on all seven continents. He and his mom also ran the Kauai half-marathon in Hawaii at the same time as us in 2016 and the Outback Half Marathon in Australia alongside us in 2015. He came in third overall in the Antarctic half—my goal was for him not to lap me during the race.

There were nine of us from the Africa trip, and a few from Easter Island. The world is huge, but if you lace up your shoes just to prove to yourself that you can, it can be pretty small. A few of us don't run as fast or as long as we used to, but one guy at seventy walks the half distance now and has done so on all seven continents. Another guy who was legally blind beat me. Along with his guide, he plans on doing all seven continents. I try to point out to folks who don't run/walk races anymore that their excuse of a sore knee or whatever just doesn't hold water when I've seen individuals like the ones I have met continue to try and sometimes fail.

Back in Argentina, we went back to Reserv Ecologica Costanera Sur park for one final run before leaving. We saw others from our group coming and going prior to their flights back home—the eleven-year-old and his mom were also doing the loop.

I decided that instead of being a life-changing experience, Antarctica was more of a once-in-a-lifetime experience. Emphasis on the word "once" since I didn't plan on doing it again.

# CHAPTER
# 24

## Live and Learn

Find life experiences and swallow them whole
Travel
Meet many people
Go down some dead ends and explore dark alleys
Try everything
Exhaust yourself in the glorious pursuit of life.

—Lawrence K. Fish

As we headed for destination number 223, one would think that I had learned a lot over time. I had made a few mistakes, but my one of goals was for us not to show up for a plane and have them say, "The flight left yesterday" or arrive at a hotel and have them say, "Your reservation is for tomorrow."

Our trip to Antarctica had gone off without a hitch. We were at the airport at 2:00 p.m. on a Saturday, three hours early for our flight from Buenos Aires to San Paulo, when the ticket agent informed us that we didn't have a visa for Brazil. We weren't getting on our flight.

During my last three years at UPS I had been responsible for this neck of the woods, so you would think I would have known better. I had a Brazilian visa in my old passport, but it had expired in the later part of last year, and it never occurred to me to get one for the new passport.

I had gone to government websites to check requirements many times, but not this time. Maybe I was becoming complacent or road-weary. We put on our sad faces and explained that we had to get to Brazil to visit Catherine's brother. The frowns and dumbfounded looks worked, and we were given the emergency phone number for the Brazilian Consulate.

I gave it a try. Lo and behold, someone answered—but she only spoke Portuguese. She handed the phone to a translator who said we had to be there by five. We jumped in a cab. and there we were on our very lucky day.

It was our lucky day because two very rich families had a sim-ilar problem, and each had brought three kids to the consulate. If it hadn't been for them, we would have had to make an appointment some time the next week. Three hours later, we were dragging our bags a half a mile back to our hotel. Luckily they had rooms, so we dropped off our bags and had the finest steak and Pisco sours to cap off the long day.

This was definitely a case of "Live and learn." I knew better but needed this real-life experience to get me back on my game. But we weren't out of the woods yet. I'm not kidding anyone when I say I spent hours on the phone with Orbitz getting our reservations squared away. At midnight, and it was still not resolved and I was thinking of throwing in the towel, but instead got six hours of sleep and pressed on.

It seems that since we didn't make our flight we were classi-fied as no-shows and it was undecided if we had a return flight with Orbitz still. I pressed the issue, and they caved and honored our flight back—but I could no longer book online.

Fees and additional cost for new flights be damned, I was not going to be denied. A slight problem was that San Paulo was not our final destination. Catherine's brother Larry and his wife Eliana live near a small airport, Ribeirao Preto, so we would either have to catch a puddle-jumper or make at four-hour drive. No matter what we were willing to pay, we weren't getting there the next day.

Marriott has a hotel near the airport in San Paulo, so we planned to arrive late at night, stay over, and fly to see Larry and Eliana the next day, refreshed. You would think I had planned it this way. We got to breathe the air of a different city and still get four nights of family time with Larry and Eliana. I didn't add up the additional cost, but as long as we were staying in nice hotels and experiencing all this together, no big deal.

As we were on our way to the airport, we had another "live and learn" experience. As we were driving down the highway, leaving the hustle and bustle of the city, on both sides of the road was green space where families were having picnics, playing soccer, and flying kites. This was along the highway the entire way to the airport. I was awestruck. There were signs saying clearly that this was forbidden, but I guess it was just one of those rules that was meant to be broken.

No matter where we traveled, everyone was trying to do the same things to enjoy life. Some just have to improvise to accomplish what others might take for granted.

It was only a fifty-minute flight, and then we could rest up for the next four days with no planes, trains, and automobiles. The ATR 172 was a great jet prop aircraft, and the flight was on time with plenty of room at our seats. It was only about a one-hour drive to Larry and Eliana's home in Bebedouro. After a first career as a chemical engineer, Larry now owns a farm there where he raises bananas and passion fruit.

I guess you could say Larry and I were on parallel tracks when it comes to retirement. He was using his experience from his previous job to fulfill his dream of farming. I was using my navigation experience from aviation to help us run all over the world. I really enjoy the challenge involved in trying to figure out how to safety get from point A to B, learning as I go along.

Living on the farm was another example of "live and learn." Larry used a drone to survey his farm. He was growing passion fruit, which farm hands had to go around and fertilize by hand, moving the pollen from plant to plant. He also grew bananas, and told me his goal was to be self-sufficient. This lifestyle was not for me, since it would require me to stay in one place, and I wasn't ready to stay put They had two puppies at the farm, including a two-year-old miniature Pinscher, and before we left we had to check Catherine's bag to make sure she didn't try to take them back to Atlanta with us.

I learned a lot on this trip. I need to stay on my A game if we are going to continue at this pace; also, just because what you're doing is the answer to your dreams doesn't necessarily mean others have the same dream.

# CHAPTER
# 25

## Here We Go Again

Time is like a river. You cannot touch the same water
twice, because the flow that has passed will never
pass again. Enjoy every moment of your life.

—Unknown

As a couple, Catherine and I don't like doing the same thing over
and over. Yes, we've done many marathons and other races, but few
in the same place, so it always makes the experience different in many
ways.

The main reason I got an artificial heart valve was that the pig
valve usually only lasts ten to fourteen years, and I didn't want to
repeat that experience. Whether I liked it or not, I was headed back
to the operating room. My surgery/procedure to repair my aneurysm had been scheduled, and I would only have two weeks before
our next trip to recover. I called it a surgery/procedure since I wasn't
exactly sure what to call it. I'd have to stay in the hospital for two days
afterward so I guess "surgery" would be more appropriate, but I liked
the way "procedure" sounded.

First, though, was a round robin trip to see some relatives and
then a trip to Springdale, Arkansas for a half-marathon. I was pleasantly surprised by our experience with the Springdale/Fayetteville/
Fort Smith area. We went there for the Hogeye Half Marathon only
because we had a free weekend and they had a race.

It was called "Hogeye" because forty years ago that was the name of the little rural town where the race started and finished. After about thirty years they moved it to Fayetteville, and this year it was moved again to Springdale. We started and finished in the quaint downtown area. There could not have been more than one thousand people for all four races: the full, half, 5K and kids' marathon. The way the kids' marathon worked was that they had to show that they had run twenty-five miles so far that year and then did the final 1.2 on race day.

We got to run a small portion of the course the day before when we did a five-miler around Lake Fayetteville. The weather was perfect on race day, packet pickup was just prior to the start, and they even had a "thirty minutes early" start for those who might need a few extra minutes on the course. They had just about as many volunteers as runners, and the police were out in full force to help us cross the few streets along the way.

I wanted to take it easy before the surgery but didn't want to walk the whole race, so I modified our run/walk routine once again. We ran during one song, then walked during the next. We continued this until the last three miles, when we ran down and walked up the rolling hills. I had planned on taking it really slow and coming in under three hours. We ended up coming in about one minute early, and I didn't even use a watch.

The food at the finish went beyond the usual bananas: there was freshly grilled chicken, hamburgers, and hot dogs, and they gave you two beer/cider tickets to redeem at either of the two local bars, which were on the same block as the finish line. We felt like we had earned it: it had been a year since we finished a half-marathon that fast.

After a few days back in Atlanta and Los Angeles, we were on to Seattle for my surgery. I had a feeling of malaise to the point that I stopped working on future trips until I could see the outcome.

To get me ready, we had to play with my INR number, which is essentially a measurement of your clotting time. To prevent blood clots around my artificial heart valve, my INR needed to be 1.5. (Normal is 1.0.) They tested my blood the day before surgery, and it was at 2.0. My surgeon wouldn't operate if my INR was above 1.7, so we could either wait a few days or they could give me a one-fourth pill of vitamin K. I took the pill and was down to 1.7 just prior to surgery.

Yes, it was surgery and not a procedure, and right before I was wheeled into the operating room, the anesthesiologist pointed out that this was, in fact, major surgery, and there was a possibility that I wouldn't live through it. I guess he had to tell everyone that fact. The surgery is called stent graft placement that extends into the bilateral common iliac and right internal/external iliac arteries. Basically, while I was under general anesthetic, they went through both sides of my groin to insert a stent around the aneurysm to keep it from bursting.

I did live through the surgery, but the recovery didn't go as I had envisioned. I had expected to be up bouncing around in a day or so, but I didn't take into account the effect the two incisions in my groin were going to have on my ability to walk. The only way I can adequately describe it is that it felt like I had been kicked in the groin by a horse with great aim.

It did slow me down a bit, but I was out of the hospital the next day and was able to walk, somewhat, back to the hotel one-half mile away. I had planned on a flight four days after surgery, but the vitamin K had stayed in my system and now my INR was too low. The medical team in recovery came up with a great plan for me to inject myself with a medication called Enoxaparin in my belly twice a day. I upped my usual dose of Warfarin from 7.5 to 10 mg a day, and lo and behold my INR was back up to 1.8 just prior to flight.

I tried to keep moving in between surgery and flight, but unfortunately, I sprung a leak on both of my entry points and had to do some serious patch jobs at the hotel between when I was discharged and before my follow-up appointment. After many days of recovery, I was back to about 80 percent and ready for the flight back to Atlanta.

I had gotten in and out of the hospital in twenty-four hours, but they still managed to find $200,000 to bill my insurance company. My out-of-pocket was about $600, but I couldn't wait to see how much of the rest insurance would be willing to pay and how much would fall my way.

I now definitely fell into the category of people with preexisting conditions, so there was no telling how this was all going to work out in the future. I did have another aneurysm on my aorta above my heart that would need to be repaired in five or so years. I would be on Medicare by then, so I didn't worry about my million-dollar lifetime cap. I really didn't have time to worry about much.

I finished putting together another month-long trip that included business class on Emirates A380, a river cruise from Saigon to Hanoi, and a two-night stay in Dubai in the largest Marriott in the world on the way back to Paris. From there we would finish up with a half-marathon in Petra Jordan.

I love when a plan comes together, and with all the successful plans in my rearview mirror, I was one happy man. My cardiologist reviewed the results of my CT scan and said that the graft, stent, and repair of my right iliac artery looked great. Our flight left that day so I didn't have a lot of wiggle room in this plan. Just the way I like it.

Our destination was Lucca, Italy, for a "land-based running cruise." I've talked about our running cruises with John Bingham and Jenny Hatfield many times. For their Marathon di Tuscany, instead of a boat, a bus would take us to different parts of the Tuscany region of Italy, where the various races over the course of a week would add up to 26.2 miles.

Since I was fully recovered from my surgery two weeks ago, we were planning on getting in a many miles as possible. Some fifty people in our group were meeting up at 7:00 a.m. on the first morning, but not us. Since we're on the road all the time, sometimes we just do our own thing. We finally got out around noon and walked back to where all the tourists are. This was our third time in Lucca, but it never gets old, and it was nice to get a good long walk in.

We were back in time for the welcome reception, where they offered delicious treats like carbine with pistachio, which I enjoyed, and Catherine's favorite, tiramisu. With our bellies full, we spent some time catching up with folks we had seen on other cruises—and getting adjusted to the new time zone. For some strange reason it is was taking longer than it usually did.

For our first run, we had a choice between 4K (once around Lucca's walls) or 8K (twice around). This area became famous for us the last time we were here back in 2011, when three ladies ended up on the opposite side of the wall when it came time for us to meet up for the bus ride back to the hotel. When then named them the "Lost in Lucca Girls" for the rest of the trip.

Since I had not run in about a month, I decided to take the two laps slowly. We mostly ran along the broad, tree-lined pathways along the tops of the massive sixteenth and seventeenth-century ramparts that encircle Lucca's historic city center and its cobblestone streets. It did feel good to once again fill my lungs with fresh air, but my legs felt like they were one hundred pounds each. We were only one minute slower than I had predicted, which was not bad for the first time out in a while.

After the run/walk we had a private guided tour of Lucca, where we discovered the living testimony to past times, kingdoms, and dominions which lies in a green valley just northwest of Florence. This almost perfectly preserved jewel of medieval architecture and buildings emanates charm and shows layers of history from every corner of its narrow, winding streets.

The next morning, we opted for the 10K versus the 5K run event in the beautiful Parco Delle Cascine, a monumental and his-torical park in the city of Florence, along the Arno river. They were having an outdoor market along a half-mile portion of the route, so we had to navigate without running over some of the local bargain seekers.

After the run/walk, our tour guide took us on a walking tour of Florence. That evening we tried our hand at becoming famous Italian pizza-makers with a Tuscan cooking class and dinner. We learned the secrets of kneading and stretching pizza dough, including the world-famous toss in the air, and sampled local wines.

It really surprised me how out of shape I got in a month. I was getting my wind back, but my legs still hadn't gotten with the program. It might have had to do with the fact that we were doing a lot of walking.

The next day was the infamous Amazing Race. This one had a one-hour time limit, so Catherine and I did a sixty-minute run together while everyone else did their best to find all the places on the map.

Afterward, we took a guided tour of the many sites that make Siena one of the most visited cities in Italy. We had time to explore this magnificent city on our own. Later that afternoon, we were treated to visit the village of Monteriggioni, which was built between 1213 and 1219. Its fourteen towers on square bases connect two portals and gates, one facing Florence and the other facing Rome.

We had put in a lot of miles, so Catherine and I welcomed a day off. The next day we were to hike along the scenic and famous Cinque Terre, a string of centuries-old seaside villages on the rugged Italian Riviera coastline. In each of the five towns, colorful houses, and ancient vineyards cling to steep terraces. The hiking trails offer glorious views of this unspoiled stretch of the Italian Riviera.

Unfortunately the route that we had planned on hiking was closed due to the rain that hit the area a few days prior to our arrival. Instead John and Jenny were able to adjust our schedule on the fly.

In Val D'Orcia we met our professional Italian guides just outside of Montalcino to begin the trek. About 9K of unpaved roads later, we arrived at the forest trails of St. Antimo. We stopped for a visit at the Abbey of St, Antimo, and had a lunch that features plentiful pasta and wild boar.

On our way home we stopped at Bagno Vignoni to visit the hamlet and its antique sulfur baths in the middle of the Roman ruins. We drove through the UNESCO world heritage site of the Val D'Orcia and saw Pienza, the touchstone of Renaissance urbanism, on the top of the hill as we made our way back to Florence.

On our last morning, we walk along the Arno River and found a great place to get a cappuccino. In the evening we gathered to receive our finisher's medals and celebrate our week together with a traditional Italian lunch featuring three kinds of pastas, antipasto, salad, dessert, and wine-tasting.

The restaurant that held the cooking class let us back in for the awards ceremony, and the night kicked off with a champagne toast. John and Jenny told us that we put in more than fifty miles if you factored in all the sightseeing, so we ended up crushing the marathon milestone. Then they selected some special awards, which included giving me another yellow hat for the "Comeback Award." It brought tears to my eyes.

Even though this was our third time in Tuscany, the sights never got old, and I was overjoyed to achieve my goal to participate in this trip so soon after my surgery.

# CHAPTER
# 26

## Searching for Aha Moments

Some moments are nice, some are nicer,
some are even worth writing about.
—Charles Bukowski

The first stop on our sixteen-day cruise from Venice to Athens and then back to Rome was Hvar, Croatia. (Some said the *h* was silent, others said it was hard). We were looking forward to our stop in Hvar, since celebrities from Prince Harry to Beyoncé have made it a go-to place for both unspoiled escape and action.

The island was covered in pine and palm trees, vineyards, gorgeous beaches, and fields that earned it the name the Lavender Island. We decided not to run while we were there, but we put in a lot of miles walking up a hill to the fortress where we had a commanding view of the Venetian Cathedral. We didn't see any celebrities, but the large yachts in the harbor indicated that some might have been in the area.

Our next stop was Dubrovnik, where we anchored right beyond the famous walled city so we could admire its beauty with every glance. No cars are allowed in Old Town, so we were hoping to get in some good running miles—and were looking forward to watching some bold divers leap off the cliffs into the crystalline sea.

We didn't see any daring divers, but we did find a rare gem of a place to run. We followed the water to the right and there was a split in the road about one mile out. We first took the split to the right that came to a dead end after about one-fourth mile. We turned around and then took the left split, onto a road with one lane and no traffic to be seen.

We continued for another mile until we joined up with a major street. The views were breathtaking, and I was able to conclude why I really enjoy going one way and returning to our original starting point another way.

With my intense sense of adventure, I'm always looking for those ah-ha moments. For me, it's like an addictive drug without any of the terrible side effects. I see them all the time and constantly look for others. The one road to a destination might provide me those moments, and so I think I might find other ones if I go a different route back.

In this case I was able to get a different perspective on the way down the road than I had on the way up. I noticed some large cruise ships in port, and throngs of buses taking visitors to the fort. This particular fort is famous as a backdrop for the HBO show *Games of Thrones*. I had never seen the show, but we did run into something unexpected: graduating students were celebrating right outside the gates of the fort. Despite a heavy police presence, they were lighting off flares and singing and dancing in the streets.

There was another large fort right on the water, but I was about forted out, so we bypassed it for the cable car to the top of a mountain for some more breathtaking views.

Our next stop was Kotor, Montenegro, one of Montenegro's most beautiful bays, and the approach offered one breathtaking fjordlike view after another. We really enjoyed the bright red rooftops of the medieval town and the blues and greens of the landscape. The charming streets of the Old Town remain car-free, filled with the twelfth-century Baroque palaces and Romanesque churches.

From the port, we set off on a long walk by following a road uphill for some great views of the bay below. When the narrow road we were walking along started to head back down to the water, I realized that I had been on this road before. The last time we had been here, we did an out-and-back run along this road, so it was great to see it from a different perspective.

Once we got back to Old Town, it was time for us to conquer the fortress on the hill for a breathtaking vista. After walking up 1,300 steps, we were able to say we made it to the Castle St. John, an Illyrian fort. About three-quarters of the way up I got into a huge fight with my quads. They were no longer into doing the steps, so I had to sit and hydrate to get them to cooperate again. The trip down was much easier, and it was well worth the walk.

The next three days we made stops in Greece. First was Katakolon, a scenic seaside town at the mouth of the Ionian Sea that was the gateway to ancient Olympia, the original home of the Olympic Games. At Magna Grecia Farm, located in the heart of a traditional agricultural region close to ancient Olympia, we visited the olive groves and learned the history of the olive tree and the tasty, peppery fruit produced there. After a short demonstration of Syrtaki dance, many actually joined in the dance, which was done by all holding hands and moving around those who stayed seated.

The food here and on the ship was exceptional, so our plan was to run/walk at least ten miles a day to balance calories in and calories out, but it became apparent to me that my body still needed some time to heal from my surgery. I would feel great one day, go for a run, and then feel like crap that afternoon and the entire next day. We were training for a half-marathon in Madagascar a month away, but if I didn't rest, my body would just force a down day.

After Delphi we transited the Corinth Canal which connects the Gulf of Corinth with the Saronic Gulf in the Aegean Sea. Most ships have to take the long way around but ships our size can take the short cut. It cuts through the narrow Isthmus of Corinth and separates the Peloponnese from the Greek mainland, thus effectively making the former peninsulas an island. The builders dug the canal through the Isthmus at sea level; no locks were employed. It is four miles in length and seventy feet wide and was built from 1881 to 1893 after various fits and starts.

Our next port of call was Nafplio, Greece. Of course they had a fort with more than nine hundred steps to the top, but we chose a much longer route by road: 2.5 miles to the Palamidi Castle/Fort, then a mile walk around—and of course I had to go back down to the ship a different way, which was well worth the four-mile walk around the base of the fort.

Nafpilo is considered one of the most beautiful and romantic towns in Greece, nestled by the sea with two mountains and the fortress overlooking the town. I had seen many a fortress/castle during our travels, but this one topped them all. In the very heart of the city stands Syntagma Square, with historic buildings, monuments, and Turkish mosques on a peninsula that juts into the Argolic Gulf.

When we arrived in Athens, there were about six other ships docking at the huge Piraeus Cruise Terminal. We departed with everyone else and got on the Big Red Bus for a three-hour tour of Athens. After a forty-five-minute tour of the seaside, we saw the Acropolis (which was packed shoulder-to-shoulder) and the Parthenon. During that portion we went by the Archaeological Museum of Piraeus, Votsalakia Beach, Mikrolimano Harbor, and the Planetarium.

Other stops were the National Library, National Archaeological Museum, Karaiskaki Square and a really funky area called Thession. It looked like an outdoor antique market on steroids. Back at the Acropolis we switched back to the bus for the trip back to Piraeus. This route took us by the Niarchos Foundation and Municipal Theatre.

Our overnight sail took us to Monemvasia, Greece. This Gibraltar-like town is tied to the mainland by a single thread of causeways and holds treasures that are old even by Mediterranean standards. Once there we tried something we had not done in a while: going for a hike. We found a trail up the mountain behind the homes in the area. After an hour of challenging climbing up, we came to the end and had to go back down the same way—which in many ways was way more challenging.

After that, we walked along the causeway to the Monemvaia Castle. Inside the confines of the castle walls we found not only shops, restaurants, and bars, but also a slew of hotels. I had never seen anything like that before.

In Gythion, Greece. we were able to get in a nice, slow, and picturesque six-mile midmorning run along the coast. I crossed my fingers that my body wouldn't impose a down day in protest.

A day at sea brought us to Giardini Naxos, a commune in the province of Messiana on the island of Sicily in southern Italy. Our visit began with a trip to Gambino Vineyards, a family-run winery that displayed a passion for perfection in all they produced. After a short tour we had a scrumptious lunch at the winery, where excellent wine pairings and live music made it a great afternoon experience. Once back to the dock, we were still able to get in our ten thousand steps along the same route we had done back in October.

Our next port of call was Lipari, which is the largest in a chain of islands in a volcanic archipelago that straddles the gap between Vesuvius and Etna. When we got ashore it became clear with the narrow streets and uneven pavements that this was going to be a long walking day. It wasn't easy to find roads that were either closed to traffic or had sidewalks. We managed it get in about seven miles, and once again found some great views of the harbor.

The next morning, we threw open the curtains and were met with the cliffs of Sorrento, Italy. The legendary Sirens, mythical provocateurs of pure voice, were said to lurk in this water off Sorrento. They would lure sailors of antiquity to their doom by singing beautiful songs and driving them mad, causing them to crash their vessels on the rocks. Homer's Ulysses (Odysseus) overcame the sirens' call by strapping himself to the mast and having his oarsmen pour wax into their ears to drown out the sweet songs.

It was a run day for us, so it didn't matter that most sidewalks were only an inch wide. We were able to get in four very slow, careful miles. After that, we walked the narrow streets where everything from limoncello to any and everything you might want or need was for sale.

When we got to our last stop of Rome, Windstar sent us off in style with an incredible wine tasting for us returning guests. The owner of a rather new winery in the area came onboard and we worked our way through eight different wines.

It was a somewhat tearful goodbye, since there was the feeling of family amongst everyone on board. It had been an extraordinary sixteen days and, we were looking forward to more trips with them over the next several years. "Running all over the world" doesn't have to mean racing. The mere fact that we could open up our curtains in the morning, see the new sights of the next port of call, then lace up our shoes and run, sometimes to the left from the port, other times to the right, meant that we were never far from our next "ah" moment.

# CHAPTER
# 27

## It Never Gets Old

Travel is fatal to prejudice, bigotry, and narrow-mindedness,
and many of our people need it sorely on these accounts. Broad,
wholesome, charitable views of men and things cannot be acquired
by vegetating in one little corner of the earth all one's lifetime.
                                                    —Mark Twain

Like a lot of other phrases, "it never gets old" has a double meaning for me. During our travels, we've seen many old churches, forts,
and museums; and no matter how many times I see them, it's like I'm
seeing them for the first time. Another way to look at it is that, even
though I might be getting older, I never really feel that way. I might
not be able to run a marathon as fast as I used to, but it doesn't stop
me from trying. Even after running a distance of at least 13.1 miles
in twenty-four different countries plus Antarctica, it never got old.

From Rome, we took the high-speed train (cruising at 186
mph) to Lake Como for the wedding of my niece, Ana. Lake Como
is indeed breathtaking, but we had seen so many views on this trip
that I believed I might be having, desensitizing syndrome, a syndrome I just made up that meant when I looked out the window of
our hotel I was clearly not as impressed as others visiting the Lake
Como area. Maybe I needed to look at a blank wall for a while to get
my senses recalibrated.

We were able to get in a great run and long walk while here. Of course, there was a castle, and lucky for us, we were able to find one way up to the Castello Di Vezio and a different route back down.

From the castle, we took in views of the town of Varenna right beneath us and Lake Como in all its splendor. The beginnings of the castle probably date back to late antiquity, a time that links it to being used as a strategic military hub during the late Roman period. From the castle, it would have been possible to keep watch over the road that went from Bellano to Esino Lario, and it was also used as a watchtower and signaling point that overlooked the whole lake.

As we headed off to Milan to get serious about training for the Madagascar half-marathon in two weeks, my right knee was giving me trouble, which was unusual for me. I was starting to understand the fact that as I got older, my cells don't regenerate like they used to, so I needed to learn to compensate.

On our first day in Milan, we got our bearings, and on the second day, we ran around nine miles. On the third day, we got in a nine-mile walk where we were able to see the third-largest church in the world, Milan Cathedral. We have seen St. Peter's Basilica in Vatican City, the largest but, not the second-largest, the Basilica of the National Shrine of Our Lady of Aparecida, a Brazilian municipality.

After visiting the church, we walked over to the huge soccer stadium, San Siro. My knee held up both days and I felt like I was ready for the off-road adventure in Madagascar.

Another first for me: After dinner, I put my credit card and receipt in the slot of my phone case. No big deal. I had done it a thousand times before. We decided to take the long way back to the hotel. Near the end of the route, I checked to see how many miles we had walked—and noticed that my credit card and receipt were gone.

I traced our way back to the restaurant where we ate, but no joy. We went back to our hotel and made a call to the credit card company to report it lost. While I was on hold, the hotel phone rang and the receptionists told me that someone had turned in my card. I told the credit card company that it had been found and went down to retrieve not only the credit card but also the receipt from the restaurant.

I was completely amazed, especially since my impression of Milan had been somewhat mixed. There were so many people out and about with their cups asking for money, but to know that someone went out of their way renewed my faith in humanity. I promised myself that the next day that I would give everyone asking for help some change.

Our next destination was Amsterdam, and during one of our walks, we can upon the famous Dam Square. When Catherine saw the adjacent buildings and structures she said, "It never gets old." I asked what she meant by that, and she explained that there are some things she didn't remember; but when she saw the square, she remembered the other two times we had been there, and her impression was that these sights never get old.

After a refreshing five-day stay in Amsterdam, we were off for the final leg of this fifty-three-day adventure to Antananarivo, Madagascar, for thirteen days. There we would run a half-marathon in our twenty-fifth country. Before we set up this trip a few months back, I had never heard of Antananarivo, which is the capital. Fortunately for those like me who might have trouble pronouncing it, it's called "Tana" for short.

I had planned this trip to start from Amsterdam, so the flights wouldn't be that brutal: a one-hour flight to Paris, a two-hour layover, then a ten-and-a-half-hour flight to Madagascar. I am not fond of flights of this duration, but luckily, the middle seat was empty so I could do some modified leg stretching. Catherine was sitting across the aisle from me, wasn't so lucky, with all four of the seats in her section taken.

My first impression of Tana was that this place was amazing, but not in a good way. There was despair everywhere: Moms and children carrying babies and begging for money everywhere you turn, especially outside the hotel, where they smile with their hands out. We did give out some money but there were so many of them. Catherine wasn't taking the whole experience very well.

They say the country has plenty of money but government corruption has kept it away from the people who need it. Whatever the reason, it was heartbreaking. Statistics indicate that 70 percent of the population was under thirty-five, life expectancy was sixty-five years old, and the leading cause of death was diarrhea. Sanitation is of great concern, so we hope we could stay healthy during this last portion of our trip.

There are large numbers of people everywhere in Tana: cars and every mode of transportation tried to share the same space. Shack and shops crowded the roadside, with food for sale in all forms and levels of preparation. On top of that, there were folks just walking along the road, and folks running alongside, pulling carts full of fruits, candy, spices, and many items I had no idea what they might be.

They have a unique multipurpose use of the land. Rice is the staple in their diet and is grown all over Tana. The other part of the rich, moist soil is used for making bricks. They dig up the soil, form them, and then set them out to dry, first in a fire pit and then back out in the sun.

To tend the soil, they use ox-type animals called Zebu. When I say "tend," it wasn't with a plow. It was just the process of the zebu walking back and forth over the land. Everything we saw the people do looked like hard manual labor. There was no mass transit here, mostly vans of all shapes and sizes fully loaded both inside and on top. They barely stopped as people jumped off and climbed on the back.

The main attraction is the Queen's royal compound high atop a mountain. In reality, it wasn't much to see. It was built back in the 1800s and has a very rich heritage. Our tour guide shared a lot of facts and figures, but in my jet-lagged state all I heard was "blah blah blah." We finished our day with a visit to a tiny museum where I learned that Madagascar split from other landmasses 165 million years ago. Another fact stuck out for me: Madagascar is the only country where everyone speaks the same language, Malagasy. They also speak French and English. They use our alphabet with five letters left out: C, Q, U, W, and X.

The race was to be in Toliara near the city of Isalo, located on the west coast of Madagascar. The five-hour van drive wasn't my favorite part of the trip, and I wasn't looking forward to getting back to the airport the same way after running a half-marathon. We went through at least a dozen villages of different sizes and levels of prosperity. Some were very organized and others were just a few huts on the side of the road.

The last hour was at night, which raised my apprehension level somewhat, especially since the two-lane road we were on was also used by large trucks and zebu-drawn carts—or zebus themselves, being herded in groups of twenty or more. When we went off-road for the last five minutes, headed to the dark as opposed to the lights of the villages we had passed, making me start to wonder.

Out of the dark we arrived at the Jardin du Roy, which was jaw-dropping, to say the least. It had been built six years before. Our room was spacious, and you could tell that a lot of time, thought and rocks went into the design and construction process. I could only imagine how much something like that would have cost back in the States.

They had plenty of folks on staff so you really didn't have to wait for anything. I felt better seeing all of them working there, knowing that they all had families that would benefit from us, tourists. It was a long-term goal of Thom, the founder of Marathon Tours and Travel, to bring a marathon to this part of the world. He and his crew really worked their tails off to make sure it was a success. I'm sure it was a logistical nightmare but they all made it look easy.

By now I was feeling the effects of the local bacteria, and even though it wasn't the worst experience in the world my GI track was not a happy camper. Zebu steaks were no longer sounding appetizing, but a lady on the tour had some miracle drugs she got from the pharmacy in Tana. It only took about five hours for Colicalm to kick in, and I no longer had to worry about finding somewhere to go out on the racecourse.

We arrived two days prior to the race and had a great four-hour hike/tour looking for their local true breadwinners, the lemurs. They say that 80 percent of Madagascar's plants and animals are found nowhere else on Earth, and tourists come from everywhere to see the lemurs, who love to congregate at this one campground site, and love to pose for all their fans.

The day before the race, we did a short hike to see the process of sapphire mining up close and personal. It was nothing like I had expected, and very labor-intensive. The process starts out with a group of men digging ten holes about twenty-five feet into the ground about ten feet apart. If any of the holes have any sapphires then they will turn the ten holes into one big crater with only shovels and the strength of their backs.

They then take all the rocks to the nearby watering hole to sift the sand out. The true experts go through the stones to find the sapphires, which are few and far between. After that, we were off to (you guessed it) the sapphire store, where I coordinated a van load of folks who had no interest in buying to leave soon after we got there.

The race itself reminded me a lot of the Amazing Masai race in Nairobi, Kenya. The half-marathon was ten miles in a park, two miles along the main road, and the last mile back off-road to the hotel with the finish line by the pool. I would say the course had every type of terrain known to man. The rocks and tall grass were not my favorites. I had to slow down to a walk to take in the beautiful scenery, since every time I took my eyes off my feet, I would trip and almost fall. My right knee really gave me problems with the uneven running surface, but that sucky feeling quickly went away as each of the marathoners came across the finish line. The last one, one of the youngest runners, came in eight hours and two minutes after she had started.

I had two goals for this race: not to fall and to enjoy a large frosty bottle of Three Horses Beer with my feet in the pool. I achieved them both. We came a long way to achieve these goals, and so far, it has been worth it. Sometimes I get so caught up in my own accomplishments that I start to believe that I've done a lot so far in my lifetime—but then I'm slapped back to reality when we go on these trips with some true overachievers. During this race, a gentleman broke the record for the highest number of countries in which someone had run a marathon, with a total of 132 countries.

We had two other super-duper overachievers in this group. One lady made a wrong turn and put in an extra three miles for her marathon, but still won her age group. And a gentleman thought someone had made a wrong turn and put in an extra hour of running to try to locate her before giving up and catching her on the course since she hadn't gotten lost after all.

After getting some good sleep back in Tana, we were on a turboprop for Morondava, which is also located on the west coast. Note to self: don't sit in row 6 on this plane unless you're in love with watching a prop spin at some mind-splitting RPM right outside your window. The flight attendant did come to tell me I could move to the exit row once the seat belt light went off. Must have been my legs sticking in the aisle that gave him that great idea.

After two more days of tours then a free day, I was looking forward to a day on the beach overlooking the Mozambique Channel. Our bungalow at Palissandre Cote Ouest Resort and Spa was only a few feet from the beach, and I did not want to leave.

But of course, we did. After a short break, we were off for Baobab Tree Alley. Our guide wanted to make sure we got to the perfect spot by sunset. It was a rough ride in our off-road vehicle, but at the end of it was another example of how traveling never gets old. It's hard to explain the spectacular beauty of the sun setting on these trees, so I will allow the following picture to speak for me.

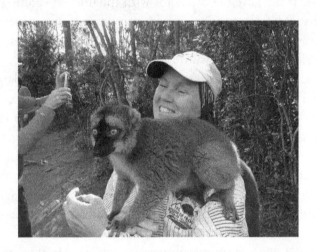

The next day, after a three-hour off-road ride we made it to Kirindy Reserve and research station and my first thought was, "Well I now know where the middle of nowhere is." We went for a two-hour hike in search of more lemurs and fossa. Little did I know that I really didn't want to find the fossa, due to the fact they looked like they would eat my ankles in one bite. They are Madagascar's largest carnivore, but we didn't see any of them. We did find brown and dancing lemurs. As an added bonus, Catherine got to give one little guy a drink of water out of a snail-shell.

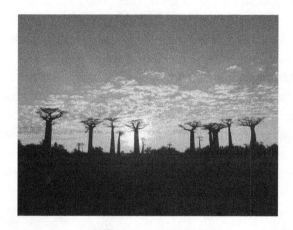

One of my favorite things to do on these trips is to have a day with no planned races or excursions. Being at a resort on the beach made it even better. After breakfast, we went for a long walk along the beach. There was a one-mile section in front of some villages that wasn't very picturesque, but the rest of it was relaxing and exhilarating at the same time.

From the porch of our bungalow, we were able to enjoy a nice bottle of South African white wine while watching a spectacular cloudy sunset over the Mozambique Channel. Cloudy sunsets can be some of the best, especially if the sun peeks out just before it goes down. One thought that came to mind was that very few folks can enjoy such an experience in this part of the world.

After a short flight back to Tana, we were prepared for a four-hour bus ride to Andasibe, where we would spend two nights looking for more lemurs in the Easter Rainforest at the Analamazotra Reserve and Lemur Island.

It was Independence weekend in Tana, and the traffic was horrendous. They were celebrating their 1960 independence from France, and everywhere you turn, people were out in the streets in force. Once you got past that fiasco, the challenge was surviving the winding pothole filed, two-lane road. I lost count of the trucks that were broken down on the side of the road, and when we got to one little town several trucks just decided to take a break for about an hour and blocked traffic in each direction. In all, our "four-hour" drive ended up taking seven and a half bone-crushing hours.

Somehow, the lemurs in the rainforest made it all worth it. We were able to experience the elusive creatures in two different settings while in Andasibe. There were twelve types of lemurs in Zahamena National Park, and on the guided tour of the we saw all but the dancing lemur up close and personal. The howling, territorial call of the black and white rings-tailed lemurs was the highlight for me. That afternoon we spent about two hours enjoying lemurs jumping from tree to tree and on everyone but me. Using a treat, the guide was able to get the dancing lemur to jump all along the bank of the river for us, so I now have lemur stories that will last a lifetime.

The drive back to Tana was uneventful, and at the same time eye-opening and stunning. I was able to focus on the beautiful terrain including the mountains as opposed to the hairpin turns. Some trucks were still broken down from the other night, and only a few were brave enough to make the passage during the day, since they are only supposed to use this road during the night.

There were patrols to pull them over outside of a few towns, but they were mostly there to offload the severely overloaded vans. People would pile out and start walking, only to squish themselves back in the same van further up the road.

After our farewell dinner, about twenty-five of us headed to the airport, way early, for our 1:25 a.m. flight. Good thing, because the Independence Day celebration was still in full swing, so once again people were walking faster than our van.

Most of the people we met in Madagascar were nice to us and had smiles on their faces. This was a unique experience, maybe even be a life-changer. As all the thoughts and sights settled in over the next few days, I knew we would have some great stories to tell. We take so many things for granted, but seeing someone with a big container on their head for their daily search for water slaps you back to reality. It's a huge world out there. I didn't think I would go back to Madagascar, but I was very happy I went.

One thing is for sure: even when Air France decides that, after boarding forty-five minutes late, the best place to do one more bag search is outside, in the dark, right at the stairs of the airplane, running all over the world never gets old.

# 28

## Live Life Large

Life is one big road with lots of signs. So when you riding
through the ruts, don't complicate your mind. Flee from
hate, mischief and jealousy. Don't bury your thoughts,
put your vision to reality. Wake Up and Live!

—Bob Marley

I try to live life large, not only because I'm six foot six but because,
all my life, everything that I have done has been on a grand scale. I
decided that what I wanted for my sixty-second birthday on July 6
was to pay a visit to all my kids.

After a few days in Atlanta, we drove down to Athens, Georgia,
to see Mariah. As a County Commissioner who also teaches at
University of Georgia, is working on her PhD in Linguistics, and is a
rap artist and has a podcast, she likes to juggle as many balls in the air
as possible. My advice to her was to keep her eye on the ball closest
to the ground.

Next we were off to Bloomington to visit Catherine's daughter,
Christie, and her family. Then we went over to Cincinnati to see
Shawn and Cassie. From there we went to Louisville where we had
an incredible dinner with Barb, Teri, and their brother, Greg. His
twin sons loved our Madagascar half-marathon medals, which we
gave them.

On my birthday, we headed to San Diego for a traditional lobster dinner with oldest son Aaron and his girlfriend Kelsey. In between runs around the Marina area and Mission Beach. We met several folks from our trip to Madagascar. One of them, Ana, met us for a great outdoor lunch at C Level, and we swapped stories and impressions of Madagascar. It's always interesting to get a different perspective on a shared experience. Ana seemed more adventurous than either of us: she totally enjoyed the entire trip, whereas we were a bit more reserved.

We both love San Diego and could see ourselves living there—sometime in the future. The real reason we were out on the West Coast in the first place was to run the Napa to Sonoma half-marathon, with my sister Gwen who was going to do the 5K.

As you might expect, the Napa to Sonoma race was all about the wine. There was a wine tasting at the hotel just as we arrive, followed by a welcome reception hosted by Marathon Tours and Travel. I was hoping my right knee would cooperate. On our last training run, it had done well for more than miles. I had to be really careful with foot placement during the race, and thought the rolling hills would be good for it.

I realized that the best practice would be to take six to eight weeks off running, but I wasn't sure that would be possible. We both find running very therapeutic. It gives us both the opportunity to take a break from the day-to-day obstacles and to completely divorce ourselves from those worries, so even if I had to limp along, it was much better than nothing.

The next day we had two wine tastings. The first was at Deerfield Ranch Winery, where they had a wine cave for the tasting. They did have some good wines, but nothing I tasted seemed worthy of my hard-earned money. The second one was at the Ledson Winery, where we had a picnic-style lunch and a tasting that turned into an all-out wine feast. The Cabernet was my favorite, but I had no need to buy any since I had plenty at the winery and there was a complimentary bottle of wine at the Fairmont Sonoma Mission Inn and Spa Hotel as well. This was an upgrade from the Marriott Sonoma Lodge and Spa Hotel, where we stayed last year. The pillow top beds and shower made me think about coming back again next year.

On the morning before the race, we hiked the area known as Lookout Trails. The switchback trails up the small mountain gave us extreme views of Sonoma below. We spent several hours there and afterward headed to the race expo for some more wine-tasting. There we did find an excellent Champagne from Meadowcroft Winery that warranted my purchase.

That evening, Destination Races put on an outdoor VIP pre-race dinner. Meadowcroft Winery was pouring their signature Champagne as we arrived, so once again, I was a very happy man. They also made a Pinot Noir wine especially for the race that complemented the outstanding chicken dinner very well.

During the race, my right knee totally cooperated—but it did have some help. I iced it before the race, and I had bought some Rock Tape from Road Runner Sports in San Diego, so I taped it up, following a video I found from KT tape. I also put a recovery Tommy Copper sleeve over my work of art. Each mile I kept expecting the pain to return, but I was really careful with foot placement and it felt great the entire race.

The temperatures rose rather quickly as we ran, so it was water over the head at every water stop. There was a wine stop near mile 10, but I decided not to take any chances with the heat. We actually heard several rescue vehicles go by, and there was one man stretched out on the course. Later we heard that he recovered from heatstroke, and a few others required some IV fluids.

To me, living life large isn't about reckless abandon. It's more remaining within your capabilities but at the same time pushing the envelope from time to time. This race was a perfect example: I could have easily dropped down to the 5K because of my knee, but instead, I came up with a workable plan to run the race that I had signed up for.

It was also a training event for our Desert Half Marathon in Petra, Jordan, in August. My plan for that race was that we would continue to train in the heat of the day to help with the acclimation.

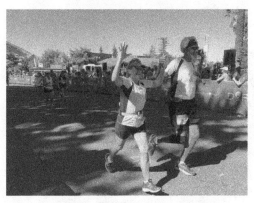

*Another hand-in-hand finish*

Where better to run in the heat than Florida in the summer? We met up with "The Crib" in Miami and drove it across the state to spend a week in Fort Myers. On our first day there, we got on a nice, hot six-mile run around the area. I have a love/hate relationship with Florida. I love the sun (even though the noon sun actually hurts), the seafood, the water, and the people. I tolerate the humidity but hate the mosquitoes and their friends called No-See-Ums. After a few days in the area, I was bitten all over. Since I'm on blood thinners, they really love me.

People often ask Catherine and me if we miss our friends as we run all over the world. Looking back at the last few weeks, I could easily say no. This month I was able to see all three of my kids and their significant others, my sister Gwen and my sister-in-law Joan, Catherine's various family members, five folks from other trips, and another half-dozen new best friends. If that's not living life large, I don't know what is.

# CHAPTER

# 29

## As the World Turns

If you travel, you are reading a book. If you don't
travel, you are only reading one page.
—Our Cambodian tour guide

I asked Catherine for a chapter title idea this time around, and after
reviewing what we would be doing for the next thirty days, she came
up with "As the World Turns." To get from the US to Vietnam, first,
we went to Paris and stayed two nights at the Marriott near the airport in an area called Roissy en France. Across the street was a small
park dedicated to Air France, which included big posters depicting
the history of the airline. They even threw in a landing gear from the
ill-fated Concord. Adjacent was a gigantic structure that made no
sense to me and turned out to be part of the ruins of the castle of the
lords of Roissy, some of which lies underneath the Marriott.

The next leg was from Paris to Dubai on Emirates. This was
my first time on this airline, and after seeing their commercials with
Jennifer Aniston, I went for the upgrade to Business class on their
A380 aircraft to see how the rich and famous travel.

They sure do know how to run an airline. Private chauffeur transportation from the hotel to the airport was included. Strangely, however, in Dubai, they had their airport lounges designated by what class of
service you were traveling on. The three-hour layover went by quickly,
and I couldn't imagine what extra benefits awaited the First-Class folks.

The next leg was another seven hours on a Boeing 777. The service once again was top notch. Getting through immigration was easy enough—I should hope so since the visas for Vietnam and Cambodia were about $1,500 including all the special handling charges since I could only be without our passports for three weeks prior to the trip.

Getting the local currency threw me for a loop. My currency exchange app kept telling me that I needed to get four million Vietnamese Dong from the ATM to have the equivalent of $200. I suddenly understood why they say most Vietnamese people are millionaires.

We picked the AMA Waterways Ama Dara river cruise in an out-of-the-ordinary way. Last October, we had been on another AMA Waterways cruise along the Rhone river from Marseilles to Lyon. During that cruise, you could fill out a card and, for a $200 deposit per person, get a 5 percent discount for a future cruise within two years plus a $100 per person shipboard credit. That seemed like a no-brainer since we didn't have a home and had to live somewhere.

Our plan was to do the Petra Half Marathon near the end of August, and we were still working on what to do prior to that when we got an email offering a deep discount for this particular cruise. After a few phone calls with AMA Waterways and looking at flights, we were able to put this cruise on the schedule. With the 5 percent discount for filling out the card and the discount for this particular trip, it ended up equaling a 2-for-1 cruise.

It was the beginning of their cruise season for this itinerary, and the owners, Rudy and Kristin, were on board the ship. They were joined by the gentleman who handles the hiring and training of all the wait and housekeeping staff. With all that oversight, the passengers were pampered beyond belief on this trip. Internet routers in each room were included and very reliable. Wine and beer were included during lunch and dinner, and house-brand beer and liquor flowed freely during other parts of the day.

Our cruise took us along the Mekong River from Vietnam to Cambodia. We got to see the floating market, nineteenth Century Gothic Cathedral, a rice paper mill, and a coconut candy workshop. There I got to sample some of their exotic snake wine. It actually tasted pretty good, but I only had a taste so I can't give any information about its rumored effect on males.

A must-see is the lively local market along the riverbanks where we found buckets of live frogs and eels and baskets of beautifully displayed skinned rats and snakes. I didn't eat a rat myself, but a member of the group had one that was fried and declared it very tasty.

The next day we were off to see the many rich green rice paddy fields of the Mekong Delta, known as Vietnam's rice basket. The district capital, Tan Chau, is famous for its silk. The products were so good we even bought one silk scarf for Catherine and one for her daughter Christie.

Local transportation while on land that day was by bike-powered rickshaw, which was a hoot to experience. It took me a while to figure out where to put my long legs, but I managed not to drag them on the ground beside me.

Back on board, they had a to-die-for local fruit demonstration. I was not fond of the stinky fruit called durian. They said it's an acquired taste, but for me, the taste was as bad as the smell. It was no big deal as long as you were upwind—and they had at least a dozen others, including passionfruit and dragon fruit.

The next day was the most emotional part of the trip. From the port of Phnom Penh, the capital city of Cambodia, we traveled south to visit two sites that recalled the dark days of the Pol Pot regime: the Khmer Rouge's grim Tuol Sleng (S21 detention center) and the Killing Fields. Everyone really needs to see these two sites in their lifetime to ponder how many people were brutally killed in those areas. One of the buildings held nothing but the skulls of people who were found in the killing fields.

In the afternoon we got to visit the Royal Palace and the spectacular Silver Pagoda. The sheer opulence and size was overwhelming. Phnom Penh is also noted for its tuk-tuks (motorcycle trailers). We had a brief tour of the city where we got to ride in one, but mostly we walked around the city. The Central Market was worth the visit just because of its sheer size. There was one area where you could pick out your fabric and then hand it to someone to take your measurements and make a suit, dress, skirt, shirt, or blouse on the spot.

The transportation system in Cambodia had a long way to go, but with China's help, there were plans afoot to keep gridlock from completely shutting it down. They had a fleet of brand-new buses and a two-year plan to put up an overhead rail system. As opposed to Vietnam where they basically use the Mekong River for transportation, Cambodia is still way behind.

Just before lunch, we headed for Koh Chen, where we experienced our first docking of the ship right along the riverbank. Prior to that, we had either dropped anchor or actually docked at a port. As we arrived, I couldn't imagine where we were going to put this thing. It turns out all they needed were two big trees to tie ropes to.

In our travels, we have seen a lot of begging by the locals, but here the kids had a unique approach. Their unemployment rate is only 1 percent since most work in the agricultural industry, so the kids approached us with something to sell. If they didn't have anything, they would pick a flower to offer us along with their huge smiles. They also practiced their English by asking us questions like salesmen do.

We had the opportunity to visit the one school for the nearby villages, and they sang "Old McDonald" to us in English. We reciprocated by doing the same to them. We also visited one of the local copper and silver shops and learned that all you need to do to tell the difference between silver-plated and real silver is toothpaste and a brush.

The next morning, we were off by motor coach to Oudong, the former capital of Cambodia. There we visited a Buddhist monastery with one of the largest pagodas in the country. We were blessed by the monks, who chanted for around fifteen minutes. We also participated in their daily lunchtime alms ceremony. Basically, we lined up and put a spoonful of rice into each of their dishes as they passed by.

Another highlight of our trip was the short ox cart ride. As we started out on the ride, the local children picked a cart to run alongside and talk to in very good English. The little girl alongside ours offered us a couple of pieces of grass.

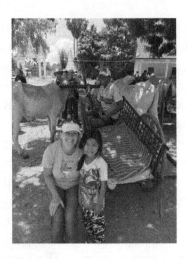

Our Cambodian tour guide had many words of wisdom. The one I thought was worth repeating was, "If you travel, you are reading a book. If you don't travel, you are only reading one page." I find that to be so true. You expand your knowledge and horizons when you travel. I must say that this trip to Vietnam and Cambodia has certainly done both for us.

One night, we had the opportunity to sit at the owners' table for dinner. It was an unlikely experience to swap stories with the folks who not only started AMA Waterways but also Viking cruise lines. I had always wondered where the "AMA" in the name came from. Turns out it was only part of the name they originally wanted, Amadeus, which in their case was a combination of the Latin words *ama* and *deus*, which together mean "love god." Another cruise line had already licensed that name, so they shortened it to AMA (pronounced "ama," not as an acronym) Waterways.

While on the cruise, we ran into another couple who had also been on the road for two-and-a-half years. They had a plethora of knowledge. They hardly ever went back to Canada, where they are from, and would be revisiting their plan after a total of five years, when the condo they were building in Panama City, Panama, was finished. They seemed a bit more adventurous than us. Whereas we usually went places we had heard of, whereas, they liked the off-the-beaten-path places.

They gave us a simple solution to the prescription drug problem we sometimes faced on extended trips. Surprisingly enough, they just show up to the local pharmacy, hand them the empty bottle, and could get as much of what they needed without a prescription—and on the cheap.

Our next stop was a floating city where about five thousand people live at the mouth of the Tonie Sap Lake, which the Mekong River flows into and out of, depending on the time of the year. Fun fact: *me* means "mother" and *kong* means "water." This mother water is the twelfth longest river in the world.

When we were there, more than 50 percent of Cambodians were younger than twenty-five, and they had an average life expectancy of only sixty-three years old. That's understandable with all they had been through over the last sixty years. They still had somewhere between two and five million unexploded land mines in the area, and two hundred people were killed by them yearly. Only half the population had electricity but 95 percent had a cell phone, so many used either solar panels or car batteries to charge them.

At the end of the river cruise portion of the trip, we took a six-hour motor coach ride to Siem Reap, the former capital of the Khmer Empire. Reflecting on all that I had seen so far, the title "As the World Turns" was becoming even more appropriate. Times had changed for the better for the people in this part of the world, and tourism played a big part in their daily lives.

With all the rich, fertile ground and abundant fish, I got the feeling that no one was going hungry there. They all seemed so happy, and I wondered if Buddhism had anything to do with that—96 percent of the population are classified as Buddhist.

Our cruise manager, Son, stayed with us and led us around for six more days: three in Siem Reap, two in Hanoi, and one in a luxury junk on Ha Long Bay.

Siem Reap's claim to fame is the renowned Angkor Wat, where we visited three different historical temple sites. We stayed at the Sofitel Royal Phokeethra, where there were large marble columns everywhere.

231

The first site was Angkor Thom, where 1.2 million folks lived over one thousand years ago. It was made with over five hundred million tons of sandstone slabs that were brought from an area over forty miles away. I called this place "Angkor Town" since it was where most people from that time period lived.

The next was Angkor Wat Temple, also known as Temple-Mountain, because it was built into a mountain. The sheer size of it was jaw-dropping. It's the largest religious monument in the world, and the carvings on the walls throughout were amazing. Each told a story, and I was surprised how much detail of the carving was still there. This site took thirty-five years to build and actually was not finished, since the ruler at the time died during the construction.

Most temples face to the east, but this was the only one that faces to the west. The thought was that this would help them go back in time and bring the dead back to life. Since the ruler died and we haven't seen him since, I guess that didn't work out for them.

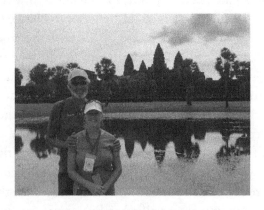

Last but not least was Ta Prohm Temple. I called that one Angkor Jungle because they decided to leave it mostly as they found it. I would have to agree with the tour guides that the contrast between the structures and the jungle that intertwined itself with the structures made it the most impressive.

While we were there, we saw a traditional Apsara Dance show, which featured dancers in masks and wildly colorful costumes performing slow, deliberate hand and foot movements to the beat of offstage bell ringing and singing. We also walked around the city, which included a night market and Pub street. We listened to some great dance music in a club that filled up by the time we left at 11:00 p.m. Unfortunately, one of the two establishments where I used my credit card decided to copy down the numbers and tried to use it while we slept that night.

Over the last two-and-a-half years of being on the road, this was the sixth time this had happened. When I woke up the next morning, I had several text messages, emails, and phone calls from Chase, asking about what they thought were fraudulent charges to my card. As in the past, Chase didn't honor the charges and I had to cut up my card and wait to get a new one until we got back to the states.

From there, we caught a very nice hour-and-thirty-minute flight to Hanoi. I thought the last hotel was something, but the Sofitel Legend Metropole Hanoi took the cake. It was recognized as among the top six Sofitel hotels in the world, thus the name "Legend." I thought that this was what it must be like to be rich and famous. When they were doing some renovation of the restaurant a few years back, they found a bomb shelter underneath the floor and now have tours of that area.

The next day, we toured the famous Hanoi Hilton where John McCain spent some time as a POW. I learned that it was originally built by the French during their occupation of Vietnam in the mid-1950s.

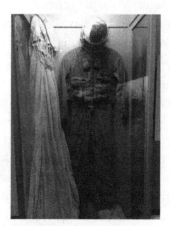

*John McCain's flight suit*

We also got to visit the Ho Chi Minh Mausoleum—from afar since it was closed to the public on Monday and Fridays. That afternoon, we experienced the real life of the people of Vietnam during a cycle tour of the Old Quarter.

The Old Quarter is somewhat hard to describe. "Uncontrolled chaos" is the best I can do. There were no stop signs or lights at intersections and thousands of motorbikes and pedestrians. Each street was named for the items sold on that street, so shops on Copper Street sold all items made of copper. That was a lot of fun to see and experience, especially, since no one got hit by any sort of vehicle.

We finished the evening with a traditional Vietnamese water puppet show. Supposedly, back in the day, the ruler wanted entertainment for the people so they came up with the idea to have this type of show in the lake. Now they do it in the nearby theater but still done in water. I was unable to figure out exactly how they were able to make all the puppets move as they did, but it was very enjoyable.

For the final leg of our AMA Waterways adventure, we spent twenty hours on what is referred to as a "luxury junk" in Halong Bay. Located in the Gulf of Tonkin, the bay is known as the Baby of the Descending Dragon and is a UNESCO World Heritage Site famous for its dramatic limestone cliffs, thousands of islands and islets, and groups of floating villages. Multiple generations live and work aboard small wooden junks dotting the bay; fishermen cast their nets and tend to pearl farms; women tend to giant woks; and curious children hang over boat railings to greet new faces.

The luxury junk was a smaller version of other cruise ships we had been on in the past. The accommodations were impeccable, and the crew bent over backward to make us feel at home during the twenty-four hours we were on board. Soon after we boarded, we had a quick safety briefing and lunch as we cruised around the bay. There are more than six hundred vessels of different shapes and sizes that routinely cruise around the nearly two thousand limestone islands in the area. Our boat, the Paradise Elegance, was docked on the only island made of soil.

Later that afternoon, we got to tour Hang Sung Sot cave, the largest cave in the bay, which locals call Surprise Cave because of an unexpected (and huge) third chamber. It was spectacular, and we had great panoramic views of the bay from the top.

Back on board, we cruised to a spot for a breathtaking sunset, followed by a cooking demonstration, wine-tasting, dinner, and dancing. We were up early the next morning for a hike up to the top of Ti, Top Island. After a quick shower and breakfast, they bid us farewell promptly at 10:30 a.m. ahead of our four-hour ride back to Hanoi so we could catch our flight on to Dubai at 1:30 a.m. It would be a long day for us—we should have planned better before we stayed up late dancing the night before.

I was not prepared for the stark difference between the sights, sounds, and smells of South East Asia and the United Arab Emirates. After experiencing a lot of poverty, we were now seeing only wealth and opulence. I have seen commercials about Dubai on TV, but to actually experience it firsthand was simply mind-blowing.

Of course, we had to stay at the tallest Marriott in the world, which was the J. W. Marriott Marquis. They had a room for us at 6:00 a.m., and we were able to get a run-in right after we arrived. There was no need to eat out since the Executive Lounge had both breakfast and dinner, each day. They also provided a shuttle to and from the Dubai mall.

There was so much to see and do, and with only two nights there, it was hard to choose. Of course you can't go to Dubai without seeing the tallest building in the world, the Burj Khalifa, standing at 1,804 feet. We opted for the fast-track tickets that took us directly to the 148th floor and the outside observation decks at floors 125 and 123.

Catherine coined the phrase, "Build it and they will come to Dubai," and this was a great example. You have to go through the largest mall in the world to get to the entrance to "At the Top," which is what they call the outdoor observatory. Dubai was noted for having the biggest, tallest, largest, fastest, and only of whatever in the world. I really enjoyed watching all the different outfits the people from this region were wearing. My favorite was the guys in their long white garbs and baseball caps. I guess that was their way of being rebels without a cause.

With so much to see and so little time, we opted for their version of the big red bus to see as much as we could. The top deck did have an enclosed air-conditioned section up-front so we got to see all the sights without being exposed to the ovenlike 109-degree heat. The two main loops took about two hours each and departed from the Dubai Mall. We also walked around the mall for a few hours, and I only think we saw about half of it. Some highlights were the waterfall, the indoor aquarium, and the ice-skating rink.

Here are some interesting facts, figures, and observations I made note of while were in Dubai:

- 98.2 percent of their drinking water is from boiled seawater.
- There are cranes and construction everywhere.
- The visibility is reduced by airborne sand particles.
- Not many people smoke, but they do allow smoking indoors.
- I didn't see a single dog or cat, and very few birds.
- There were no beggars or any signs of poverty.
- The locals were not very friendly.
- The Palms Island where Atlantis resides is a man-made island from reclaimed sand that they call the eighth wonder of the world.
- They have another mall that is adjacent to the only indoor ski slope.
- Foreigners can only buy alcohol at the duty-free store at the airport.
- All bars must be in a hotel.
- They are building another mall that will be finished by 2020 and will be a city within a city. In other words, you could live, work, shop, and play without ever going outside.

With all that said, I really don't understand why anyone would want to live here. The service industry folks at the Marriott were like cruise ship workers. They were all from somewhere else and were provided housing, food, and transportation. They got one month off a year to go back home.

The Executive Lounge folks presented us with a handwritten thank-you note they all signed and a really nice fruit plate on our last night there. We topped off the evening (pun intended) at a place called the Vault. Our room was on the sixty-seventh floor, so we took one elevator to the sixty-eighth floor and another to the rooftop bar, which had windows all around so you could get a panoramic view of the city. The drink that I ordered came in a box, and when I opened it, a light inside came on to illuminate the one huge ice cube inside.

Back at the airport, we discovered that in Dubai, Emirates has a special area to drop off First and Business Class passengers where someone is waiting to take your bags to the ticket counter and their own customs and security screening area.

We opted to spend the night in Paris before we continuing on to Petra for the half-marathon on Saturday. We were using a different tour company, Albatros, whose slogan is "Pushing your limits" since they were the ones organizing this race.

The weather forecast was calling for seventy degrees at the start and around eighty by the time we finished. The heat would be the easy part since there was a mountain we had to climb for about two miles in some pretty challenging terrain.

Overseas, in order to save on electricity, you have to use your room key to turn on the lights and AC. When we arrived in our room at the Dead Sea, it was hot as hell since the AC had been off and it had gotten up to almost one hundred degrees during the day. It was all worth it when we got to float effortlessly the next day in the Dead Sea.

We even put sediments they dig up from the bottom all over our bodies and faces. Here we were 1,377 feet below sea level. Not many people can say they were at the tallest building one day and the lowest point in the world a few days later—a change of 3,182 feet.

We met a couple who had been living in Dubai for the last seven years and asked them why anyone would live there. They said that there is a lot to do there and, most importantly, it's a very safe place to live—so safe that the current ruler of Dubai drives himself around town without any bodyguards.

To put it simply, the race in Petra was the hardest half-marathon I had ever done. I had prepared for the heat, but unfortunately not the terrain or the climb of the mountain. We started the day meeting at the Petra Visitor Center. As the sun rose, the two hundred of us walked to the very famous Treasury, which is one of the new Seven Wonders of the world. We stopped there for some pictures, then continued on to the start line. That was the moment when I really started to wonder if we had adequately trained for this adventure race. It was already seventy-five degrees.

They had a very strict seven-hour cutoff for the marathon, and if you weren't at the 30K point in five hours, the medical team was there to pull you off the course. That was not a problem for us since we were only doing the half, but I know there was no way I could have completed the full, even in my prime.

I don't really like trails, since for me, I like to keep my head up and watch the scenery instead of having to watch my feet. Our goal was to stay upright the entire race, so I was very pleased that neither of us took a spill. The downside was that some of the hardest terrains were coming down off the mountain, mostly rocks and gravel, so, unfortunately, we had to walk most of that portion. We started at 2,870 feet and climbed to 4,839. The elevation gain was only 1,968 feet, but the 20-degree plus grade both up and down was unlike anything I had ever experienced before.

Catherine was very apprehensive about running in the desert during the summer but was a real trooper and kept moving forward. I do think I saw her head spin completely around once and she cracked me up by saying, "I'm never running again."

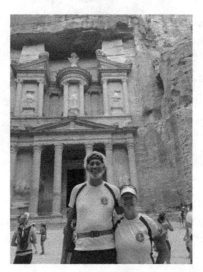

*The Treasury in the background*

I, on the other hand, felt that this was a great training run for the two full marathons we were to do at the end of September and the first of October. It had been over a year since our last marathon in Prague. Whatever doesn't kill you makes you stronger, but you still have to prepare and be very careful.

Of course, we met and made friends with some great people and had fun swapping stories with them. This was probably the most diverse group of folks on one of these racing tours. There were thirty-eight different countries represented, and it was fun to listen to all the different languages around the table during meals.

The day after the race we had the official four-hour tour of all the historical sites. Some members of the group continued on to see some sights that required seven hundred to eight hundred steps for some incredible views, but we opted for the view from the pool and rooftop bar.

We ended the evening with a gala dinner in Little Petra, where they had all the surrounding caves lit up and a rock formation light show. The tour group put together a slide presentation, and one of the slides was of Catherine and me crossing the finish line, once again hand in hand.

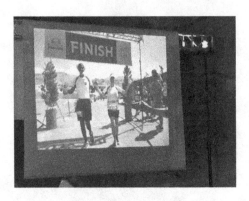

The following day there were two tours provided: Adventure and Cultural. We were getting a bit too old for Adventure tours, so we opted for the Cultural tour. First up was Mt. Nebo, the mountain where Moses saw the Holy Land before finding his final resting place on the mountain. It had great views of Israel and the Jordan Valley. Then we saw the historic city of Madaba, famous for the ancient "Mosaic of Jerusalem," which is one of the oldest pictured testimonies of the Holy City.

From the hotel the next day we went down the Jordan Valley to Bethany Beyond the Jordan, better known as the Baptism Site. The place has been identified as the site where John the Baptist preached and where Jesus was baptized by John.

We then went to the small town, As-Salt, which featured dazzling houses from the late Ottoman period. A walking tour through this inviting community showcased some of Jordan's most charming buildings and bazaars. In As-Salt, many traditional businesses and skilled artisans enrich the city's cultural life, and as we walked down the street, we saw a variety of shops, including blacksmiths, shoemakers, barbershops, Arabic sweet stores, and herbalists. For lunch, we were fed a delicious traditional lunch by a local family. The main dish was called upside down. The mother of the family started by cooking the meal in a pot, and when it was finished cooking, she put another pan on top and then turned it upside down as she raised it over her head. She then removed the pot and served all the cooked items from the pan.

On the final day of this tour, we headed north through the Jordan Valley to the city ruins of Jerash. These well-preserved ruins were once the ground pillars of a Roman Decapolis city built in approximately 330 BC. During its peak, the city flourished from trade with the Nabateans from Petra and was one of the most important cities in the Roman province. In AD 747, Jerash was hit by an earthquake, and the city was slowly abandoned.

As the years went by, the sand covered the columns and buildings, which is why everything was so well preserved when a Russian expedition excavated the city in 1878. After our visit to Jerash, we drove back to Amman for a tour of the capital's most prominent sites and buildings.

Their yearly festival was coming up when everyone would be sacrificing goats and sheep as Mohammad did back in the day. That was why we saw so many pens of them along the streets for all to buy. The food here was the best out of all the places we had visited so far. My favorite dessert was called umm ali, a type of bread pudding served hot and made with flaky pastry, nuts, and raisins.

The men here loved them some women. They mostly stared at me but were constantly chatting up all the women on the tour. I guessed it was because they don't get to see so much skin on a daily basis since their women are covered up from head to toe.

During this thirty-day jaunt, we got to see and hear about several different religions and taste a variety of foods. I was all toured out and glad to be heading back to the States, where we would just be running from place to place.

I was really looking forward to only having to set an alarm occasionally instead of daily. It was a bit difficult to get our runs in too, so I was really looking forward to that also. Once again, we met some interesting people and made some new best friends.

Thinking back to the title of this chapter, "As the World Turns," it was very clear in my mind how two very different societies dealt with the everyday challenge of trying to find something to eat, someplace to work, and someplace to live.

Back in Halong Bay, the Executive Vice President of AMA Waterways, Kristin, left us with some words of wisdom. She said if more people traveled, then this would be a much friendlier world. It's hard to hate someone when they offer their home to you for a meal. You don't have to travel in as intense a fashion as us, but getting outside of your comfort zone is good for your mind and soul. No matter where you are, what time zone you might be in, what your religion or beliefs might have, everyone is trying to accomplish the same things. Some are more successful than others, and it's a lot of fun to watch and experience firsthand.

# CHAPTER

# 30

## In Pursuit of Seven Continents and Fifty States

The idea was to die young as late as possible.

—Ashley Montagu

I've set goals for myself all my life, and as we ran around the world, Catherine and I agreed that we would aim to run a marathon or half-marathon on every continent and in all fifty states. We were headed to New Zealand to get the last continent in November. As for states, Catherine only had five left, and I was seven behind her. Whereas she insisted that her races must be marathons, I had conceded to the last twelve being a combination of full and half-marathons. I would run the full marathons with Catherine and do the rest as half-marathons.

After a few days to recover from our thirty-day escapade in Vietnam, Cambodia, Dubai, Paris, and Jordan, we are on our way to Detroit Lakes, Minnesota, where I would get my next state with a half-marathon and be one step (pun intended) closer to my goal of all fifty states. After that one, we were headed to Bismarck, North Dakota, for another half-marathon.

We had two great days walking around Detroit Lakes prior to the Dick Beardsley Marathon and Half Marathon. All was perfect for a great race on Saturday. Sometimes, however, things don't always go as planned. The course was once around the huge Detroit Lake for half-marathoners and twice for marathoners.

At mile 5, I was two minutes ahead of plan, and while my right foot was in the air, it felt like my right knee-joint separated. When the foot came back down, it was as if I had just gotten shot in the knee. At this point, stopping wasn't an option, so I shifted to speed walking and finished the race.

Afterward, I tended to myself with RICE (rest, ice, compression, and elevation), but our plan to complete a race in North Dakota a week later wasn't so certain. Ironically, before Detroit Lakes, Catherine had an epiphany where she decided to finish her fifty states by doing the rest as half-marathons. She said she was worried about my health—and now we had solidified that decision by me screwing up my knee. I only hoped I could even get a half-marathon done now. On a positive note, I realized that since we had both done a half-marathon in Colorado, we were one step closer to getting all fifty states done.

The four-hour drive back to Bismarck was boring as hell. We went straight eastbound on ninety-four and all there was to see was farmland and bales of hay. My knee was taking forever to recover, and with only two days before the race, it was fifty-fifty that I would even be able to walk the course. I did buy some trek poles to help out.

As I got older, I had to adjust to not being able to do things I used to be able to do. When I went to pick up my number for the Bismarck Half Marathon the day before the race, my right knee was 80/20. It felt okay as long as I iced it down every thirty minutes and kept Tylenol in my system every five hours. There was some question in my mind if I would do more damage if I did the race, but I was not really looking forward to having to come back here next year to try again. No time like the present, and I would have two weeks to recover before our next race.

On race day, I got up an hour before the alarm went off and put some more ice on my sore knee. I used some KT tape on it and then put a Copper Fit compression sleeve over my work of art. With my Trek Poles in hand, I headed out the door to arrive at the start in time to ice the knee down one last time.

When I was a pilot, I used to say that you must continuously update your decision to land the aircraft right up to the time the main gear touches down. The same was true here. I kept updating whether I was going to do this race right up to the moment the horn went off.

My knee still was hurting a bit, but actually felt better the longer the race went on. To keep my mind off my knee the last few miles, I concentrated on folks ahead of me as I passed them one by one. As I went by, I would pick someone off to distance to see if I could catch them. I actually got faster as time went on and I learned the different ways to use the trek poles.

I came up with three different ways. For speed, I would use the left pole to strike the ground as my right foot hit the ground, which was how it was suggested to be used in a video I found on the web. That was a real upper-body workout, and I couldn't keep that up for very long. When the knee would start to bother me, I would then switch up to both poles hitting the ground with each right foot strike. That was also good when I was going up or down an incline or uneven terrain. When I was feeling good, I would use both poles after a few foot strikes and would alternate to help either left or right foot. It was a great race and the scenery was outstanding, with the route going through many parks, trails, and nice neighborhoods.

Forty-one states plus DC down, and nine to go. I wasn't sure what was wrong with my right knee, but rather than dwelling on the why I would just concentrate on taking care of it between now and the next race.

During our downtime in Kissimmee, Florida, we were able to get some great walks in, since that was all I was able to do. I wasn't sure if I would ever have the guts to run again. It worried me that my right knee was doing fine one second and just gave out the next. But I found that I could racewalk only about one minute slower per mile than I could run, so maybe running wasn't worth the risk. Even with my knee coming along just fine, I had a minor setback with my right wrist. I was a bit aggressive with the trek pole usage, and that tweaked my wrist a bit. Nothing major, just bothersome. It sucks getting old but beats the alternative every time.

The weather was perfect when we arrived in the Plymouth/ Bristol New Hampshire area and got on some nice walks around the area. Unfortunately, that wasn't the case on race day when cold, light rain was with us the whole 13.1 miles. The course took us halfway around Newfound Lake and the rolling hills were nice, but I wasn't a big fan of running against traffic the entire way on the shoulder of the road. Most folks, but not all, pulled over to give us some room, but it was somewhat unnerving. Of course, the sun came back out the day after the race, when we were on our way to Rhode Island.

The Amica Newport Marathon and Half Marathon hit it out of the park. The course was gorgeous, and the race was extremely well-organized. The parking lot was only about two miles from our Residence Inn, and the race start was only about a mile from the parking lot. There were plenty of buses to the start, and we got there in time to witness another spectacular sunrise.

My knee felt great, but I decided I was going to racewalk this one. Two miles into the race it felt so good I thought I would give running a try, but my knee wasn't having any of that. With racewalk-ing now the firm plan, I had my sights on trying to beat my PR (per-sonal record), time of 2:44 for racewalking a half-marathon. That was a stretch goal since the race where I set my PR was all downhill and this one had numerous rolling hills. A more realistic goal was a 13:00 minute pace that would have me finish around 2:50.

With those two times in mind, I set off to keep up with the 2:45 pacer group. I moved far ahead of them at mile two, and since I wasn't wearing a watch, I didn't much think more about it. My plan was just to spot someone ahead of me and see if I could catch them.

At mile 5, the 2:45 pacer group went by me like I was standing still and steadily moved out of sight. I had started my timer on my phone, so I looked at that and figured I was on a 2:45 pace, so I just kept going.

The course took us along the ocean and past some huge man-sions that occupied my time for the next four miles. This was where it really got fun. By now those who started out running or even run/ walking were breaking down, so one by one I would catch and pass them. I could see most of them saying to themselves, "Hell no, I'm not letting this guy walk by me," so they would start running or pick up the pace to pass me. Experience had shown that was going to be short-lived.

As I went by each for the final time, I would say to myself, "May I have some of your energy, since you don't look like you'll be needing it anymore." At mile 12, I checked my phone one last time and it looked like 2:45 was within reach. Lo and behold, the 2:45 pacer was standing about a quarter-mile ahead since she had figured out she was well ahead of her designated pace. I had to laugh as I crossed the finish right behind her.

Catherine, on the other hand, had to run to keep up with me, even if it was a slow pace for her. We usually took walk breaks every half-mile but instead, she just kept running. She did walk up some of the hills and would simply catch up on the downhill. Near the end, she would run past me, walk till I caught up, and then run ahead. We did, however, cross the finish line hand in hand as always, with me walking and her running beside me.

Changing the subject for a bit, a running buddy of ours, Kayna, suggested a word that fits us to a tee. The word was "peregrinate," which means "travel or wander around from place to place." People who peregrinate are constantly on the move, traveling from one location to another. Instead of telling people were homeless or nomads, I liked to think of us as peregrinates. Now I just needed to learn how to pronounce it properly.

As we headed to Florida for destination number 283, we were averaging a little more than 3.6 days per stop. My goal was to get that number up to about four to five days to cut down on our expenses since the airfare was our biggest expense, and I really don't like driving that much. It still didn't make sense for us to get an apartment in Atlanta. We did go through there a lot but didn't stay there long enough to justify the extra expense.

I continued to give my knees a rest and concentrate on improving my race-walking form, but I was going through running withdrawals. I remembered having the same feeling after my open-heart surgery and couldn't wait to get back to running. As I would see other people running by, I just wanted to trip them.

On to Portland, Oregon, for the Columbia Gorge half-marathon, it rained the entire day before the race, and on race day, the skies opened up and we saw a dramatic rainbow in the distance.

One of the things I love about our travels was that a month and sometimes a week didn't go by without witnessing something I hadn't experienced before. This time around it was the wave start for people who were running with dogs. The race was mostly in a park with grass on both sides of the paved trail, so it was perfect for the fifty or so four-legged friends.

The walkers, which included me, were in the last wave after the dogs, so it worked out well for Catherine. After a few miles, we were able to catch most of the group of dogs, so Catherine would run ahead and pat some of them, and I would eventually catch up to her. This went on the entire race. She was in doggie heaven.

The fall colors were in full bloom, and even though the area had experienced a terrible fire a few months prior, you really couldn't tell during the run portion. It was more evident during the drive from Portland. This concluded our pursuit of all fifty states for the year. I had the six that I needed and, more importantly, the two remaining for Catherine mapped out for next year.

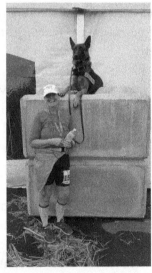

*Doggie heaven*

It was now time for us to transition to some follow-up exams dealing with my surgery six months ago for my gut aneurysm, so off we went to Seattle. After a quick CT scan and doctor visit, I got a partial clean bill of health. The aneurysm repair looked good, with the stent in a good position, but I had a tiny blood leak caused by incomplete sealing of the aneurysm sac, which I was told was typical for someone on blood thinners. I was due back in six months.

For the moment, I was glad that no one said I needed another operation in the near future. I planned on being around for another thirty or so years like my parents did, so I tried to put everything into perspective. It helped that we were relaxing before the final half-marathon for the year with a great week in Puerto Vallarta, Mexico. I was really ready to get back to running again. I missed the feeling of being completely airborne as you are when you run, no matter how slow it might be. It must have been the pilot in me.

We were going to New Zealand for two weeks so both of us could reach the goal of running at least a half-marathon on all seven continents. I wasn't looking forward to the trip there and back. Since we were already on the West Coast, the flight to Auckland consisted of a fifteen-hour flight to Sydney, a two-hour layover, then another three-hour flight into Auckland.

With our Diamond Medallion status with Delta, we each got four global upgrades a year. This doesn't mean that we will actually get an upgrade on each flight we designate them for, but it does give us an advantage over those who are only trying to upgrade with their current status. For the flight to Auckland, we used Catherine's last global upgrade, and since I had already qualified for Diamond status for next year, I was able to apply for my next year's award for this flight. Unfortunately, when I checked in, someone else had gotten the two upgrade seats we were hoping for. I hadn't seen that happen very often. I guess they paid more for their original seat than we did, or else had million-mile status.

The flight wasn't that bad, and with our first hotel, the Sebel Quay West, being two blocks from the Harbor, we couldn't wait to get out and do our usual walking tour of the area.

A few first impressions: Based on the sheer number of boats of all kinds, I called Auckland "The Boating Capital of the World." I was also surprised by the multitude of Asians living in and touring New Zealand. Last but not least, the amount of construction taking place was mind-blowing. They said there were more than seventy cranes operating on various construction sites.

After five nights, we moved a few blocks to the Rydges Hotel, which was right next to the sky tower that people jump off of all day long. At the Rydges, we met up with the other clients of Marathon Tours. On the second day with the group, we enjoyed a trip over the Harbor Bridge and visited the famous Auckland landmark of Mount Eden, a dormant volcano whose summit offers excellent panoramic views of the city and harbors. From that extreme vantage point, we saw evidence of Auckland's volcanic history, the most significant being the youngest volcano of Rangitoto Island at the entrance to the Waitemata harbor. The sightseeing tour also took us to the Auckland Domain, the city's oldest park, which was situated on a sixty-two-thousand-year-old volcano. In addition to the natural features, the city's sights tour also took in the trendy shopping area of Parnell Village with its historical buildings that have been transformed into boutiques, antique, craft and specialty shops.

The next day we caught the Fullers Harbor ferry to nearby Waiheke Island in Auckland Harbor. There we met a very knowledgeable tour guide who drove us around the island for both an olive oil and wine-tasting tour. The views from the Batch winery were phenomenal and an unexpected nature hike featuring llamas and sheep was an added treat.

We could hear thunder in the distance, but the light rain could barely make it through the thick canopy. By the time we made it back to the boat, the skies opened up for the only time during our two-week trip. The locals said that the lack of rain was unusual for this time of year, but we really enjoyed the blue skies.

We enjoyed a leisurely start to the next day with a two-hour flight to Queenstown, where the race was held. Catherine and I stayed at the Heritage Hotel on top of a hill, so we had a lakeside view from our room, which included a kitchen and washer/dryer combo unit.

Lake Wakatipu was gorgeous and was one of the deepest (averaging 300 meters) and coldest (averaging 54ºF) lakes in the world.

I joked that Queenstown was like Disney World on steroids. Open up your wallet and let them take what they want. We went overboard with the budget, but you only live once. I did notice that their credit card machines were the fastest in the world. I guess they don't want to give you enough time to change your mind.

That being said the prices for food and drinks seemed reasonable and the people were super friendly—they'll talk your ear off if you let them. Another surprise was the sheer volume of young adults backpacking their way around the island. I guess most are doing their traditional gap year or just trust-funding their adventures. To each their own, but I did find it a bit odd.

A must-do in Queenstown was taking the gondola to the top of the mountain for the views and plenty of other excitement. Many in our group went bungee jumping. I decided that the time I did that in my forties was enough for me. I came here to run the half-marathon to achieve my goal of running on all seven continents, so a broken back or neck would have thrown a wrench in the plan. It was a hoot to watch, though.

Another must-do was the TSS Earnslaw, the only commercial passenger-carrying coal-fired, twin-screw steamship in the Southern Hemisphere. Clocking in at more than one hundred years old, the Earnslaw still works fourteen-hour days during the summer. They call it the Lady of the Lake, and for eleven months a year, it makes its way from Center City to Walter Peak several times a day.

Back in the late 1800s, the Mackenzie family took over Walter Peak, and now provide a variety of activities: horseback riding, sheep-shearing, and round-up demonstration by two breeds of dogs. They also offered tea and crumpets and an area where you can feed some of the local animals.

By now it was time for some thrill-seeking, so we went out on the speedboats that are famous for their ability to do 360-degree spins at top speeds. The tour of the lake lasted an hour and it was hair-raising, to say the least. Catherine loved it so much she was too excited to be seasick.

Back in town, I was keeping my eye on the lines at the Fergburger, which was famous for its many tantalizing varieties of hamburgers. It was so popular that it often had hour-long lines from first thing in the morning to the wee hours of the next day. I was sure there was a veggie burger with my name on it, and I had a plan. I figured that right after the race the line might not be that long—but I would have to wait.

All the food we had was outstanding, and the different varieties of beer kept my whistle wet. They also had a great winery right in town where you could pour a half or a full glass of whatever taste you fancied. Toss in some cheese and crackers in some great comfy chairs, and we were in heaven.

With all the wining and dining behind us, it was time to get busy and complete the Queenstown Half-Marathon. The expo had limited supplies of apparel to buy, and this was only the second race we had run where you had to buy a race T-shirt. We also had to buy a sticker for the bus to the start.

The course itself was on well-groomed trails with both rolling and undulating hills. I had to stop to take the rocks out of my shoes about halfway and some of the downhills on the rocky surface kept it interesting. The views of the mountains and the lake kept my mind occupied, so overall it was a great race.

My right knee wasn't fond of me running this race but I couldn't bring myself to simply walk this one. I did take walk breaks when my knee would scream bloody murder for me to simply stop. I just kept thinking about all the folks I had seen in wheelchairs with prosthetic legs or on crutches during races and kept reminding myself that if they could do it, so could I. Once again, we crossed the finish line hand in hand, and another goal of ours was completed.

Back to my plan for Fergburger. We had to walk right by the place on our way back to the hotel, and there were only a few people in line by the time we got there. I got an amazing veggie burger called Holier Than Thou. It was made with tofu, and I devoured it on our leisurely lakeside walk back to the hotel.

That evening, Marathon Tours had a small celebration for the seven of us who had completed all seven continents. Catherine and I were the only couple.

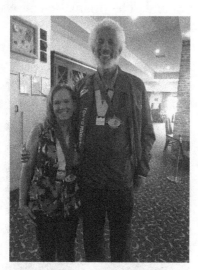

Sporting both or our medals for the race and the seven continents

The next day's adventure took me back forty years to when I first became a pilot. There were two options to go tour the famous Milford Sound. One was to get there and back by bus, which took about twelve hours including the ninety-minute tour of the fords. The other option, which we took, was by small plane. We flew on the same type of aircraft, Piper Lance, that I first flew for Wheeler Airlines back when I carried canceled checks, in the middle of the night, in and around the Carolinas and Virginia. The thirty-minute flight each way gave us a bird's eye view of the glaciers and mountain peaks. Often we flew between the peaks. I must admit that the five of us on board were pretty quiet during the trip. The pilot did a great job pointing out the incredible landmarks.

About eighty thousand years ago, the last big freeze (known as the Otiran Glaciation) began. It kept the southern mountains ice-bound until about ten thousand to thirteen thousand years ago. Ice descended the mountains and down the valleys, forming rivers of ice up to two thousand meters thick. Icebergs calved from floating ice cliffs where they met the surging sea. After the glaciers receded, leaving behind sheer cliffs, hanging valleys, and spectacular waterfalls, the ocean flooded the Milford Valley, forming a fjord that has been misnamed Milford Sound. The original name was Milford Haven, after Captain Cook's birthplace in Wales.

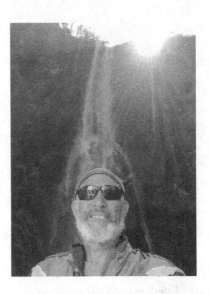

The captain of the *Jucy* ship took us up close and personal with Stirling Falls, a beautiful waterfall was named after Captain Stirling who brought the HMS Cleo into Milford Sound during the 1870s. With a 146-meter drop, it was the second-largest permanent waterfall in the fjord and was fed by glaciers situated in the mountains behind.

The captain's seafood restaurant had won awards for its lamb and New Zealand was famous for lamb dishes, so I went off the rails and temporarily ditched my pescovegetarian diet to enjoy a rack of lamb. It was very tasty, but surprisingly enough, I enjoyed the apple walnut salad much more.

Instead of going straight back to the States after the race, we spent two more days in Auckland. On the first day, we went for another long walk around the city. It was easy to get around on foot by just keeping the Sky Tower in sight. On the second and final day, we caught a harbor ferry to another island called Rangitoto. Sitting majestically just off the coast of Auckland, this 5.5-kilometer-wide volcanic island was an iconic landmark on the city's skyline, with its distinctive symmetrical cone rising 850 feet high over the Hauraki Gulf. The climb to the top through the volcanic remnants along the summit track was a bit harder than I had expected but well worth it for the views of the city.

Rangitoto erupted from the sea between 550 and 600 years ago in two dramatic explosions ten to fifty years apart. Both are thought to have lasted for several years. This makes it the youngest island in the Hauraki Gulf, and the last and largest volcano to have erupted in the Auckland volcanic field.

This trip taught me a couple of things about myself. First and foremost was that one of the reasons I travel was because I don't like to do the same thing more than once. Using New Zealand as an example, even though I'd like to return I realized that I probably won't. It just wouldn't be as good as the first time.

The other realization was that we were ready to move on to someplace new when we run out of new places to eat, drink, and—most importantly—someplace new to run or walk. Queenstown was a bit of an anomaly, with plenty more great restaurants to try out and trails going every which way. The flights there and back were a bit much but doable.

When we got back to our hotel in Atlanta, a throw pillow waiting for us said, "Travel: the only thing you can spend money on that will make you richer."

# CHAPTER
# 31

## Three Years and Counting

Don't listen to what they say/Go see.

—Chinese Proverb

During the last three years, we had been to three hundred different destinations. Every 3.65 days we unpacked and packed up our bags. We had spent seventeen weeks on boats: nine weeks on Windstar Cruises ships, four weeks on AMA Waterways river cruises, and four weeks on the Royal Caribbean cruise line. Last but not least, we had run ten marathons and twenty-five half-marathons, which brought the total of countries where we had run at least a half-marathon to twenty-seven plus Antarctica.

Many runners talk about how many miles they have run each year. Unfortunately, since my right knee has been giving me a problem on and off since last September, I have had to include my race-walking miles. In 2017, I walked or ran 1,525 miles.

It was rather sad to go back to San Juan after the hurricanes had ravaged the area back in September. I used to fly into San Juan for many years, and always enjoyed visiting the area. We were able to get in a couple of long walks, and we saw that some progress had been made, but there was still a lot that needed to be done. Vacationers had yet to return to the area.

Unfortunately, with some other islands also heavily damaged, the itinerary for our Windstar cruise had to be changed. We were now experiencing a rather rough day at sea on the way to Martinique. Simply put, Catherine wasn't faring well.

We ran into another couple that spends about twelve weeks a year on cruise ships. I was sure that would take our cash burn rate well above the $500 a day that I strive for. However, they mentioned a cruise that goes around the world in about six months. I didn't think Catherine was up for being on a big ship that long.

My knee was starting to cooperate, but now I had challenges with one of my blood pressure meds. My cardiologist had doubled the dose of Losartan Potassium, and now my blood pressure was so low that it was very difficult to run without passing out. He told me this would probably happen, but since I still have another aneurysm above my heart on my aorta, he felt it would be best to keep my BP down.

Since we routinely ran in the morning, I was taking that med after I exercised each day. If we're allowed to wake up every morning, we must all learn to deal with personal health issues that crop up from time to time. As a pilot, I got a full physical every six months, and it looked like the routine would continue throughout my life.

The final day of this week's cruise finished up with the island of Saint Barthelemy, often called St. Barts. The capital city of Gustavia was under repair from the hurricanes. They were in much better shape than Little Bay where we were yesterday which was under construction. The official capital of Montserrat at Plymouth in the south of the island was abandoned in 1997 after it was buried by the eruption of the Soufriere Hills volcano. So the plan was for Little Bay to be the future capital.

We pulled anchor at 1:30 p.m. and made our way back to San Juan to finish up the first week of cruising the Caribbean. For immigration reasons, everyone had to leave the ship by 9:00 a.m. With that in mind, we decided to go for a nice long, walk from Old San Juan back to the Marriott Hotel area where we stayed before the cruise. There were areas that looked like there was no plan of ever fixing the damage done by the storms. Most of the traffic lights were inoperative, which made crossing some intersections a bit hazardous.

During our second week, I learned how best to handle the first day at sea: Dramamine, Dramamine, Dramamine. Catherine did a much better job. During our first stop in Martinique, we decided to catch the ferry from Anse Mitan over to Fort-de-France and walk around the area. The weather once again was perfect so this week in the Caribbean was getting off to a great start. We had dinner at the Captain's table. I always appreciate the behind-the-scenes information about the cruise line, the ship, and crew; and since I flew airplanes for all those years as a Captain, I really enjoy getting a different perspective from someone doing what I used to do in a different mode of transportation.

In Les Saintes, Guadeloupe, we decided to actually go on an excursion, something we didn't typically do. I had heard from other guests last week that the speedboat tour of the island was a great trip. The water was a bit choppy but that made the excursion even more fun as we whipped around the island. We did stop for about an hour to snorkel, have a bite to eat, and sip some homemade rum drinks.

After that, we were able to make the walk up to the top of the nearby mountain for the views from Fort Napoleon. On the way back down, we took a side trip over to a very secluded beach. We ended the day with a great swim off the back of the ship. These ships have a platform that they can lower into the water.

We finished off the week back in Gustavia, St. Barthelemy for a short stop there. This time around we decided to walk over a mountain to get to the local airport. It was great watching the small passenger planes fly between the two hilltops and then drop into a very short landing strip. Back on the ship, we had our last sail away. Now all we need to do was figure out a way to stow away for another week in the Caribbean.

As we closed in on three years on the road, a couple of things came to mind. First and foremost was the fact that there are people much older than us who love to travel just as much as we do. They might not be as active as us, but they seem to get around pretty well, and are all enjoying life within their limitations.

The second one concerns my take on why we were still on the road. Many people we met continued to tell us stories about places we still hadn't been to, and why those places should be on our list. It seemed like we would never run out of places to go but just run out of money to travel on.

We finished off our third year of running all over the world on Tybee Island outside of Savannah, Georgia. At the Airbnb we rented on the island, we were able to enjoy the New Year's fireworks show right off the deck. I had hoped for moderate weather for our family get-together, but it was bitter cold. Luckily, I put together an extra bag of warm clothes for our trip there.

My New Year's resolution this year was to not sweat the small stuff. With our health issues, airplane departures, and new and exciting destinations, life was way too short to dwell on the fact that there wasn't a mint on my pillow.

I asked Catherine if it felt like we had been three years on the road. She replied, "It feels like this has been our lifestyle forever."

"True happiness is...to enjoy the present, without anxious dependence upon the future" (Lucius Annaeus Seneca).

*****

Our first destination of January 2018 was Utila, a tiny island off the mainland of Honduras. Before we arrived, I wasn't exactly sure where it was—but that was how we rolled. We're not the type to buy books on how to best tour an area. I really don't do much research on the internet either. We just arrive and let our feet do the touring. We hit the street; some days we turn left, and other days we turn right.

To get there, first, we had to fly to the relatively big city of Roatan, Honduras. Our friend, Jen, lives there and arranged the small plane ride from Roatan to Utila on Island Air Honduras.

Jen typifies the quote above. She was enjoying the present on her private island where everyone knew her name. The folk on Utila were very diverse. The local Utilians had a thick, somewhat Irish/British accent. Others transplanted from the mainland spoke Spanish freely, and then there are the numerous tourist/expats here to escape the rat race or frequent the thirteen dive shops. They were all very laid back, happy, friendly, and accommodating.

Our Airbnb accommodation allowed us to fall asleep to the water lapping at the shore and the sounds of local music and laughter in the distance. It was rainy season here, but that fact really didn't keep us from our daily activities. The sunrises and sunsets from the 360-degree deck were spectacular and our landlord, Fiona, was very attentive: she even invited us to her private birthday dinner party by the water. Catherine was happy as a clam since Fiona's dog came up to our deck daily so she could get her doggie fix. Dogs here were numerous and not aggressive at all. We rarely even heard any barking, which was out of the ordinary.

We had some extraordinary meals, which for us was saying a lot since we eat out all the time. Looking at some of the restaurants from the street, we were sometimes uncertain about what to expect, but we weren't disappointed once. At the last restaurant, they were cutting up the fresh catch of the day. When I ordered the whole fish, the man doing the gutting held up two to ask which one I wanted for my meal.

A must-see area was Neptunes at Coral Beach Village. A free water taxi took us to a secluded stretch of beach that can only be accessed by boat. There was a rocky beach and a dock for those who have come to enjoy the sun, along with a couple of hammocks tied to trees. Trip Advisor lists their grill and bar number one on the island, and we enjoyed both.

We went for a long walk while there, and a mile down from paradise was an area where all the plastics have washed up on the shore. I understood that last year, some residents had a daylong campaign when they bagged up hundreds of pounds of trash. It was sad to see, but this was a worldwide problem.

We were able to get in some great runs along the narrow streets as the tuk-tuks, golf carts, and motorbikes managed to dodge us. The numerous speed bumps did slow them down somewhat. Most people walk the streets with the vehicles coming from behind but I could not seem to adjust to running in that traffic pattern. I want to see the eyes of the person who might run me down.

Yes, I did say "running." I had a new contraption to keep my knee from killing me with each step. It was called the X-Trap Dual

Strap Knee Support. It straps above and below the kneecap to keep it on track, and so far, so good. Taking my morning blood pressure meds after I run has also helped a lot. Our next race was in March so that should give me the time to getting my stamina back to where it used to be.

It always amazes me how out of shape I can get when taking time off to recover from an injury. Our last half-marathon was less than two months ago in Queenstown, but in the heat of Utila, I felt like I had never run one before. Hopefully, my knee and the rest of my old body would cooperate so I could run a half-marathon in Jerusalem two months from now and in Cypress a week later.

Just like many other places in the world, visitors have to leave this piece of paradise every three months or pay a penalty in cash. That is, unless you get hired by a local company, as Jen was trying to do, or could show $1,500 per month in retirement income.

As Catherine and I ran all over the world, we were always looking for someplace to settle down. We weren't looking for mints on our pillows, just hot water; plenty of sunshine; and reliable internet, cable, and healthcare.

Utila wasn't our cup of tea, even though this little gem had a lot to offer. It was also a bit unnerving when an earthquake was reported nearby the other night. There were no tremors where we were, but for about two hours, there was a tsunami warning for our island. I stayed awake to see if the lapping and calming waves were going to change to a tidal wave of water.

Another reason we came here was to get over my fear of scuba diving. I tackled my fear of being around wild animals back in July 2016. Our guide assured me that these animals don't eat Jeeps or tents, so if I stayed inside them, I would be okay. Unfortunately I couldn't stay inside while scuba diving. That fact didn't help my unfounded fear of being getting eaten by a shark.

My bottom-line impression of scuba diving was that I'm one and done. It was very unnerving. Like all others, I had to show some simple underwater skills. I didn't much like the one where you take out your regulator and then put it back in your mouth. The fear of gasping in the Caribbean Sea was overwhelming.

I can see why others love scuba so much. My instructor at Parrots Dive Shop, who started diving at the age of five, did a great job. It was a good form of exercise, but I would rather just put my running shoes on and either go left or right. Also, I didn't much like signing my life away just to see some beautiful things at the bottom of the sea.

After they dropped me off the rest went out for a second dive, and from their description, the enormous urchin that came out of a sunken ship they were diving around would have made me pee my wetsuit. Speaking of which, with the tank, weights, and all I was surprised how hard it was to go down. My instructor had to push down on my tank. It might have had something to do with the fact that I really didn't want to go any closer to the wildlife, either alive or dead.

Utila wasn't for everyone but was for anyone, especially if you're the type that can recognize true happiness. Going back to Seneca's definition, I had trips planned for this year and the next, but we mostly took it one day at a time. We both took our health situations seriously but didn't obsess over them. We were enjoying our way of life while trying not to be anxious about the future.

# CHAPTER
# 32

## Can We Live Here?

Coddiwomple (V.) To travel purposefully
toward an as-yet unknown destination.

—English slang

This is a question we often discuss while enjoying our new destination as we run all over the world. First, I need to describe what I mean by the word "live."

For Catherine and me, who had been on the road for over three years, "live" was a relative word. Some could say we were living now on the Island of St. Kitts. Granted we would only be here for seven days, but for us, this was where we were living now. For sake of discussion, when I ask, "Can we live here?" I'm thinking more long-term.

We'll probably be on the road until we can no longer do so. I can't imagine being pushed around in a wheelchair with an oxygen tank but hope to be able to run/walk all over the world well into my eighties. Both my parents did so, and Catherine's Mom, who is eighty-two, just met us on Tybee Island last month. She also ran a faster half-marathon at sixty-three than I can do now at sixty-two. Catherine and I both have pensions, and with Social Security and great health care, we can live somewhere very comfortably with the occasional trips to visit our grown children.

I was thinking after five years maybe we could live somewhere for a month or two at a time. St. Kitts is definitely on the shortlist.

As a matter of fact, we were already planning on coming back for a week and staying at the nearby St. Kitts Marriott Resort. We had stayed there before and just found out that they have a senior rate for those over sixty-two.

Our trip here started with a fun-filled morning sailing with Miles on his yacht in Cockleshell Bay. He gave us some time to go snorkeling and see the island of Nevis up close. We spent some time on Reggae Beach and Spice Mill Beach prior to ending the day with afternoon tea at the Park Hyatt Hotel. I had my first experience with a sugar coma from the three-tower dessert extravaganza.

We had another over-the-top meal at a fabulous resort on the other side of the island called Kittitian Hill. The restaurant was called Farm to Table. We were met alongside this very long table with a glass of wine as we overlooked the adjacent farm where the chef could be seen picking some herbs for the upcoming twelve-course meal.

When we all took our seats, the chef described what he and his assistants had prepared for us, and then the feast began. There were several types of meat and veggies flavored with locally grown herbs and spices and presented beautifully. I had to be careful about taking appropriate portion sizes since I didn't want to miss anything. That was probably one of the finest meals I have ever had. The two couples adjacent to us invited us all to their place for an after-dinner drink, and all that I can say is that it was a jaw-dropping two-bedroom complex including both outdoor and indoor showers.

Gwen and Joan own a place at Oceans Edge Resort on Frigate Bay, so another option was to simply house-sit their place while we were there. The area around their property, which was just down the road from the Marriott, had it all: beaches, restaurants, bars, and grocery stores. The only drawback was the lack of sidewalks.

There was an adjacent golf course, and we didn't get chased off their cart paths during our morning runs. We were able to get in some great runs and walks around the area. I was starting to get my stamina back, and with my new strap, my right knee was still cooperating.

When we finished up our seven days here, I would say we both agreed that we could live here—maybe not for the rest of our lives but at least for a month or two at a time. It had all the things that I look for:

- It was warm.
- We had the ability to run there.
- It had reliable cable and internet.
- Heat wasn't much needed, but they did have great AC units in their indoor facilities.
- They had drinkable water and lots of places to eat out, along with many grocery stores nearby.

Even though we don't usually swim in big bodies of water, we do love to watch and hear the waves nearby. Friar's Bay with Timothy Beach was nearby, as was Carambola Beach Club. I would rather live someplace that had a great mass transportation system, but the fact that their cabs have set zone pricing and were everywhere worked for me.

Both of the Marriott complexes had great exercise equipment and pools I could actually do laps in. It goes without saying that the locals and tourists were both very nice to each other. Last but not least for me is the fact that I didn't get bitten by mosquitoes once while here. That was a big plus for me since everywhere else we seemed to get bitten a lot.

The answer to the question "Can we live here?" was a resounding YES.

Then again, the Windsurf cruise ship was a perfect place for us to live too. We would be cruising the Caribbean for two weeks. It really didn't matter to us what islands we would be visiting. It was the experience that counts, and it was the people on board that made it special. There were half-dozen crew members with who we had been on a cruise before.

Over half the folks on this cruise were repeat customers with Windstar. There were so many repeat cruisers that we didn't even make the cut to have dinner with one of the staff members. We would return to the Windsurf in April when we went from Lisbon to Rome, and I was sure most of the crew members would still be working on this ship.

As we went through Montserrat, the highlight for us was the local duo who came on board to play a full two-hour set. By the time they left, they had everyone dancing to familiar reggae tunes.

We got some great walks and run/walks in during the first week of the cruise. During our stay at our favorite port of St. Kitts, we walked to and from the Marriott Resort, a very hilly eight-mile round trip that was well worth it since the spring race season was right around the corner.

The second week was epic. A few friends from our running cruise adventures, along with Gwen, joined us. You can never be sure how others would like the small ship, family atmosphere of the Windstar Cruises Line, but the eleven of us all had a great time on the Windsurf. We had long walks, some runs, and a lot of laughs during the week.

The highlight each night was for everybody to dine together and compare notes on what we all did during the day. Some went snorkeling, some simply went to the nearby beach to suntan, and others went sailing off the back of the ship. None of us were big on organized excursions, but we all managed to keep busy and get some much-needed sun.

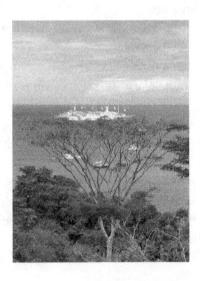

We hadn't had enough of the sun and fun of the Caribbean, so we went to Puerto Rico to catch a big ship for yet another week with some different long-time running cruise friends, Mike, Kay, Deborah, and Kim, otherwise known as the Band. Since I had been to most of the islands over the last two weeks, I conducted "Tony Tours" for the Band, where I took them on walking routes that included all the highlights of the area.

Over the last three weeks, thinking about the question, "Can we live here?" I found myself paying attention to the various reasons why people were living where they were. Often it was to be near where they worked. Others wanted to be close to family—I saw this with a lot of retirees who moved to be close to their grandchildren so they could help raise them. We preferred to visit our grown children from time to time. Some stayed near where they went to college or never left the town they grew up in. The seminomadic seniors known as Snowbirds basically follow the warmth of the sun.

Rather than sticking with the known, the routine, or nearby family support, Catherine and I had found it beneficial, so far, to embrace our life of running all over the world. As my daughter, Mariah, said to me once, "Everybody is where they want to be." For now, that included us, one day at a time.

"I haven't been everywhere, but it's on my list" (Susan Sontag).

I heard this quote from Ana, who we met last year on a Marathon Tours adventure in Madagascar. She had talked about going someplace you had never been before once a year. I commented on the fact that we were seeing someplace new about every month. Every time I thought I had been to a lot of places—seventy countries so far in my lifetime—we ran into someone who had been nearly everywhere.

On this thirty-day trip to Europe, we would run a half-marathon in Cyprus, someplace we hadn't been before. We were presently in Paris. It had taken us almost two days to get here. We took this route to get a first-class seat to Europe and only pay for the economy.

To make this happen, we flew to Detroit, then on to Paris. That seemed simple enough, but not so fast. Our plane had a slight mechanical issue, so we started out behind the eight ball for a one-hour connection. Since Detroit was experiencing a minor snowstorm, we had to hold and by the time we landed, our plane to Paris had already left the gate. The computer had already found us first-class seats to Minneapolis and then to Paris the next day.

After a short thirty-minute wait in line, we were on the shuttle to the Sheraton Hotel complete with dinner vouchers. The next day we made it fine, but Catherine's bag didn't. We arrived a day late and a bag short. This was the fourth time in three years our bags hadn't made the trip, and each time it was Catherine's. The last time it was on a flight to Hawaii, and she got some nice dresses compliments of Delta. Ironically, two of those dresses were in Catherine's current lost bag.

According to the crackpot tracking system, the bag got off the plane from Detroit to Minneapolis, and that was where the trail went cold. Air France (or as I liked to call my least favorite Airline, Air Chance) at the Charles DeGaul airport insisted that the bag was at the airport, but since they had a lot of bags it was going to take them awhile to find it.

We were on our way from Paris to Tel Aviv one bag short. This wasn't our first rodeo, so we were replacing items one-by-one at fifty bucks a day. The Air Chance agent advised us that, since the tickets were bought on my American Express, we could basically go hog wild with my replacement plan.

Lots of bags were a major headache for us because, unlike vacationers who might be away from home for a week, we might be gone from our home base for a month or two. In some cases, we might be running/walking or swimming in various different climates. Everything in our bags had been chosen with care.

Also, some of the items we carried with us had sentimental value for Catherine, such as her Boston Marathon jacket from 2003. People with Alzheimer's tend to have more attachment to these items and people with a home tend to leave these items at home. It tended to help Catherine to carry comfort items like her jacket with us, but when they got lost, it was hard for her to handle, and she didn't have a positive attitude about the prospects of the bag eventually being returned.

This trip was shaping up to be a real doozy. We were all lined up for the flight to Tel Aviv when we were informed that our plane had technical issues, so we ended up being over an hour late. That was after getting the most extensive body and bag check ever since our tickets said "Israel."

We arrived a day before the rest of the Marathon Tours group and stayed at one of my favorite Marriott properties, Renaissance Tel Aviv, for the first two days. The hotel is located right on the Mediterranean Sea with a paved running and biking path right out the back door.

I was somewhat distracted by trying to find Catherine's suit-case, which entailed several phone calls a day plus shopping for some must-have items. Delta now thought that the tag came off the bag when it came off the plane from Detroit and went to a holding area in Minneapolis. The only problem with proving that theory is that Delta's delayed bag department in Minneapolis wouldn't answer the phone or return any messages to them.

I had spent about $1,000 so far replacing things for Catherine, and if it didn't show by the time we got to Amsterdam, I would replace all the rest of the items, which should be about another $2,000. I truly thought it would turn up, but I did learn that for fifty bucks per flight you can get excess insurance at the ticket counter up to $5,000.

Here's the rundown of what we did and saw on our second trip to Israel.

### Day 1: Tel Aviv
Marathon Tours hosted a fabulous welcome dinner at the Abrage Restaurant in Yaffo.

### Day 2: Tel Aviv | Jerusalem
We started the day with a guided tour of Tel Aviv, which began in Rabin Square and continued to Old Jaffa, one of the oldest port cities in the world, where we visited the ancient ruins and walked along the Artist's Quarter. The next stop was Neve Tzedek, the first neighborhood of Tel Aviv, built in 1887, and Nahalat Benyamin, the

pedestrian mall of the city with a stop at Sheinkin, the lively and colorful street known for its unique shops, café life, and youthful ambiance. After lunch and some free time, we made our way to Jerusalem and checked in at the hotel.

Day 3: Jerusalem

We toured the Old City and the New City. We drove to the Mount of Olives for a panoramic view of the city, visited the Tomb of King David and the Room of Last Supper on Mt. Zion. Upon entering the walled city, we visited the Roman Cardo and the famous Western Wall. Next, we walked via Dolorosa to the Church of the Holy Sepulchre. Following the tour, we made our way to the expo for our bibs and race packets. Immediately after that, we enjoyed a great pasta buffet dinner, which was organized by the race and was served at the expo venue. At the same time, I had to buy some needed items that were in Catherine's bag for the race.

Day 4: Jerusalem

Race day was a bit much. We did manage to once again finish hand in hand, but it was a very tough course and Catherine had to drag me across the finish line. We actually ran into the old city and the course was extremely hilly. You were either going up or down the entire 13.1 miles. My right knee was very unhappy with me on the downhill portions. It was a very organized race, and since Shabbat was that afternoon, closing off the roads to traffic was not a problem.

That evening we gathered for a celebration dinner at a local Mediterranean restaurant called the Lavan with amazing views of the Old City and Mount Zion. We had run right by this place during the race.

Day 5: Jerusalem | Dead Sea

We had a full-day excursion to the ancient ruins of Masada and the Dead Sea. We stopped at the world-famous Dead Sea cosmetics company AHAVA where we saw an informative multimedia presentation and received expert advice from one of the many cosmetologists on hand.

Day 6: Jerusalem | Tel Aviv

We visited the Yad Vashem, the memorial to the Holocaust, and continued to the Machne Yehuda Market. We had time there to explore on your own before we departed Jerusalem and made our way back to Tel Aviv.

Day 7: Tel Aviv Biblical Highlights of the North Tour

We departed Tel Aviv via the coastal road and drove through the landscape of Lower Galilee to Nazareth, the town where Jesus spent his childhood. We visited the Basilica of Annunciation and the Church of St. Joseph. We continued, via Kana, to Tiberias, the lively resort town on the Sea of Galilee. We drove along the Kineret Lake to Capernaum and view the ruins of the ancient synagogue where Jesus taught, then continued to Tabgha and visited the Church of Multiplication of the Loaves and Fish, with its beautiful mosaic floor. We then proceeded to Yardenit, the famous baptismal site located where the Jordan River flows out from the Sea of Galilee to the Dead Sea.

Day 8: Pearls of Western Galilee Tour

We drove along the coastal road to Caesarea, the ancient Roman capital and port; then enjoyed a walking tour of the theatre and the archaeological ruins and excavations. In Rosh Hanikra, we descended by cable car into the underwater grottoes and admired the spectacular natural formations. In Acre, we visited the Old City, recognized by UNESCO as a world heritage site; walked through the market, the mosque, and the old port; and visited the remarkable underground Crusader City and crypt, with its pillared dining hall and storerooms, an orderly latrine, and a dungeon whose stone walls still had holes for attaching shackles. We then continued to Haifa for a scenic view of the city, the port, and the magnificent Bahai Gardens and Shrine on our way back to Tel Aviv for the last night of our tour here.

As the quote above suggests, we haven't been everywhere, but I thought we could say we had seen it all in Israel and there was no need for us to return. There was a lot of rich history here, but they just tried to kill the Palestinian prime minister while he was visiting a water treatment plant in the Gaza Strip. We were ready for some R and R in Cyprus.

We had another half-marathon to run while there, but besides that, I planned on enjoying the sun and sand along the Mediterranean. Cyprus would be our twenty-eighth country where we have run a least a half-marathon and our twenty-seventh half-marathon on this venture to run all over the world.

Quick bag update: During my twice-daily call to Delta, the automated system said that they had located the bag and it was being forwarded. Since we were once again on the move, I stayed on the line to give them our new address. The agent said that she didn't understand why the system said the bag was being forwarded since her system showed that they still didn't know where the bag was and neither Minneapolis nor Detroit had returned their request for information.

In the meantime, we were enjoying the sun and food in Cyprus. The organization of this trip was a bit different than what I was used to. It was like being on a Marathon Tours trip without the organizer with you. When you go online to sign up for the race, you get to pick your hotel, your transportation to and from the airport, etc. Our race packets were waiting for us in our room, so we only needed to go to the race site for the pasta dinner and the start. We were staying at the Mediterranean Beach Hotel. There were plenty of great places to eat in the nearby area, but it was off-season here, so there was a lot of construction going on, and some places were closed.

It kind of irked me that we had to pay for water, even at the fitness center, and for ice. I couldn't really complain, though, because the price per night was only about eighty bucks. There was a nice walking path along the water and an archeological site to visit nearby.

The internet at the hotel kicked me off each time I put my phone down and asked me to reenter my password to get back online. I bought a device for about two hundred bucks a while back called Skyroam. For nine bucks it provides high-speed internet for twenty-four hours. I used it some while we were cruising the Caribbean and a few times during this trip when we were away from the hotel and airport, and it worked well.

The race itself was out and back and flat as a pancake. The main road was closed all day, but they did have a bus do several trips from the hotels to the race start, so it was easy enough for us to get there. Getting back to the hotel was a different story, but after about a two-mile walk, we were able to find a taxi stand for the ride back.

There were some elite runners for both the half and the marathon, but the total size of those races was only a couple thousand—quite a contrast to the more than twenty thousand we had in Jerusalem. There weren't many folks to cheer us on, but there was plenty of water along the route. Just like in Jerusalem, they handed out regular-size bottles of water, which seemed like such a waste since most people took a few sips and threw the bottle on the ground. The poor volunteers had to first empty them before they could throw them away.

The frigid pool water felt great on my knees after the race, and we relaxed by it each day until we left. We don't normally do this, but there was one restaurant, Nama, that we liked so much we ate there twice. The food each night was simply amazing, and there was not a so-so meal for the whole week.

We did get some long walks in and were able to take a tour of the nearby archeological site called Amathous. The first occupation of this site dates back to the eleventh-century BC. After changing hands numerous times, the city was destroyed by Arab raids and abandoned in the AD seventh century.

It's a toss-up as to if we will come back to Cyprus. The weather, food, and people were great; but there are still so many other places, everywhere, to visit in our lifetime. Maybe we'll put it on our short list of places to stay for a month or so when we slow down ten years down the road.

I love to set short-term and long-term goals for myself, and at this point, I had my sights on running at least a half-marathon in fifty different countries and visiting one hundred countries. I might have to change that to at least a 10K since I plan on dropping down to that distance when I turn seventy. Down the road, I'll probably drop down to 5K at eighty until I die. You never know with me since my running and speed-walking half-marathon times are less than five minutes apart. The stress on my body is much less when I speed-walk them.

Final bag update: When I called in, the woman I spoke to pretty much said that they might find the bag one day, but for now, I should plan on not seeing it again. She figured the bag tag came off, and it had gone to the warehouse for those type bags in either Minneapolis or Charles de Gaulle. She said it might show up in a couple of months since both warehouses are huge.

So the plan now was for us to do some serious shopping in Amsterdam during our five days there. I made a complete list of what was needed and could visualize all the stores that would have those items. I was kind of looking forward to shopping for Catherine and updating her wardrobe. We were going on a river cruise on AMA Waterways to tiptoe through the tulips, so she would need some nice blouses and dresses.

I was interested to see how Delta handles this claim since we were going to be well over what they were required to pay us. However they decided to handle this wouldn't sway our airline of choice since they have reliable service to most of the places we go. It was sad that a bag tag can come off a bag, and it had to go to the Land of Misfit Bags for the rest of its life. I remembered seeing an episode of the reality show "Baggage Wars" where people bid on bags that hadn't been returned to their owners. The thought of Catherine's items being auctioned off creeped me out.

When all the shopping was done and I downloaded the last of the thirty-four receipts totaling $2,000, lo and behold, I saw that Catherine's bag had been put on a plane from Atlanta to Amsterdam that morning. No call, no nothing from Delta.

I now had three bags and a bunch of clothes to deal with until we get back to Atlanta in a week. I wasn't sure where Catherine's bag had been—or when and how it got to Atlanta prior to the flight here—but it had at least six different bag tags on it.

I learned more than I ever thought I would about how Delta calculates the replacement value of a lost bag. They actually have a currency called Special Drawing Rights (SDR), and their rate of reimbursement for international flights is 1131 SDR, which was $1644.10 USD. That was a bit short of the $2000 I spent on replacement items, but Delta came through with $250 each in credits for future flights, which is like cash for us. No complaints here, but I did write them a long comment on the survey they sent us about how they can improve their delayed/lost bag procedures.

After losing her bag multiple times, Catherine decided that from now on she was going to carry most of her clothes on board. That would require some changes to both what we carry and how we pack. We would still check my bag and another one with all our replaceable products.

During the seven days on the *AmaKristina*, I thought a lot about "going everywhere" since we went to a number of places I had never even heard of before. It was a bit colder than we had expected, but since Catherine now had twice the amount of clothes we usually carry, keeping warm was not that hard to do. The cold also meant that the flowers were not in full bloom, but they were gorgeous just the same.

I really liked the way AMAWaterways does their cruises. All our guided tours, daily bike tours, and excursions were included; and all we had to do was give a small tip to the very knowledgeable guides and experienced drivers. They had a sip and sail an hour prior to dinner where they offered a drink of the day. It was a great way to bring everyone to the lounge to socialize and be there for the daily port talk.

The tulip arrangement in each cabin was a nice touch, and the blue light that would come on only at night in the bathroom when you opened the door was a feature I really liked. Nothing worse than a bright light in the middle of the night when you just want to go and then go back to sleep.

The cruise started with an overnight stay in Amsterdam before we made our way to Hoorn and Middelburg. From there we continued on to Antwerp.

Before we left Antwerp, we walked by way of the underwater tunnel to Linkeroever and back. It was about a half-mile walk each way and can go down and up from the tunnel by elevator or wooden escalator.

The trip back was a bit stressful. Since we used global upgrades, we had to go from Amsterdam to Paris, then on to Atlanta, with the first flight leaving at 6:45 a.m. Since I'm getting too old for multiple flights, we stayed at a very nice Marriott near the airport.

We were now nice and comfy on our flatbed, nine-hour day flight to Atlanta. It was a nice touch to be given a handwritten personalized card thanking us for our business as we settled into our seats, but we could only wonder if our bags would be there in Atlanta to meet us. No luck. We were now in Atlanta three bags short—and of course, Delta had no idea where they were. Their tracking system showed that two of them got on the plane with us in Paris and the third was missing in action

Hooray! Our bags showed up at the hotel twelve hours before we had to leave for our trip to Bloomington. That did not give us much time to rearrange our bags and drop off all the extra clothes at our storage unit, but I got it done. Delta was still our favorite airline but, they needed to fix their baggage tracking system.

# CHAPTER
# 33

## Enjoy Life to the Fullest—It Has an Expiration Date

*Live your life, and forget your age.*

—Jean Paul

The quote above was written on the wall as you get off the elevator on the sixth floor of the Marriott Renaissance hotel in Atlanta. This hotel had become one of our favorites for a number of reasons.

It's located on the first stop of the airport sky train and everyone there makes you feel like family. The only drawback is that they have valet parking for twenty-nine bucks a day, and their cost per night is a bit pricey but to compensate we usually stay there on points. They also have an executive lounge, so breakfast and dinner are on them.

We definitely live our lives, and—except for birthdays—we don't think about our ages. It might have to do with the fact that both of us have some health issues.

Our latest twenty-eight-day jaunt would start with us going to Amsterdam for a night. I do show my age, sometimes, when we're going to Europe and I need a stop to recuperate before going on to Lisbon, which is another one of our favorite destinations. This will be my fourth trip there, second for Catherine.

If anyone knows about the area of Lisbon called Bairro Alto you definitely know about the attraction of the city. I'm always intrigued by the level of detail of the stonework of the sidewalks. We enjoyed some of the best food and drinks we'd ever had. One restaurant didn't have much curb appeal. but when I asked the man standing out front with menus in hand if they had salmon, Catherine's favorite, he pointed to the fresh display of seafood inside. Not only was the salmon prepared to perfection, but it was complemented well by homemade Sangria. After two nights in Lisbon, we met up with our favorite cruise ship, Windstar's Windsurf.

We had been aboard in the Caribbean back in February. Most of the crew would still be on the ship, and I understood that twelve out of the fourteen days of the Atlantic crossing were smooth as silk. The last two days had been a different story while they navigated around some storms in the area. Two rogue waves hit the ship broadside, and the passengers' accounts were hair-raising.

They had to bring on a special crew and supplies in Lisbon to do some cosmetic repairs, but within days the ship was once again like brand new. Some of the two hundred passengers that did the crossing were still on board, and they wore the experience like a badge of honor. One account came from a man who showed off the bruise he got from being shot out of his bed and across his room all the way to the door at 4:00 a.m. With that in mind, I guess an Atlantic crossing is now off our life list. Our first day was a sea day, and with our fingers crossed, it was the smoothest sailing ever.

As always, we needed to get our steps in, so we went around and around and up and down among the three decks, and in no time ten thousand steps were in the books. It was really nice to give all the familiar crew members high fives. Our first stop was Tangier, Morocco, and that was a much nicer experience than we had in Casablanca a couple of years ago.

As we were traversing the Straits of Gibraltar, we could actually see Spain in the distance, a mere seven miles away. The next stop of Malaga, Spain, is a must-see if you are ever in the area. The Botanical Gardens called Jardin Botanico Historico La Concepcion was well worth the four-mile walk each way. I'm sure everyone else on the ship saw the breathtaking site either on a tour or by taxi but for us, sightseeing by foot is the only way to go.

When we arrived at our next stop in Almeria, Spain, we decided it was time to do a two-a-day. We took a morning walk along the boulevard that runs from the port to the surrounding mountains and came back by the only functioning bullfighting arena in the area, Plaza De Toros. After a quick bite to eat back on the ship, we were off again, this time along the beautiful beach.

While we were there, they brought on the ship a very talented flamenco dancing troupe, and I was spellbound. The couple was exceptional and the other three who accompanied them were also outstanding. Picture if you can the night ending with a deck barbecue as we sailed away with the sails out and the sun setting in the distance.

I must admit that had to be my favorite meal ever. The sheer number of different entrées, salads, and desserts for you to feast on are too numerous to mention but suffice it to say that many were taking pictures of the beautiful presentations.

Life always seems to have twists and turns, and now that my right knee was doing much better my left foot thought it would be appropriate to raise some Cain. The toe joints were giving me problems for no good reason. Usually I can figure out what I did to aggravate whatever body part wasn't happy with me at the time, but in this case, I had no clue. Old age, I guess. Another possibility was a simple overuse. We had been putting in a lot of steps/miles these days.

As I usually do on these cruises, I too an assessment of our fellow passengers and their abilities or lack thereof. I like to take a gander at what lies ahead of me. Some passengers had canes and others were leaning on others, but they were all living by the adage, "live your life and forget your age."

It always amazes me that people who are ten or more years older than me are still working full time or have been winding down their work schedule over the last several years. Many say they love their jobs, but I think they love the steady income even more. Who am I to judge? They're simply living their lives as they see fit, no matter their age.

Off we went to another city that I had never heard of: Cartagena, Spain. Surprise, surprise, they had a famous, fort, church, amphitheater, etc.

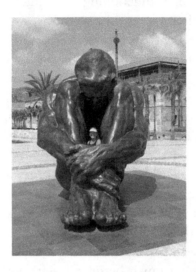

Overnight we were sailing to Ibiza, Spain. The last time I was there I was in college, and I understood that not much has changed in forty years. The experience would be completely different since we would only be there during the day and would not be able to go to the largest nightclub in the world. I understood that most people there wouldn't even be up during the day.

Our mission for the day was to find some replacement running shoes for Catherine. Her six-month-old New Balance shoes had a blowout the other day, and with my Wi-Fi in my pocket and iPhone in hand, my GPS took us from running store to store until we found some reasonably priced Nikes that will work for our race in Geneva in two weeks.

After lunch on the ship, we were off to a nearby lighthouse and massive fort, Puig de Missa, that I didn't even know existed forty years ago. I'm not sure how I missed it, but I imagine I really wasn't interested in something like that back then.

Southern Spain turned out to be very special, and Tarragona, Spain, was another gem all should visit. It's only sixty miles from

Barcelona, and I understand that many people who live in Barcelona often make the hour drive to the beautiful beaches here. Just like anywhere else along the Mediterranean coast, there was a fort, a Roman Amphitheater, and a Cathedral. We were able to hit them all, and we walked many miles along the beach.

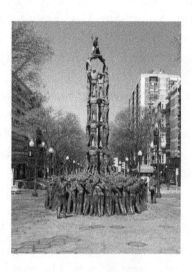

I thought I might have figured out the big toe joint pain. I found some relief by sticking some cotton balls between the two toes causing all the uproar. We had walked a lot of miles so far, and I feared trying to run since my right knee was doing so well.

We had run a marathon in Barcelona four years before, so except for seeing the famous Columbus Monument and traversing La` Ramblas boulevard, our search was to get some much-needed supplies. We were then off for another unheard-of landing point at Port-Vendres, France. One of the things I loved about Windstar was that their ships could slip into ports that the large ships cannot so we could see the hidden gems of the world.

The challenge for us in Port-Vendres was to go to the nearby city called Collioure, the gem of the Catalonian coast, of course by foot, and then make our way safely up and down to the nearby fort called Saint-Elme which was originally a signal tower. The trek up was steep and rocky, but I'm a vista junky and was not disappointed by the views from this fort. They even had a grand museum inside that was well worth the hike up and down along with the small entrance fee. We were very diligent in getting at least ten thousand steps in a day, which equates to about five miles. This past week we had doubled that average which was great since the food on this ship had been, as always, exceptional.

Our next stop, Sanary-Sur-Mer, France, was a quaint town about twenty miles south of Marseille. It's where the pioneers of diving Jacques Cousteau, Frederic Dumas, and Phillipe Thailliez learned their skills.

We just did a nice slow walk around the area from the pier to the nearby beach called Le Levant, then in the opposite direction to a hideaway beach called Place de Portissol. It was a large crescent-shaped, mainly sand beach fringed by tamarisk trees and sheltered from the wind.

We were then off to our fifth country on this fifteen-day cruise: Monaco. The city of Monte Carlo was all abuzz with the construction of the stands for the upcoming Grand Prix. Monaco covers just 1.95 square kilometers and would fit comfortably inside New York's Central Park or a family farm in Iowa. The goal I had set myself was to see the Grand Casino and Japanese Garden, walk up into nearby foothills and make the last stop at the Prince's Palace. We were able to stay in Monte Carlo until midnight, and the night lights were magnificent.

Our next port of call was Cannes, where we had been three years ago, so the plan for this port was plain and simple: a six-mile fast run/walk along the Mediterranean.

Our path took us right past the site of the Cannes Film Festival, the JW Marriott where we had stayed three years ago, and the famous Carlton Hotel. We were loving this cruise so much we went ahead and booked the cruise in the opposite direction in June of next year. By doing so, I was able to take advantage of their reduced deposit policy that includes 5 percent savings as a returning guest, an additional 5 percent discount for booking within sixty days of taking a Windstar Cruises, free laundry, and $500 per person shipboard credit.

As we were coming into Portofino, Italy, I looked at the landscape from the ship and reviewed the material provided on the port and came up with another very energetic game plan. First, climb the mountain in the rear of the port, then make our way to Santa Margherita, once again by foot.

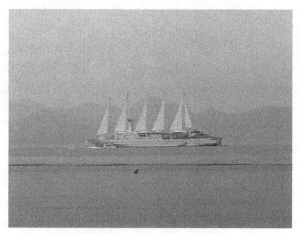

*Our ship with the sails out*

I thought my heart was going to explode as we climbed the well-marked trail. It had numerous branches going off to different places I had never heard of, but my mission was to the top. Catherine took the very steep trail and steps like the billy goat that she is, and I had to stop numerous times to catch my breath. It actually felt good to press the envelope, and the views were also well worth the effort. We made our way back down by another well-marked road barely wide enough for a small vehicle, and the last stage in the descent was along with an extremely narrow set of steps to the street.

Next up was to find our way to the next port, called Santa Margherita, but since the street didn't have sidewalks, I found a trail system that was well-paved and sat right above the road below. The 2.5-mile walk each way was once again well worth it for the views.

Our last stop before they were going to kick us off in Rome was Portoferraio, Italy. I believe this port held the record for the most forts (three), but I had decided that I was forted out, so we just took a leisurely walk around the busy port. The ferries were plentiful and constant. Watching the well-orchestrated offloading and loading of hundreds of vehicles, including large buses, was fun.

Just like clockwork, we were kicked to the curb in the Roman port of Civitavecchia, Italy. For a small fee, a bus was provided for those of us going straight to the airport. Instead of saying goodbye, we said "see you next time" to the wonderful crew, knowing that we would be back on this ship in the Caribbean next February.

Alitalia was our next mode of transportation, taking us to Cagliari, Sardegna, a small island off the coast of Italy. Picking this stop was very scientific. We finished the cruise in Rome and had to be in Geneva in five days for a race. We looked at a map and asked ourselves, "What's nearby that we haven't been to before?" Sardegna fit the bill.

Often your first impression is your lasting impression. Through Orbitz, the hotel, La Villa del Mare, had arranged for our transportation from the airport. As we arrived, the street adjacent to the beach was full of activity with people walking, running, and biking.

The owner met us at the gate, and we felt right at home. The room/apartment was spacious and had everything we could ask for. The sky was blue and the beach and water were very inviting, but I couldn't wait to walk the boulevard in front of the hotel to explore the area. The owner gave us a map of the area, the bus schedule to the center city/port, and a list of the recommended restaurants both nearby and in the city.

They had bikes and beach towels to rent and even sold bus tickets. Very reliable and fast internet was included; and I woke up each morning with anticipation for the beloved chocolate croissants, freshly prepared fruit, and the best-ever cappuccinos. This was a great transition since we had come off a cruise ship where bacon and eggs were the staples for breakfast.

For Catherine's birthday, we got in a very long walk around the nearby park that was home to thousands of pink flamingos, followed by a very tasty dinner at a nearby restaurant. The next few days were a bit challenging since the rain gods had found us, but the hotel gave us a list of indoor activities in the area.

We did make it to the port one day. As we walked along trying to find someplace to eat, the sidewalk cafes were not very appealing, but lo and behold we saw a sign for a rooftop bar and restaurant. Once again, the food was good, the place was empty, and the cost above average.

I guess the owners of the hotel felt sorry for us because of the washout because when we got back to the room, they had left a bottle of Prosecco, cheese, and olives while we were gone.

We were then off to Geneva in Switzerland, which was my seventy-first country to visit. I truly didn't know what to expect since my recollection of Switzerland was the Alps. For a runner, all that came to mind was hills or mountains.

Since I don't do a lot of research before we go somewhere, I was pleasantly surprised by the basically flat course. There were a few rolling hills through the farmland portion of the race early on, but I really enjoyed the downhill after the tunnel down to the lake at around mile 8. The race started off in a beautiful park and finished right next to their majestic lake. I can say that was one of the best half-marathon courses I had ever been on. The weather was perfect, and getting to the start and back from the finish to the hotel was effortless.

The weekend was full of different races for every member of the family. The half started at 8:30, with the full at 9:45. That worked well since we were able to still be at the finish to see the men's and women's marathon winners come flying by.

Our hotel was only a few blocks away. The race website suggested hotels in the area, but the one that I picked because of price and location gave me great pause when we arrived, so we checked in at the Novotel around the corner. The hotel had absolutely no curb appeal, but the area itself was very interesting, with all the hookers in the city forming their very own red-light district in the six square blocks surrounding the hotel. They didn't harass us as we walked by, and every now and then the police would show up—not to pick them up, but to merely ward off their clients. With two laundromats within blocks of the hotel, there was plenty of work for the ladies of the day and night.

The room itself was clean and even had a kitchenette, which came in handy. The food was very expensive, and in some restaurants, the portions were a bit small—maybe I was still adjusting after two weeks of cruising. There were several parks and a wonderful botanical garden adjacent to the lake, and I couldn't believe the number of people running around the area. We could see the Alps off in the distance, and I couldn't resist a Swiss boat tour of Lake Geneva so I could get up close and personal with the world's tallest water fountain.

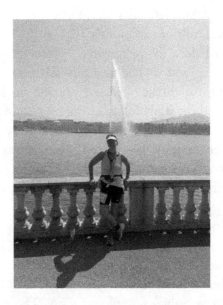

Here are the stats: It draws the water from the lake and shoots 500 liters of water per second to a height of 140 meters, at a speed of 200 kilometers per hour. The column of water weighs 8 tons and the pumps generate 1360 hp. The fountain operates only when the wind blows at less than 20 kilometers per hour.

There were more than forty political cartoons from around the world in an area near the Lake, and the US was the butt of some of their jokes.

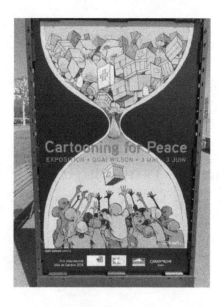

I learned a number of things about Switzerland that I hadn't known. I didn't realize how diverse it is, and the fact that they speak four official languages. No matter my age, I would not come back since this trip and race were near perfect, and I would like to keep it that way in my mind.

The bottom line is that I refused to let my age determine what Catherine and I were going to do with the rest of our lives. Even as we got older and things didn't work like they used to, it still beats the alternative.

# CHAPTER
# 34

# Nomads (Noun): People Who Wander from Place to Place

Home is the here and now.

—Buddhism

After our bad experiences with our bags getting delayed and or lost recently, for our latest two-week trip, we decided to try to carry on bags instead of checking our usual two fifty-pound bags. This was going to take some getting used to.

After three-and-half years as a nomad, I thought I might be getting travel fatigue. I now had a tendency to just drop in somewhere without doing the research like I used to do. This trip was a prime example. First, we went to Seattle to have a follow-up exam for my right iliac artery aneurysm repair, then we had flights to Seoul (twelve hours) and Bangkok (five hours). We got the upgrade to Delta One (what they call First Class on their international flights), which was nice, but the fare didn't allow us to pick our seats on Korean Air. I hadn't done my due diligence during the booking process, and the agent hadn't pointed it out, either. After hours on the phone, I was able to get seats close to each other, but we would have the same problem coming back.

Three years ago, I would have figured that out right away and would have made the change within the twenty-four-hour change window. Maybe I just had a lot on my mind with our health issues or the fact that Bangkok would be stop number 333. That's a lot of planes, trains, taxis, rental cars, hotels, race registrations, and simple logistics to find someplace to eat for anyone to coordinate. If it was easy, anyone could do it. But would they?

The next snafu was that, while I was concentrating on the carry-on bag issue, I had failed to read all the material on exactly where we were going and what we might wear. I was thinking, "It's near Bangkok so it'll be warm, no brainer."

Yes, we would be in Bangkok for six nights and it would be warm—but Paro, Bhutan, where the race would take place and where we would be for a week is at seven thousand feet and would be in the midforties. We would be doing three tough hikes to around ten thousand feet, and last but not least, there was rain in the forecast.

Having worked in management for one of the largest logistic companies in the world for twenty-seven years, I do love logistics, so figuring out at the last minute how to solve this problem was right up my alley. The hotel we would be staying at in Bangkok was a Marriott Executive Apartments, and our mission while there was to find some appropriate clothes for the Bhutan experience and still be able to do carry-on on the way back.

Thinking about it, I was sure I would find what I needed there and would get my belly full at the same time. Maybe in retrospect, it wasn't travel fatigue, but I just needed to keep things interesting. That would also explain our nomadic lifestyle.

"All that and a bag of chips" is the best way to describe the Bangkok experience. For me, going someplace we have been before, especially when it was great the first time, has a tendency to make me apprehensive. Could our second trip to Bangkok be as good as our first time three years ago?

Our walks in Lumpini Park were a bit warm and steamy but as pristine as I remembered. When it came to shopping for outerwear, the nearby mall had everything we needed. As we explored, we came across another mall complex that took up several square miles. Since the sidewalks are usually filled with street vendors we went for the overhead skywalks, whenever possible, to get from place to place. It made it easy to get from one part of the mall complex to the other and made crossing the street a piece of cake. Above the skywalks was the rail system that, for some reason, I hadn't noticed either during our first trip.

I really love the customary Thai greeting of pressing their hands together as you would for a prayer and making a slight bow. Thailand is noted as the country of smiles, so a big smile is a must when greeting someone. It's considered disrespectful for someone not to return a bow, but I noticed that many foreigners didn't.

Catherine had decided to do a half Ironman in New Orleans in October, so we made good use of the great hotel pool while we were there. After four nights at the Marriott, we transitioned to the Marathon Tours designated hotel, a Novotel at the airport, which made it convenient for our 5:00 a.m. flight to Paro, Bhutan, the next morning. Most of the folks in the group didn't arrive until late that night, and I felt sorry for those who had to turn right around with the 2:00 a.m. wake-up call. I try not to schedule us like that anymore. We found that we had been on trips before with about half the people in our group.

Apparently the Paro Airport is listed as the world's sixth-most dangerous airport to fly in and out of. Before that hair-raising experience, we made a short stop in Kolkata, India, where we got a glimpse of Mt. Everest off in the distance. As we came into Para, there were mountains everywhere, and we had to make some pretty sharp turns to follow the required path into the airport. I wasn't scared but more intrigued by the terrain.

After our flight, we drove to the old capital city, Punakha, visiting the historic Iron Bridge on the way. We then drove over the spectacular Dochu La Pass, with amazing views of the Southern Himalayas, and into the Punakha Valley. We were on our way to the Temple of Fertility and Punakha Dzong, which is the historic capital of Bhutan. The drive over to Punakha Dzong was much scarier than the flight: we went up and down the mountain passes without any guard rails and occasional piles of rocks at the curves did nothing to calm my nerves.

After a good night's sleep, we were off to hike the Himalayan Mountains for more than eight hours. A 20K hike to Soela Gompa via Khamsum Yuelley Namgyel Chor was a great acclimatization activity. We stopped by one of the many temples we would see on this trip as we made our way to the summit some ten thousand feet into the clouds.

We started our trek at seven thousand feet, but you would have thought I was on top of Mt. Everest the way I was sucking wind. On our way back across and down the mountain, we thought this hike was going to end. As an added treat, many of us (including myself) had to have leaches pulled out of our feet by the guides. It was surreal to see my three stowaways sliver off into the grass with their bellies full of my blood.

Since I'm on blood thinners for my artificial mechanical heart valve, it took me a while to get the flow of blood to stop. It was a pretty gross scene but just another day in the life of the locals here in Bhutan. That hike was the hardest thing I had done in the two years since we stopped doing marathons. As my heart was beating out of my chest, I kept telling myself that this was a good way to prepare me for the half-marathon in three days.

They call Bhutan "the land of happiness," and the people do all seem to be pretty happy. I'm sure their Buddhist faith has a lot to do with it. The symbols inside their temples were unlike any other: they have one monk they pray to called the Madman. They do love to pray here and give you plenty of opportunities to do so. Besides their numerous temples, there were prayer wheels, prayer flags, and poles. Another clue as to what makes them so happy: we found marijuana growing on the side of the roads—and there are a root and leaf, Betel nut, that everyone chewed on to get a buzz.

The next day we were off to the capital city, Thimphu, where we hiked up to Buddha Point and the giant seated Buddha. At the Takin Reserve, we saw herds of Bhutan's national animal, the Takin, otherwise known as the Goat Antelope. We visited Thimphu Dzong and craft workshops. After lunch, we drove back to Paro to visit the Drukgyel Dzong and Kichu Lhakhang, a very important Himalayan Buddhist temple. We also had the chance to hike part of the marathon route before visiting the Paro Dzong.

Dzongs are huge fortress-looking buildings that used to be defensive structures but were now Bhutan government buildings in the front and monasteries in the rear. They were all lit up at night for all to see.

The next day was a bit easier, as we hiked for five hours up and down to the famous Taktshang Tiger's Nest monastery. The hike was fairly demanding, The UK's Prince William and Kate, Duchess of Cambridge had recently done the same hike. The final portion included 756 steps each way.

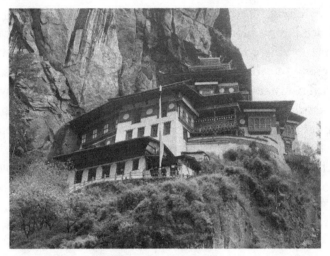

*Tiger's Nest*

As we were instructed to take our shoes off and put away cameras before entering the temple, I thought that, unless you come to these places yourself, you'll never see what those who have made the trip will see. There aren't even any pictures on the internet, and after all the hiking, it felt like their goal was to put each temple or dzong in the most remote and hard-to-reach places.

Here are some fun facts about Bhutan:

- More than 90 percent of people wear the traditional shirt and skirt outfit called a Kira for women and a Gho for men. Since most people are employed by the government, they can be fined if caught not wearing them.

- Most, if not all, restaurants have the same meals for tourists since they were all trained by the same master chef and the government wants consistency for those visiting their country.
- People traveling from India, Bangladesh, and the Maldives do not need visas to enter Bhutan, whereas it is required by everyone else.
- Blue Poppy is the national flower and the name of the government-owned company that provides tours of the country.
- You see the name "Druk" everywhere, and it is their dragon symbol on their flag.
- Dogs are plentiful. You can't go a few feet without seeing one or more everywhere.
- The houses are spectacular, covered in very colorful artwork, and draped in prayer flags.

We had a rest day scheduled the next day; but instead, we went shopping, had lunch in town, and enjoyed a hot stone bath. We sat in a trough, and they put hot stones in a separate chamber. The stones would crack open and release minerals into the water we were sitting in. They added an herb called artemisia to enhance the experience. I rubbed the herbs on the bites from the first hike, and it seemed to help.

All that was left now was race day. The marathoners had to climb more than three thousand feet. We only had to do half that, but it was hard as hell for me. The only saving grace was the sights and the fact that it stayed cloudy while we ran. Fun fact: they only allow women to run the half-marathon. A local marathoner finished in 3:05, whereas the first Westerner in our group came in more than thirty minutes behind him.

When I turned fifty, I decided to run the JFK fifty-miler. The first half was along the Appalachian Trail, and I used to joke that the only thing we didn't do was rappel during that race. I had the same feeling in Bhutan. We went way off-road and had to cross two suspension bridges. There were water hazards and extremely narrow paths with steep descents. Their idea of rolling hills was half-mile climbs and quarter-mile gradual descents, but at least I won my age group.

Overall, it was a great trip but definitely not for the faint of heart. This was a good training run for Catherine's state of Wyoming half-marathon next Sunday in Casper. We met folks who we had seen on prior Marathon Tours in Africa, Petra, and Madagascar, and also made some new best friends.

When we got to the airport, the agent told us we couldn't check in for the Seoul to Atlanta leg of our trip and that they had already assigned our seats for the five-hour flight from Bangkok to Seoul. She showed us on her seat map what they were and asked if they were okay.

The Airbus A330 is configured 2, 4, and 2, and our seats were aisle to aisle, so that was fine with me. When we got to our assigned seats, the flight attendant advised me that my monitor didn't work and that I was going to have to take the window seat. That allowed me to use the space of both seats and made me one happy man.

Well, we had to do the airport 5K to make our connecting flight back to Atlanta. We taxied in right on time, but there was a plane at our gate so we had to wait fifteen minutes on the ramp. At the same time, Delta sent me a text message letting me know that our flight was now leaving fifteen minutes early.

Since we hadn't been able to check in, we didn't have boarding passed for the next flight, so we had to stop at the transfer desk to get them, which took an additional five minutes. Lo and behold, when we were handed our boarding passes, the nice lady advised us that Catherine had been selected for additional screening.

After security gave us the once-over, we were met by an agent with a walkie-talkie in hand and directed to the other side of the terminal to gate number 255. I used my thirteen-minute racewalking pace, and we ended dropping the agent somewhere around gate number 250.

We arrived at the gate with six minutes to spare and our carry-ons in tow. I knew there was a reason we chose to carry on for this trip. We arrived out of breath but with our dignity, and then waited for the original departure time. It turned out they send out "leaving early" messages to connecting passengers so we would all do the airport 5K and they wouldn't have to wait for people taking their time or shopping on the way to the aircraft. It was a learning experience for us here in Korea.

No complaints from me since it makes for a good story, and we were not disappointed at all with the layout in Delta One. We each had our own little suite, but I still needed to figure out how to manage our sleep since we were going to arrive in the Atlantic one hour after we departed Seoul.

Our good friend Kayna often wore a sweatshirt that had the words, "Not all who wander are lost" on it. As a nomad, I can agree with that statement. Being on the road for the last three-and-a-half years had taught me to be very flexible and also not take life too seriously. We had met some great people, and I had learned a little from all of them.

One thing I learned on this trip was that difficult challenges are good for Catherine. The mental challenge of climbing the mountains during the hikes and the race seemed to forge connections in her brain that were at one time broken.

I had read about how music and dancing help those with early-onset Alzheimer's; and I could see how the concentration necessary to not trip and fall while trying to balance on rocks, roots, and uneven surfaces could only benefit her. I don't like trail runs but would be looking for some good places to hike during future trips.

Short-term memory is damaged by Alzheimer's, and my hope was that these exciting experiences would go into long-term memory so that, instead of Catherine being frustrated on a daily basis about forgetting what she had for breakfast, we could reminisce about our extraordinary trek of the Himalayas.

The socialization of being on tours like these is also very beneficial since folks with Alzheimer's want to withdraw from others, which only exacerbates the disease. Last but not least, physical activity, endorphins boost, and her desire to meet or exceed her goal of at least ten thousand steps per day can only enhance her mood.

With Father's Day around the corner, I was reminded that the four-year anniversary of my surgery was approaching. I remember like it was yesterday the feeling I had when I woke up from my surgery. I couldn't see since vision is the last sense to return, but I could hear Catherine in one ear and the nurse in the other telling me to wake up. I thought I had died—and technically I had since they had to stop my heart during the surgery.

I knew at that moment that my life, as I knew it, was going to be completely different, but also that staying active was going to continue to be a great part of my life. I had run twelve marathons since my surgery, but half-marathons were more to my liking now.

I have had several occasions in my life where things that seemed bad turned out to be blessings in disguise. My flight surgeon told me at the height of my career that I had a heart murmur, which was devastating news. As the need for surgery became a reality, I didn't realize that it was just what I needed to get off the merry-go-round of work. Always trying to grab for the brass ring and the realization that it was time for me to get off.

Now that we had been at this for three years and 176 days and had unpacked our bags 342 times I wouldn't have done anything differently. I have learned a lot. For example: just because you might need something one day didn't mean you should carry it around in your suitcase every day.

Time would only tell how long we would continue as nomads, but until then, we were going to enjoy the ride.

# CHAPTER
# 35

## This Is a First

Happiness is not a destination, it is a way of life.
—Anonymous

Pretty much everything we do is a first. We really don't like to do the same thing more than once, unless you count marathons (sixty-four for me and seventy-eight for Catherine). However we rarely do them more than once in the same place.

The "first" in this chapter was that I didn't write it as the trip developed. I decided to wait until we got back to Atlanta and write it from my memory. I loved writing about our adventures as we ran all over the world, but I was finding myself thinking about what I was going to say about wherever we were instead of totally enjoying the experience. It was as if I was writing each experience in my head. I also found that I was taking time out of the day that I could have used to do something exciting rather than sitting down at the computer writing.

Someone once asked me what the hardest and easiest things were about traveling all the time. For me, the hardest thing was always thinking about money. Most of the folks we spent time with were on vacation, but this was our lifestyle, so I needed to keep track of every expense. When the savings were gone, we would have to settle down and live on our pensions and Social Security. I wasn't ready for that to start next year, so I kept a close eye on the almighty dollar bill.

I did have a pretty good system, however. Instead of just enjoying the meal, I tended to think about how much it was costing. I'm not a penny pincher by any means, but I did make decisions based on cost most times. As an example: Is that excursion for $179 per person worth it to see another castle on a hill?

For Catherine, the hardest thing is the food choices. Her digestive system is a bit tricky, so going from place to place is somewhat difficult. If they have salmon and sweet potato fries, she is good to go. I can eat just about anything just as long as you tell me exactly what it is—and no "meat" is not enough detail.

The easiest part is talking about our travels. We used to just tell people that we were from Atlanta, and if they seemed interesting, then we would go into more detail about our nomadic lifestyle. On this trip, we switched it up and told everyone who asked where we were from and that we were nomads.

Catherine pointed out after a few days that we were meeting and talking to a lot more people than usual. I guess we seemed interesting to them, so they hung around to hear more. I sometimes come across as aloof when I first meet people, so I also tried to be more inviting. Catherine was also more engaged, so that was a plus.

Over the years, we have gone back and forth on how to tackle the trip to Europe. When we first started, we would just press on with a connecting flight to our final destination in Europe, but over time, we realized it was easier on the body to stop over for a few days before pushing on. Since time was usually not a factor, we would sometimes stop in Paris or Amsterdam.

For this trip, we stopped in Amsterdam in both directions. We stayed at the Renaissance in the center city for three days going and the one near the airport on the way back to the States. From Amsterdam, we were off to Athens Greece to meet up with our all-time favorite cruise line, Windstar. On this cruise, they were using one of their smaller sail ships, which holds about 148 of our closest friends.

During this cruise, we met up with Gwen and Joan, and Catherine had been looking forward to visiting Santorini as long as I've known her. We also visited the islands of Nafplio, Mykonos,

Kusadasi, Patmos, and Monemvasia. On the island of Kusadasi, Turkey, we had our signature dinner outside the library of Ephesus. That was a once-in-a-lifetime experience. Windstar had the library closed off to the public and the sunset during the event was over the top.

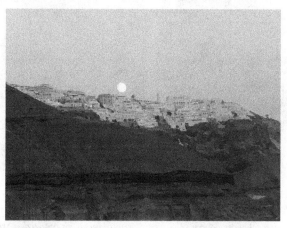

*Moonrise over Santorini as we sail away*

After the cruise, we met up with two of Gwen and Joan's friends and rented an Airbnb on the island of Crete. The area we stayed in was called Rethymno. While there we enjoyed two farm-to-table dinners. One at Arkadi, which included dancers. There, the meal included twenty-three different dishes to sample, all from their farm. The other one was just as good and was cooked by a local family. They didn't speak much English, but our neighbor was there to translate.

One day we took a ferry to two very popular beaches, Gramvousa and Balos, in the area. They were both uninhabited and pristine, and we spent a few hours at each. Several large ferries make the trip each day, and there was not an empty seat on our boat. At the first stop, you could hike up to a fort to some incredible views of the beach below.

We were able to get in some good runs and walks while in Crete before we moved on to our next destination of Copenhagen for an eleven-day cruise through the fjords and the Shetland Islands to Edinburgh.

The hotel in Copenhagen was unlike anything I had ever seen before: it had two separate buildings that leaned out as they went up, with a small section at the top and on the second floor that connects the two buildings. Once again there was a nearby park for us to run in.

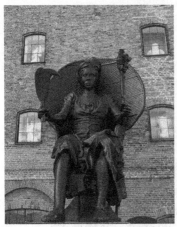
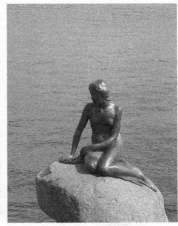

*I am Queen Mary*     *the famous mermaid statue*

On the ship, there were a dozen crew members who remembered us from previous cruises. I would say most of the folks on this cruise were there to trace their ancestors from the area. I stuck out like a sore thumb even though my twenty-three and Me DNA test says I'm twenty-something percent British and Irish.

I had people come up to me and ask the usual: "Do you play basketball?" "Are you seven feet tall?" One person thought I was Italian while another asked if I spoke English. Still another thought I was an African royalty. As usual, I took it in stride and just chalked it to the fact that they need to get out more.

We made stops in Oslo, Bergen, and Flam, Norway followed by Lerwick, Stornoway, Kirkwall, and Invergordon in the UK. These folks in their '70s and '80s sure did get around. They didn't miss an excursion. On the other hand, Catherine and I saw the countryside on foot. I'm sure we missed many a castle or fort, but that was okay by me. We were glad we got to see that part of the world, but doubt if we would ever go back.

When we arrived in Edinburgh, the Festival Fringe was going on. Every year, all sorts of bands and acts perform all over town during the month of August. Banners for such acts are everywhere, and they even have a thick free guide to list all the times and places.

You can't visit Edinburgh and not walk the Royal Mile, visit the Edinburgh Castle, or see the world-famous Royal Edinburgh Military Tattoo, a performance in the temporary stadium they build each year. For the budget reasons I mentioned earlier, the $30 admission fee to the Castle and the several hundred dollars to watch marching bagpipers in Tattoo didn't make the cut.

Edinburgh has great public transportation. They have busses everywhere going every which way, including an airport bus that runs right by our Marriott hotel near the airport to the center city. Our bus on the way to the airport displayed flight information, which was handy.

With two days under our belt, it was back to Amsterdam for two nights at the airport Marriott. They were completing their merger with SPG, so the website was not up to snuff; but we soon forgot that when they offered an upgrade to a corner room, free welcome drinks, and $40 food and drink vouchers for the two nights.

I'm undecided about how I like this new way of writing this chapter. It was nice to just experience the trip, but I must admit I couldn't help myself from thinking about what I was going to say about each experience.

I had mentioned that this trip was full of firsts, but I realized we had them several times a day. On the other side, we were running out of places to go. I ran into a couple who told me about a cruise that goes up and down the Nile from Cairo to Cairo, and I probably have a dozen other places I would like to visit. I'm big into places whose names I know—I'm not that adventurous to do on my own.

# CHAPTER
# 36

## Can We Live Here? (Part 2)

Quit grinding your gears to fit where you
are—go, instead, to where you fit.

—Sean Keenan,
Managing Editor,
International Living Magazine

Back in Atlanta, we found an Olympic-distance race in nearby
Pine Mountain, Georgia, where Catherine could train for the Half
Ironman she was running in October. The swim was one thousand
meters, which was about half the distance of the race in New Orleans.
The bike was nineteen miles (about a third the distance), and the run
was an 8K (less than half the 13.1 miles for the run portion).

In many respects, the race in Georgia went better than I had
hoped. As a matter of fact, Catherine came in third in her age group.
She was still beaming from ear to ear days later.

I was able to assist Catherine with the transition, which gave me
some great insight into what she needed to do it entirely by herself.
First thing: a triathlon suit. That's a suit you swim in, bike in, and
run in. No changing required. All you have to do is put on and take
off your helmet and take off your bike shoes and replace them with
running shoes.

We were able to find a great purple, pink, and white two-piece
triathlon suit. (Purple is the color for Alzheimer's). We were now at

the Martin Luther King Recreation and Aquatic Center in Atlanta. After thirty minutes in the pool, she was banging out twenty miles on a stationary bike. I was enjoying the role of a coach. It brought back memories of coaching my kids when they played soccer as kids. I do participate in some of Catherine's training sessions, just not at the same intensity. Another benefit of all this intense training is that she's so worn out that she gets plenty of sleep.

As we ran all over the world, we used Atlanta as our home base since Delta has their hub there, and as far as I was concerned, they were the best Airline. We also liked Atlanta as a city: there's quality health care and the people are friendly—with many looking just like me.

At the end of each year, I look at if we could live there. Each year the financials show that staying in Marriott makes more sense, so we kept looking for other places to live. We were at it again as we headed to Loreto, Mexico. A very good friend of ours, Kim, had lived there since she retired in June. She referred to it as the Land of Misfit Toys.

Many expats had made Loreto their home, and Kim says we'll either love it or hate the city. It's located on the east coast of the Baja Peninsula, so the best way to get there from Atlanta was to go to LA first and then connect via an Alaska Airlines flight that arrives several times a week. That was a negative, but we kept an open mind. We hadn't made a list of things required for us to settle in one place. We would probably ease into it over the next few years. Maybe we would spend a month here and a month there, with an occasional visit to our motorhome. The list of places we want to visit is getting shorter and shorter.

I hope I have not set my hopes too high for Loreto. One person's cup of tea is another person's gallon of Flint water. Kim made it sound wonderful, and I knew that I'd get to do something I had always wanted to do: deep-sea fishing. Catching some fish and having someone clean and cook it for me is on my life list.

We were off to stop number 360 in 1360 days, still on the pace of moving on every 3.77 days. With the airfare being our largest expense, if we slow down the change of location, then maybe we can keep at this longer.

My mother traveled a lot after she retired until age eighty. She would visit her three kids for a few months at a time. She also had relatives in Florida and North Carolina who she would visit, so you could say travel is in my blood. My dad traveled way into his '90s but not at the same pace as my mom. Being a retired airline pilot makes travel more of a way of life for me.

The flight from Los Angeles to Loreto was easy enough. The pool at Kim's apartment complex came in handy for Catherine's Ironman training, and there was a mile-and-a-half stretch along the beach which was perfect for running, so we got some great workouts in while there. Since Catherine is much faster than me, I had her run to the end of the walkway along the beach while I walked/ran. She then turned around at the end of the pavement and met up with me. I would then turn around and let her take a walk break before she ran to the other end. On a couple of days, I had her do some open-water swims while I timed her.

I wondered what Loreto would look like during the high season. The prices for everything were so cheap while we were there, but expect they would be higher then. Many expats leave during the summer months, so I was sure it would be much nicer when it cooled down in the fall and winter. Overall, we had a great time, and I looked forward to our return. Catherine agreed that Loreto made it to the "We Can Live Here" list right next to St. Kitts and Amsterdam.

Something unexpected happened when we joined up with our running cruise cohorts for the Hawaiian Cruise: one or more of the Islands might have made it onto the "We Can Live Here" list.

Prior to the cruise, we met up with the group for a three-night pre-cruise on the island of Honolulu. We stayed on Waikiki Beach, which is the surfboard mecca, and since a tropical storm paid a visit the day before we arrived, the surf was up. The first day was somewhat of a washout: because of the storm Pearl Harbor was closed, but as I always say, you can't do and see it all. We did get to make the trek up to the top of Diamond Head.

We also did some touring by bus to famous spots like the Hawaii Supreme Court where Hawaii 5-0 was filmed, the Kamehameha Statue, and the Iolani Palace, which is the only royal palace in the US. Of course, we went to a Luau, visited the Aquarium, and went snorkeling. We finished up the precruise with a 5K fun run that included a unique take on the guided tour. About every mile, there was someone to go over the highlights of the area. We finished up with shave ice in the park. After a quick shower, we were off to the Norwegian Cruise Line's Pride of America, our home for the next seven days.

This was the only ship that did the five-island tour with two overnights one in Maui and the other in Kauai. It was a bit strange (and somewhat refreshing) to be on a cruise ship where everyone was American. There were plenty of familiar faces among the group, and we had plenty of time to catch up.

With the "We Can Live Here" list in mind, I paid close attention to each island during the cruise. Just like in Mexico, my phone worked great and data was included in my rate plan with Verizon, which was a plus. However, unlike Mexico prices were high for just about everything. That wasn't a dealbreaker, but the sheer distance from our kids did make it questionable.

During our day off in Maui, many of us went for a very informative hike in the nearby rainforest where our guide showed us all the things we could eat along the way. We then swam in the chilly water underneath a waterfall. Swimming underneath a waterfall was also on my life list, and it felt like a great deep tissue massage. It was well worth the freezing temperatures.

Our next stop was my least favorite, Hilo. Commonly referred to as the Big Island is the wettest of all the islands and was the site of the traditional Amazing Race. Catherine and I just ran/walked to and from the farmers market for nine miles and had her put in another thirty minutes in the ship's pool. On a free day, she also did eighty minutes on the ship's stationary bike. I thought she was ready for the half Ironman in October.

We had the honor to run a half-marathon on the Iron Man course in Kona. I had Catherine do it by herself since she needed the confidence to be able to do it on her own. She beat me by eighteen minutes in all that heat and humidity. It was a great training race for her.

On the last day of the cruise, we took an island tour of Kauai. It was kind of funny since we simply revisited areas that we had seen before in 2016. This included the Kilauea Point Lighthouse and National Wildlife Refuge Lookout, Hanalei Valley Overlook, Opeaka's Falls, and Wailua River Overlook.

The cruise ended with an awards event where John and Jenny gave out yellow hats and water bottles to the special few they had selected. They call them the Perspiration, Dedication, Celebration, and Inspiration awards. The crowning moment for me was when Jenny called up Catherine for the Inspiration award. Everyone in the room stood and cheered Catherine for her inspiration to others as she struggles and at the same time embraces the hand she was dealt with by early-onset Alzheimer's.

We then went out to the deck as we cruised along the dramatic coastline of Kauai's Napali Coast. The night ended after dinner with long goodbyes at the back-deck bar. We all had our own fond memories of the trip, and we added the islands of Kona and Maui made it onto the "We Can Live Here" list.

While we were in this part of the world, we asked ourselves if we could live in LA. The answer was a resounding NO. It's too expensive but a nice place to visit and a nice jumping-off spot for visiting the West Coast, Hawaii, or Mexico. I couldn't imagine being there for more than three days max.

We did find some nice places to consider on this twenty-three-day trip, but now it was back to Atlanta for three days then off to Portland Maine to run another half-marathon. This would be the fiftieth state where Catherine had run at least a half-marathon, but that wasn't good enough for her.

She had done a marathon in forty-five states plus DC and a marathon in all fifty was her original goal. I thought I had her convinced that the last five could be half-marathons since I really don't like to do full marathons anymore. Now she had decided to finish up the last five as full marathons.

I worked on the schedule for next year for her to get them done. I tried to find races that do two loops so I could do the half while she does the second loop herself.

After we finished our latest twenty-three-day trip, I made a comment to my son, Aaron about slowing down and he laughed and said, "You have been on the road as long as I have known you." He had a good point. Even though I was a pilot, I worked mostly in the office but every weekend we were off to some soccer field, basketball court, or concert hall, across the country to watch one of my kids, compete at the highest level possible.

You often hear of people dropping dead after they retire. That would probably be me if I ever stayed put. My plans for 2019 included a big trip to South Africa, with races in Cape Town and Patagonia.

Meanwhile, Catherine had been training for the half Ironman as we ran all over the world the last three months. As her coach, it has been very interesting since, during that time, we have been to Amsterdam, Athens Greece; cruised the Greek Isles; visited Crete, Copenhagen; cruised Norway, Scotland; visited Edinburgh, Loreto, LA, Honolulu; and cruised the Hawaiian Islands. This does not include numerous states along the way. Some might say, including Catherine, that this has been a truly international training plan.

I felt she was ready, so all she had to do now was stay healthy and do it. Better her than me. I would be a nervous wreck, but it would be well worth it. I've learned over the last eighteen years of long-distance racing, that no matter how prepared you are, the important thing is how you handle the unexpected.

# CHAPTER
## 37

# Sometimes It's a Little Better to Travel than to Arrive

Travel.
As much as you can
As far as you can
As long as you can.
Life's not meant
to be lived in one place.

—Anonymous

Catherine and I had been having more discussions about settling down but not for the reason you might think. Sometimes I just got tired of dealing with bad customer service. We were always buying a service from someone, whether it was a hotel, a rental car, a flight, or a meal at a restaurant.

In general, I had become pretty nonchalant when it came to customer service. I used to write a number of reviews on Trip Advisor. I thought I should make others aware of the situation so that they didn't make the same mistake, but that only made me think about the experience longer, which ate away at me. Now I just made a note to myself not to give my money to a given establishment again—most times, we would never be back there anyway.

I never asked for the manager; I just sucked it up and moved on. I did have a pretty bad experience at a restaurant in Seattle the other night. The waiter knew we weren't enjoying the situation. He tried his best to make it up to us by giving us dessert, soup, and beer on the house. We took the dessert back to the hotel, and I mused that it was the best $100 carrot cake I had ever had.

We were now settled in at the Town Place Suites, New Orleans Metairie, only eighteen miles from the site of the Half Ironman. Catherine and I finished up a day of working on transitions and got in some biking and running in the nearby parking lot, so all that was left now was for her to do it in four days.

We had tried to do this event back in 2011, and they had had to cancel the swim due to the weather. They had to cancel the entire event last year and moved it from April to October this year.

During the practice swim the day before the race, I was upset that they didn't have any crafts in the water. They did keep track of athletes as they went in and out of the water, but if someone had a problem during the practice swim, they had no way to rescue them. I had witnessed a person drown during the Ironman that we finished back in 2011, even with crafts nearby.

It has been my experience that to successfully complete long-distance races, you have to expect the unexpected and adjust on the fly. I tried my best to anticipate as much as I could, but unfortunately, due to the high winds on the race day, they had to cut the swim portion short. The swim also ran over thirty minutes late so they could get all the rescue crafts in place, and it took Catherine thirty minutes to start the swim.

During the bike, she had to climb a bridge four times, complete a five-mile climb in twenty-mile winds twice, navigate a highway overpass twice and make it up a steep ramp to the transition area. The run was a bit easier since she only had to climb the bridge twice. By then, it had warmed up and with the sun high overhead, there was no shade along the route.

We usually did this type of event together, but unfortunately, I was unable to compete at that level and wouldn't have made the cutoff. Ironman competitions don't allow outside help from friends, coaches, and family during the event, so that was something I needed to work around. I chose to ask for forgiveness rather than permission. Most of the course was closed to traffic, but I was able to track Catherine using the Find My Phone function on our phones.

A couple of times I did catch up with her during transitions and on the course to fill her hydration pack, which was also not allowed by their rules. One lady actually complained to me about offering outside help to Catherine. Because of the closed course, there was no fan support, and I had to park over a mile away. I ended up clocking ten miles myself that day.

Catherine managed to complete the race within the eight-hour time limit. I was very proud of Catherine and amazed that she had the guts to start and the sheer determination to finish. I was also inspired by watching the other athletes. I observed a seventy-seven-year-old man finish, and at sixty-three I felt like such a wimp. I don't like riding my bike long distances, but I figured I could handle twenty-eight miles. With some training, I was sure I could do the one-mile swim and finish up with five or more miles running.

The last time I did a triathlon was more than seven years before. I often joked that I used to do them when I was Catherine's age. She promised me that this was her last Half Ironman, but we were considering a small Olympic-distance race like the one she did in Pine Mountain, Georgia, a few months ago.

We were disappointed that they ran out of medals by the time Catherine crossed the finish, but I was so overjoyed by her accomplishment that I didn't think twice about it. Another lady was giving them hell as we verified that they had Catherine's information so they could mail it to her.

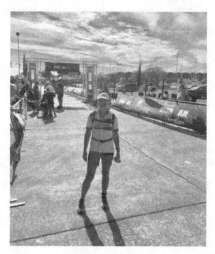

*So proud of her*

The next day we enjoyed a relaxing day walking around the French Quarter, then we were off to Ocean Beach, Alabama, tomorrow for a few days in the Gulf Shores area. I was somewhat disappointed that they don't have a boardwalk along the beach, but we did find a great trail near the huge Gulf State Park, which made its way over the nearby marshes and past a gorgeous campground.

After a brief overnight stop in Montgomery, we were off to Athens, Georgia, to take part in their annual Halloween Parade with my daughter Mariah. I had never done one of those before and highly recommend it if you ever get a chance. I donned a cape and hood to dress up as a sorcerer, and Catherine was a cat, complete with ears and a tail. ("Cat" is also my pet name for her.)

It was a bit chilly, but with layers and thousands of participants and spectators, it was well worth it. As we wound our way through downtown Athens, there were adults, students, and kids of all ages. They had bands that lined the streets as we made our way to the courthouse where the party was just getting started. I had never seen anything like it and enjoyed trying to figure out who each person was dressed up as.

Back to the title of this chapter, which is a quote from Robert Pirsig. It was a good reminder to keep things in perspective. We were presently en route to Seoul, South Korea. The destination was important, but it was really the experience of travel that I truly loved. We had to be somewhere, so on our way to Bagan, Myanmar (Burma) to run a half-marathon there, Seoul sounded like a great place to stop and experience.

I was sure there would be some missteps, but that gave me more opportunities to learn and keep the old gray matter in tiptop shape. People often say "use it or lose it" when it comes to exercise, but it's also true for the brain, the most important muscle we have.

I loved trying to figure out the best places to stay, the best way to get there, and the best places to eat when we got there. I don't like playing board or card games, but figuring out the travel puzzle really intrigues me.

We were on the move every three to four days on average. That was a lot of puzzle pieces to put in the proper place, but that was the best part. Sometimes I hit a home run and other times there were foul balls. There was always another day to plan right around the corner, and I'm a glass-half-full type of guy, so I just learn from my mistakes and moved on.

There were three hours left on our twelve-hour flight from Seattle to Seoul. We went to Seattle first for several reasons. First, I needed my six-month check on my gut aneurysm repair. Everything looked good, so I wouldn't need to go back for another year. Second, it was actually cheaper to go from Atlanta to Seattle to Seoul than directly from Atlanta to Seoul. Third, the last time we were in Seattle, Catherine got her hair done at a shop across the street from our hotel. With the Marriott Courtyard only being a block from the Sky Line station, I saved about ninety bucks in transportation costs from and to the airport.

We learned a number of things during our three-day stay in Seoul. One was that black taxis cost twice as much, but no one tells you this before you arrive. We hopped into one and the meter was racking up KRW (South Korean Won) as fast as it could. The traffic was horrible, and the driver decided to employ the time-tested trick of going the long way.

I pulled up the transportation page for the Marriott we were staying at, and it said the fare was going to be about $60, so when that equivalent came up on the meter, I put in the location to find out that our driver had passed one of many bridges to cross the river to where we were staying. I pointed it out, and he assured me this was the quickest way, then caught the next bridge over the river. No big deal since we were enjoying the sights.

Eighty-five bucks (and no tip for the driver) later, we were at the Courtyard by Marriott Seoul Namdaemun. They had an executive lounge with all-you-can-drink wine, beer, and spirits; so I forgot quickly about the taxi ride to the hotel. The hotel was centrally located so getting around was a breeze.

Namdaemun area is a very famous part of Seoul that features the South Great Gate, officially known as the Sungnyemunthe, one of the largest underground shopping areas and outdoor street market and YTN Seoul Tower, commonly known as the Namsan Tower.

The DMZ is a must-visit. According to our guide, the North Korean leadership is very determined to take over the South while the South still believes there is a possibility of reunification. I found that doubtful as we toured the DMZ and one of the four tunnels that had been dug from the North to the South.

The history was extensive. On one occasion, troops were sent over the nearby mountainside in an effort to evade the royal palace. There's no telling what the North has up their sleeves for the overthrow in the future. You read about such things in history books, but really getting up close and personal really caused those facts and figures to sink in.

On our second day, our tour took us to see City Hall, Jogyesa (Temple), and the Royal Guard Changing at the Gyeongbokgung Palace, a fifteen-minute ceremony in which a cast of about one hundred replaced guards at the main gate and throughout the Palace. We also saw the Presidential Blue House, Cheongwadae, the official residence of the Republic of Korea's head of state. True to its name, it was a pavilion of blue tiles.

Both days we were picked up and dropped off at our hotel, which was well worth the money. With the N Seoul Tower within walking distance, we had to make the trek up the mountain to see and experience the observation tower.

Overall the stay was worth the stopover, and it helped us to adjust to the fourteen-hour time change prior to meeting up with our tour group in Yangon, Myanmar. Once again, we arrived a day before the rest of our group from Albatros Adventure Marathons to further help with the acclimation. This was when I noticed a distinct difference between those who travel while still working and those who travel in retirement.

People like ourselves can take a winding road to the final destination and still arrive plenty early, whereas those who are just on vacation must get it all done in the time they have off from work. They usually arrive the night before the tour begins, after taking the most direct route. They look like hell. They sometimes arrive without their bags, and they may be a day late.

The Melia hotel that we stayed at for two nights was only an $8 taxi ride away from the Yangon airport and was next door to a mall and across a street from a lake where many people jogged and strolled. They had a great gym and a lovely pool, so getting in some exercise while we were there was a breeze.

Another puzzle piece on this trip was dressing for the weather. It had been in the '50s in Seattle and Seoul, but in the '90s in Myanmar. The smaller planes that we took around Myanmar had a weight restriction, so I left some of the warmer clothes at the Yangon hotel, which I did wish we had when we were out on the lake later on.

A very short history lesson: In 1989, the largest nation of mainland Southeast Asia changed its name from Burma to Myanmar and the name of its capital from Rangoon to Yangon. The name changes were made by an unelected military regime, and many people continue to use the old names. Yangon is the legislative capital, while Nay Pyi Taw is the administrative capital.

Our eight-hour tour began with a city tour of Yangon in an air-conditioned coach. Our first stop was one of the most iconic symbols of Yangon, the Shwedagon Pagoda, which is considered by many to be the "heart of Myanmar." The pagoda is believed to be more than 2,500 years old, and the central stupa is surrounded by dozens of intricately decorated buildings and statues. Next, we paid a visit to the Chauk Htat Gyi Pagoda to see the magnificent reclining Buddha. From there we went to the floating Karaweik Royal Barge and enjoyed the quiet settings around the lake. After lunch, we headed to the airport to catch our flight to Mandalay.

The next day we headed off for more exploration of Mandalay and its surroundings. Starting from the ancient royal capital of Amarapura, we went to the world's longest wooden bridge, the U Bein Bridge, which was built in 1782 and spans 1.2 kilometers.

We also paid a visit to Burma's largest Buddhist monastery, Mahagandayon Monastery, home to more than one thousand monks and monks to be. Our journey continued to the highly revered Mahamuni Pagoda where we saw the work of local wood-carvers and other craftsmen, followed by a visit to what is known as the world's largest "book," the Kuthodaw Pagoda, which houses the entire collection of Buddhist scriptures.

The following day, our group drove to the Ayeyarwady River, where a boat took us on a relaxing eight-hour journey to one of southwest Asia's finest treasures, Bagan. While underway, we witnessed life along the river and cruised past cities, monasteries, and pagodas. We arrived early in the evening, just in time to witness a beautiful sight: the golden rays of light as the sun set over the forty-two-square-meter grassy plains of Bagan and its more than three thousand historic Buddhist temples.

Our exploration started with a visit to Old Bagan, the center of the ancient kingdom. Here we took a closer look at the Bupaya pagoda, which offers great views to the Ayeyarwady River and nearby mountains. We continued to the Shwezigon Pagoda, built in the eleventh century by King Anawratha. Still an active place of worship, it stood as one of the most astonishing and well-kept pagodas in all of Bagan. We finished our sightseeing with a visit to the less-visited pagodas at Tayok Pyi Paya and the village of Minnanthu, both part of the running course.

The next day was race day, and it was like nothing I had ever experienced before. The route took us around and through the numerous temples, pagodas, and other religious structures. We ran alongside goats and ox-drawn carts and gave high fives to many of the village kids. The terrain was relatively flat, but we did experience all sorts of different surfaces including rather deep sand.

The race started with a beautiful sunrise, with hot-air balloons floating by outside the Htilominlo Temple. After the race, we enjoyed some snacks on the steps of the temple.

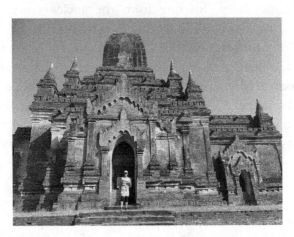

The next day we had a chance to experience a hot-air balloon firsthand. The day began with a predawn ride from our hotel on one of the vintage buses dedicated to the journey; and upon arrival at the location, we found snacks, coffee, and tea waiting for us. As we enjoyed the refreshments, we watched as the balloons were inflated. This was followed by a safety briefing and then, at dawn, it was time for takeoff.

The balloons were piloted at no more than fifteen miles per hour by skilled professionals with years of experience, who also enjoyed narrating the speed/direction strategies of steering the balloon. This experience provided an ever-changing perspective on the archeological sites and beauty of Bagan that you won't be able to seize otherwise. After a graceful landing of the balloons, the staff was waiting for us with fresh pastries, fruits, and a glass or two of sparkling wine to conclude this excursion with a celebration of our flight.

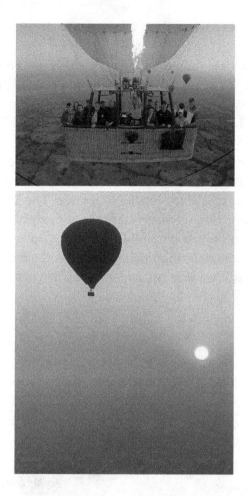

The captain took pictures of the group while in flight that could be downloaded at no cost. I had done balloon rides before but never in a sixteen-passenger basket. The experience was remarkable and well worth the very early wake-up call.

That evening was dedicated to celebrating our achievements of yesterday. The evening began with another sunset boat ride to a secluded island that was transformed just for us for the highly antic-ipated awards celebration. They basically took a deserted island and brought everything for dinner and drinks for a group of several hundred. It must have taken them all day to set it up and all night to break it down.

The next day, the group split up. After we checked out, we flew to Heho. En route to Nyaung Shwe, we visited the Shew Yan Pyae Monastery. Then we strolled through the local morning market before sailing by longboat to Inle to check in to our hotel, Serenity Resort.

Inle Lake is the home of the Inle people, one of several hill tribes living in and around Myanmar's second-largest lake, who are famous for their special leg-rowing technique. The beautiful floating gardens that dot this vast lake made for a meditative landscape to sail around. Onshore, a crumbling dome-shaped monument called stupas at the foot of the mountains enhanced the dreamlike scenery. It was almost as if we were on a different planet.

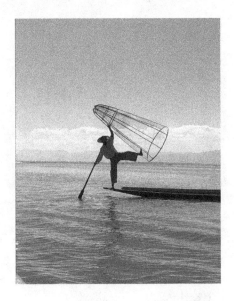

We woke up to these serene surroundings and enjoyed a full-day boat tour on the lake. Its calm waters were dotted with floating vegetation and fishing canoes. We experienced the lake's unique "leg rowers." The Inle fishermen use a special technique, where they row standing up with one leg wrapped around a single oar, leaving their hands free to work their conical fishing net. We stopped at Phaung Daw Oo Pagoda, the holiest religious site in southern Shan State.

We visited a traditional silk-weaving workshop which uses wooden handlooms and a blacksmith's forge. We passed endless floating gardens, where Inle lake dwellers grew fruit and vegetables. We continued by boat to Nga Phe Kyaung Monastery, one of the oldest on the lake, where we saw exquisite Buddha statues which are more than two hundred years old.

The next day we took a long-tailed boat across the lake to Indein, at the western end of Inle, for one of the most scenic trips on the lake. Passing through the busy village of Ywama, the largest on the lake, with many channels and tall teak houses on stilts, we entered a long tree-lined canal on either side of which farmers cultivated their land against the backdrop of the Shan Hills. We disembarked at the jetty and walked for fifteen minutes through Indein village to reach the fourteenth-to-eighteenth-century pagoda ruins of Nyaung Ohak. A covered walkway popular with souvenir stallholders led up to Shwe Inn Thein Paya, a complex of weather-beaten seventeenth-to-eighteenth-century pagodas; some of which were newly reconstructed.

The Serenity resort was nice, but there were two things that I didn't account for. The first was that two bats decided to pay a visit to our bathroom for about an hour. I have always been scared to death of bats, so I was very thankful that they left and didn't return.

The second was that the temperature really dropped overnight, and even though the A/C unit had a heat option, it didn't work. They say that you sleep much better when there's a chill in the room, but it does make it difficult to get out of bed in the morning.

The entire nineteen-day trip was memorable, but after two visits to Asia in a year, I didn't think we would be back for a while. I did learn that taking small bites of the elephant both going and coming proved to be more tolerable for the old body.

Since we really didn't have to be anywhere, I piecemeal the trip home to see how it works out. We finished the tour on Inle Lake with a morning flight back to Yangon then got a day room at the hotel for eight hours to hit the gym and take a nap. Our Korean Air flight back to Seoul left at 11:30 p.m. and arrived at 7:30 a.m.

In a first for us, we stayed at the airport transit hotel for the ten-hour layover. We were able to get a few more hours of sleep and a shower. The terminal is huge, so it was pretty easy to get in our ten thousand steps just getting to the gate.

After a ten-hour flight back to Seattle, and an eighteen-hour layover, our last flight took us back to Atlanta. We had four days before we headed out to Charleston, South Carolina, for a half-marathon on Kiawah Island.

As you can see, we loved to travel, and the destination was just a reason to do so. As our fourth year as nomads came to an end and 2019 approached, it looked like many more destinations and opportunities to travel were just around the corner.

# CHAPTER
# 38

## Old Friends and New Best Friends

Traveling carries with it the curse of being at home
everywhere and yet nowhere, for wherever one is, some
part of oneself remains on another continent.
—Margot Fonteyn

San Juan, Puerto Rico, has a special place in my heart. Over the
years at UPS, flying to and from there was one of my favorite flights.

Our fifth year of running all over the world began in San Juan
on a two-week Windstar Cruises, which was classified as a James
Beard Foundation cruise. The idea was that the cruise line would
offer an elevated culinary experience.

On this cruise, they brought onboard Chef Jose Mendin, who
had restaurants in both San Juan and Miami, who held a cooking
demonstration during our sea day. Windstar also brought on board a
mixologist and freelance bartender, Tiffanie, who referred to herself
as the Drinking Coach. She held three tastings during the cruise: a
late-morning rum tasting and afternoon wine and beer tastings. All
the wines from the tastings were available at no cost during dinner.

When we landed in Grenada, I decided to find the beach there,
so instead of turning left off the boat as we usually did when we're
there, we turned right. As we were walking along, a car pulled up
with its horn blowing, but I didn't recognize the woman on the passenger side and didn't notice the driver.

As we kept walking, the driver turned around, and I noticed that I knew him. Frank was a retired UPS pilot and someone I used to work with at Wheeler Airlines, a commuter airline we both worked at back in the '70s and the '80s.

It turned out that Frank and his wife grew up in Grenada and came back every year. It was great seeing him and brought back memories of our time working together.

I'll take this opportunity to tell you a bit about where I started my flight career. Warren Wheeler, along with his father and my grandfather, started one of the first Black-owned banks, Mechanics and Farmers Bank, which is still in business in Durham, NC. In 1969, he was a captain at Piedmont when he founded Wheeler Airlines, the first Black-owned airline certificated by the FAA. Wheeler helped integrate the pilots at major US airlines by qualifying many Black pilots who were subsequently hired by the nation's major airlines.

This was where the seeds of me wanting to go everywhere were planted. I have so many fond memories of my eight years at Wheeler Airlines. I started as Copilot of the Beech 99, on to twin-engine night flights carrying canceled checks for the Federal Reserve System. I advanced to Captain on the Beech 99 and then moved into management before I left as vice president, director of operations in 1988 to begin my twenty-seven-year career at UPS.

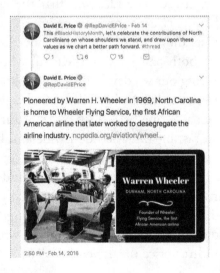

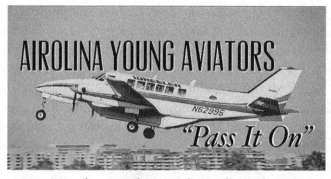

*Many hours on this type of aircraft, Beach 99*

Not many pilots can say they had only had two airline jobs, and even fewer can say they didn't miss many big family events. I always say I'm a blessed man and don't take anything for granted, but plan on trying to go everywhere for as long as I can.

I still remember my leather garment bag that held an extra pilot uniform, a pair of jeans, and sneakers. It had four pockets on the outside for my rolled-up white T-shirt, underwear, socks, and my toiletries kit. That was all I needed for a week out on the road. Now my suitcase had a bit more in it, but the concept was the same.

The first week of the cruise went off without a hitch. After a thirty-six-hour journey back to San Juan, we dropped off most of the people on board, but Catherine and I headed back out for another week of sun and fun. The second week was fabulous. It being Christmas week, there were a number of families on board, which made the group a bit more lively than usual. The ship's staff really outdid themselves this year with all the decorations throughout the ship.

One of my favorite islands is Montserrat, even though half the island was covered in volcanic ash back in 1995. Here two guys came on board and performed local music for the passengers. They had us all up and dancing. Catherine and I also took a hike over a mountain to a secluded beach that was well worth the trek.

The cruise's barbecue was held on the island of Virgin Gorda, which is famous for the area called the Baths. Unlike everyone else, we ran the one mile each way to take a gander. There was a section where you can swim, walk, or wade to get from one point to the other. I would have had to do a lot of bending over, so we bypassed that part, but the views along the path there and back were breathtaking.

When we landed in St. Kitts. It was our four-hundredth destination. We were still averaging packing up every 3.5 days. Back in Miami, we met up with our old running buddies, Kim and Debra. We were soon joined by Mike and Kay. This was the group we called the Band, and we had all met on a running cruise with Marathon Expeditions.

After a seven-day Royal Caribbean cruise out of Miami, we headed to Key West. Two more running cruise buddies, Pam and Tom, met us there, where we all participated in the Key West Half-Marathon. This was a momentous occasion for me since I had been trying to break 2:30 for a half-marathon for more than two years now.

For some reason, I decided I wanted to run a pace I had not run in over five years, and this seemed like the time to do it. It's a very flat course and a front had just gone by, so during most of the race temperatures were in the high sixties. I passed the 2:30 pacer about halfway through the race and was able to come in at 2:28. Needless to say, I was overjoyed. I counted that as a personal record (PR) for myself over sixty.

After Key West, The Band went our separate ways. Catherine and I then headed to St. Kitts, then on another two-week Windstar Cruises of the Caribbean. This would be the fifteenth week so far we had spent cruising with them.

The crew did a great job making the three hundred passengers feel like family. It helped that there were 190 of them. On a sea day when we were cruising on wind power alone, Catherine used some of our shipboard credit to get her nails and hair done—but only after she got her ten thousand steps on the open decks. She needed the training miles since wanted to do her last five states as full marathons. We just finished them up as half-marathons last year. In the first half of the year, we had five half and two full Marathons on the schedule.

I thought we loved Windstar, but we had conversations with a couple who was spending eight straight weeks on board. Gail was seventy-five and Dan had just turned eighty, and they looked like what I aspire to look like at their age. For this cruise, they became our new best friends.

One highlight of our trip was that we got to meet the owner of Windstar and his wife. Actually, they own the parent company Xanterra, which is a conglomeration of travel-related companies with a slant toward the adventurist type. Phil asked me what I was going to do when we couldn't run anymore. I told him that I would have to put Catherine down like they do horses when she can't run anymore, but I would probably just racewalk.

Nancy looked very familiar to me, and it turned out her picture is on board the Star Pride ship, which we had been on several times. She is the godmother of that ship: when a ship is christened, the owner has someone hit the hull with a bottle of champagne. That person, typically a woman, is selected because she usually has some significance to the ship or cruise line, and as Godmother is charged with bringing good luck and protection to the vessel.

Phil and Nancy were a very interesting couple who used to run marathons. They traveled together all the time and mentioned that they were envious of how we approach life. They both worked all the time to manage their many endeavors, but he still found the time to exercise every day, even though his marathon days were behind him. I tried to convince him that his walking pace would bring him in well within the usual time cutoffs for most marathons.

Phil asked me how many times I had been around the earth. I do keep track of all my mileage, and at that point, I had made it once around the earth in the last nineteen years of running, biking, and swimming. It was really cool to meet a couple that in many other circumstances we would have had nothing in common with, but our love of travel and running was our common bond.

# CHAPTER
# 39

## Run Like an Egyptian

At the end of your comfort zone, explore.
—Neale Donald Walsch

After eight days in Hotlanta, which was not very hot, we were off to Cairo, Egypt, to tour and run. I had heard about a cruise line called Uniworld that had cruises and tours of the area, but by the time, I was ready to pull the trigger the ship was sold out. I went to marathonguide.com; and lo and behold, there was a marathon, a half-marathon, and 10K in Cairo on the days I was thinking of visiting there.

On Trip Advisor, I found a seven-day tour that included a cruise of the Nile at a very reasonable price and with great reviews. A few keystrokes later, I had our entire sixteen-day trip organized and booked.

Originally, Gwen and Joan were going to join us, but they ended up getting cold feet after reports of a bombing in the area. At my age and after all I have seen and done, I don't really worry about things like that anymore. I flew planes for many years and have had two major surgeries where I was told that there was a possibility I wouldn't wake up, so now I have a tendency to take life events in stride. I do keep my head on a swivel everywhere we go and realize that in most places I stick out like a sore thumb.

Instead of flying to Cairo in one very long day, I had us over-night in Paris. I was really getting much too old to make those thir-ty-six to forty-eight-hour trips anymore, and they're also very taxing for Catherine. Our Delta flight arrived a few minutes early and we got through customs without any problems. Right after we got to the hotel shuttle area, a Marriott van arrived and tried to depart without us. I actually had to chase it down.

It was a bit cold outside, so the warm van was very inviting. As we drove off, something told me that something was amiss. The van had Marriott on the side along with Charles de Gaul and Poissy, which is the area near the airport, but I remembered the hotel van previously being black.

We had stayed at the Marriott near the airport half a dozen times over the years, so maybe I was just mistaken. The route to the hotel now seemed different, but I didn't remember there being more than one Marriott in the area. As we pulled up, I knew we weren't at the right hotel—but I had a backup plan.

I told the front desk clerk that we were probably at the wrong hotel, but with my elite status, I was pretty sure they would find me a room and then I was going to have them cancel my booking at the other hotel. She looked up my reservation and said that I was in the right place and that they had upgraded us to a suite.

I did some research and found the hotel I thought I had booked. It was merely a Marriott hotel, whereas this one was a Courtyard Marriott. I've been in some cities where there are six different Marriott brands in the same complex. These two hotels are about three miles apart, and I must say I liked the other one better. It had more choices of places to eat, and there was a mall nearby, but no harm, no foul.

Traveling to Europe is always a challenge when it comes to sleep, and this trip was no different. Our flight left Atlanta at 4:00 p.m., and we arrived around 6:00 a.m. local time. Since it was still dark and neither of us got much, if any, sleep on the plane, to bed we went. Surprisingly we both got a good day's sleep, but when to sleep next was going to be an issue.

The overnight news was that several small bombs had gone off at the London airport and train station. In today's world, there's no telling where terror or natural disaster might strike, but I refused to let it stop me from running all over the world—at least for now.

In Cairo, we got to see the Pyramids of Cheops, Chephren, and Mykerinus, as well as the Great Sphinx. We went inside one of the pyramids called Khafre's complex. I'm glad I picked the smaller one since I had to bend way over to make it down and up the ramp to the chamber where the empty crypt was located.

We then flew to Luxor, where we met our guide for a tour of the Luxor Temple at sunset. By now I was starting to get used to the sheer size and scale of the architectural feats involved in building these massive structures and understand that no one really knows how they did it but are able to tell us exactly when. So many facts and figures.

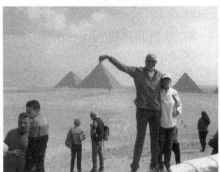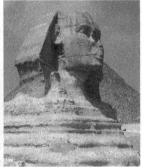

We boarded the ship that would take us down the Nile, MS Miriam, in time for dinner, but unfortunately, they had the AC going full blast in our cabin. By now the outside temperature had dropped to the high fifties and when I asked how to warm up our cabin, I was told to turn off the AC. I hate when that happens, but it's something you have to deal with when you run all over the world.

We spent the night in Luxor so we could visit the Colossi of Memnon, Temple of Queen Hatshepsut, Valley of the Kings, and the Karnak Temple. At the Karnak Temple, we saw two of the three Obelisks. The original three were made in Aswan and transported by boat to this location in just seven months. The third was recently moved to Paris in a process that took them five years. They say the technology to make most of these magnificent structures has been lost forever.

The Nile is the second-longest river in the world at five thousand miles. More than 250 cruise ships travel the Nile each day between Luxor and Aswan. We had originally signed up for a three-day cruise from Aswan to Luxor but, because of our arrival day, they upgraded us to the four-day cruise in the opposite direction for no additional cost.

After the tours were over, we headed for our next stop, Edfu. We enjoyed a beautiful sunset on one side of the ship and the glow of the sunset shining off the Esta mountain range on the other. That was when Catherine joked that she never wants to retire from retirement. In Edfu, we visited the Ptolemaic Temple dedicated to Horus. We got there and back by horse-drawn carriage, which was pretty cool.

After the tour, we then sailed to Kom Ombo to visit the Temple of Sobek, the crocodile god. One of the treasures of the temple was a cylinder that was used back in the day to track the water level of the Nile. The higher the water, the higher the tax that citizens had to pay, since it was figured that everyone would be growing greater crops.

Right next door was the Crocodile Museum, where they had twenty mummified crocodiles on display. Getting to and from some of these sites, we had to go through the gauntlet of sales folks, and here they were the most aggressive, even using kids. Since I don't usually buy anything, Catherine came up with the idea that we pretend we couldn't hear or speak, and we would start using fake sign language as they approached us.

That evening we sailed on to Aswan. It was Egyptian night for dinner, and afterward, many of our fellow passengers partied in the lounge wearing their new Galabias, a loose-fitting hooded gown or robe worn by men in North Africa. With another early start to our tour day in the morning, we took a pass.

While in Aswan we visited the High and Low dams. The Russians helped finance the high dam, and a lovely structure was erected in their honor. From there we moved on to the Philae Temple. This Temple is located on an island, so we had to ride in a motorboat to get there. The temple was recently moved piece by piece since its original site was going to be underwater when they built the High dam.

We also got to see an unfinished Obelisk. The craftsmen had found a huge crack in it, so they left it in the quarry. In the afternoon we visited a Nubian village where we toured a local school and learned how to write our names in Arabic.

Back in Cairo, we dropped off our bags at the Hilton and went to visit the Cairo Museum. They say to see the entire museum could take two weeks, but we did it in a little less than two hours. The place was full of kids, some of whom were sitting on the floor drawing the most famous exhibits, which included the gold mask of Tutankhamun, which is made of eleven kilograms of solid gold. We were also able to sneak a picture of Catherine in front of the statue of Hatshepsut, who was the second historically confirmed female pharaoh.

When we first arrived at the hotel, they said they only had smoking rooms, but when we got back from the museum, they were able to find us a very nice nonsmoking suite.

That afternoon we went on an Islamic and Coptic tour, which included seeing the military facility/mosque knows as the Citadel, as well as a place where Jesus hung out for three months and the adjacent church.

The next day, we toured an open-air museum called Memphis and Saqqara, which is the oldest cemetery in the region. We finished off the morning with a short visit to an Oriental carpet school. Students start there as young as ten. I didn't think they had many child labor laws here.

The evening was a highlight for me, seeing the hour-long sound and light show in the area of the Pyramids. The narration gave us a complete history lesson of that time period. This tour included dinner where we enjoyed the local specialty, a lentil and rice stew called Koshary, and a rice pudding-type dish for dessert.

We had the following morning free, with a plan to run by the expo to pick up our race numbers. The expo was only open in the evening, so instead, we did a few miles on the treadmill and found our way to the start line. It was only 1.5 miles from our new hotel, a

Marriott. The hotel in Cairo was incredible. It was like a city within a city. The executive lounge had full meals for both breakfast and dinner. They even had very nice waiters to fill your glass of wine or beer.

Our final evening of touring Cairo was topped off with another walking tour of an area called Al Orzo street, located within the original walls of medieval Cairo going back 1050 years. This is where the locals come to buy just about anything you can think of. On our way there, we passed numerous streets filled with makeshift carts where vendors were selling their wares.

We got our money's worth on all these tours, and except for a hot-air balloon ride in Luxor and a visit to Alexandria, which was a three-hour car ride each way, we got to experience all that Egypt had to offer.

Our last tour once again finished up with dinner, this time at a local chain called Gad, where we watched the cooks toss the pizzalike dough as they made their famous Egyptian pancakes. After dinner, I had our guide drop us off at the packet pickup location. At the expo, people were jumping around to the very loud music playing. Fortunately, all our information was listed by our phone number, so it didn't take long to get in and out of there. Since the venue was only 1.5 miles away, we elected to walk back to the hotel.

With a day of rest on Thursday, all that was left to do was to run 13.1 miles on Friday. One would think that, with an early morning race start on a Friday, there would be minimal traffic since it is Shabbat in this neck of the woods. The traffic might have been lighter, but it was still an exhilarating experience to run among the vehicles like an Egyptian. These folks didn't joke around when it came to crossing streets. They did it anywhere and everywhere. They were fearless and relentless.

My overall impression of Egypt was very positive. They really like to hustle/hassle you when it comes to selling you something, but they don't actually have beggars. Everyone asking for money is trying to sell you something, the most popular being small packages of Kleenex.

Traffic lines were purely decorative. People usually drove like a snake in and out of traffic, constantly blowing their horns, either to tell someone to move over or to let someone know they are next to them. They also blow their horns at the pedestrians dodging traffic.

Taxis and small private vans used for public transportation also blow their horns to ask if you want a ride. I wouldn't miss the constant sound of those horns. There were few street signs or traffic lights, so they had people at intersections trying their best to control the flow of traffic, which there is a lot of. On some streets, they had a guy with a gun on his belt controlling who came and went down that street. Like Mexico, they also have a multitude of speed bumps to slow traffic down.

The race itself started in a park across from the Opera House, and they only allowed the runners plus one into the park after you went through a metal detector. Speaking of which, there were metal detectors everywhere in Egypt: hotels, malls, and all of our tour sites. On top of metal detectors, at some sites, they registered every vehicle that came in the area, in some cases searching them with bomb-sniffing dogs. There were armed guards everywhere, some behind barricades and some sitting on tanks.

The marathon with 284 participants started at 6:00 a.m. with a fifteen-minute warmup to music in front of the stage. They then announced the pacers, and one by one they filed off to the start line, which was a quarter-mile away. The half was up next with a 6:30 start time. We had the same starting process, and by the time we got to the start line the race had just started, so there was no waiting for the 2,800 of us.

There wasn't much fan support, but the water stations were well-stocked and the dates at each of them were very tasty. I never really noticed how high their curbs were until I had to jump up and down them during the race.

Their solution to runners crossing multiple intersections was something they certainly would not have allowed back in the States. They just threw twenty or so teenagers at each intersection. As you approach, they would yell at approaching cars to slow down, swerve, or sometimes even stop for a hot second. They were also yelling at you to quickly cross the street. It was controlled chaos. At first, it was a bit intimidating, but after a few miles, you got used to it.

The course was flat as a pancake, and I noticed that Catherine was the only female wearing shorts. As a matter of fact, I didn't see another female in shorts the entire time we were there. It was fun to watch all the little kids coming into the finish area as we were leaving.

The weather was perfect, and if running the race itself wasn't enough, between the 1.5 miles to and from the hotel, we put in another seven miles of walking after the race. Since we were in training for a full marathon in May, I thought it would be a good idea to get in as many miles as possible.

After a day of rest, we made it to our 4:30 a.m. flight to Rome and on to Amsterdam. We did have a bit of a snafu on the way to the airport. With only two hundred Egyptian pounds left, I elected to use Uber back to the airport. After requesting a car, I got the usual "meet your driver" message but no car. I replied "I'm here" and got a message back in Arabic. I typed in my name and asked them to answer in English. At that time, a car pulled up. The driver rolled down the window, and I called out my name. He nodded his head yes, and off we went.

I had decided I wasn't going to give this guy five stars since he almost ran someone off the road while on the phone. When we arrived, he started asking me for money. Looking puzzled, he looked down at his phone and started saying what sounded like curse words in Arabic. It turned out that he had picked up the wrong fare and we had gotten into the wrong car.

By then, he started rattling off figures of how much he wanted, and I kept telling him how much I had. His figure was up to about five hundred pounds when I showed him that if I got a ride from the airport to the hotel it was only around 180 pounds. I gave him the two hundred and he went on his way. Lo and behold, Uber charged me a ten-pound (or fifty-seven-cent) cancellation fee, which they refunded when I asked them to. I would be sure to verify the license plate number from now on.

Maybe that was a scam they used in Cairo or just dumb luck on both our parts. I'll be much more careful in the future. Speaking of which, I saw that they were exchanging fire in Jerusalem, where we're this time last year; and someone shot up a mosque in Australia where we also ran a race last year.

A few final thoughts about Cairo: Parts of it were very dirty, with garbage piles everywhere, and in other places, numerous people sweeping the streets by the curb. You can walk down the street and pass a herd of goats or get passed up by a horse- or donkey-drawn cart. There were cars broken down everywhere, and people hailed cabs and vans on the side of the highway.

They call Cairo the City of 1000 Minorities, and it truly is a melting pot. Some men had a dark spot on their foreheads showing that they were Muslims who took praying five times a day very seriously. The more verses they recited, the longer each prayer took, and the more occasions for their forehead to hit the carpet they were kneeling on.

This was our seventy-sixth country to visit and our thirty-second to run a race in, so I had seen just about everything, but Egypt had two things I had never seen before: (1) The sheer number of stray cats and dogs. They both seemed very scared of humans. I'm not going to speculate why. (2) They charged a 12 percent service charge on everything. It did make it easier when eating out, but it was a bit ridiculous when it came to our hotel bill.

I was glad we went to Egypt but seriously doubt I would ever go back. We would be in Amsterdam for three nights to help with the transition back to the States. That flight departure was a bit more reasonable, at 1:00 p.m. After one night in Atlanta, we were headed on to Connecticut for my forty-eighth state where I have run a least a half-marathon. I planned to be finished with all fifty states by the end of April, then we would move on to getting some more of Catherine's marathons done, with Colorado in May and Wyoming in June. Then she would only have three marathons left to do.

# CHAPTER
# 40

## In Pursuit of All Fifty States (Part 2)

Life is not measured by the number of breaths we take,
but by the moments that take our breath away.
—George Carlin

With Catherine's goal of completing marathons in five more states in mind, our plan now was to do Colorado in May and Wyoming in June, followed by three more next year. We would end with Maine because Catherine had very fond memories of camping in Maine with her family when she was a kid.

As for me, I had three more states to conquer, starting with Connecticut. It was going to be a cold one. We had been in the Caribbean just about all winter, so our blood was still pretty thin. Neither of us likes the cold, but the plan was to layer up and suck it up. I was just hoping it didn't rain or snow.

My knees were holding up okay, but I had resigned myself to running with a knee brace on each one. I told myself I didn't need them, but I would hate to have another injury. I knew I looked pretty goofy, but who cared? Over the years, I had seen people on blades since they lost one or both legs and even saw one guy doing a marathon in a hospital wheelchair.

There was no rain or snow, but it was cold and windy. The "feels like" temperature was twenty-four, with a fifteen-mile per hour wind. The packet pick-up and race start and finish were at the Savin conference center, which was only two miles from our Marriott Courtyard Hotel. That was perfect since baby, it was cold outside.

The course started out on a path along the water, which didn't help matters, but after two miles, we started running around the city of West Haven. The rolling hills started around mile 4 and ended at mile 9. They weren't bad, just a nuisance.

They handed out GU energy gel every two miles or so, and I took some at every opportunity since we have three more half-marathons and two full marathons in the next three months. There wasn't much fan support, but I didn't blame them, due to the chill in the air. I usually take walk breaks, but I decided to try to run nonstop for the first six miles. Since we were downhill at that point, I decided to go the extra mile.

This was a bad idea for two reasons. First, my right knee was not very happy, and to compensate my back started to act up around mile 10. Second, I actually had a faster time in the second half. (We call that a negative split, and that was all good.)

At mile 11 we were back to the water and followed the coast back to the finish. We got our medals then headed straight back inside the conference center. In addition to the usual bananas and bagels, you could get your time and place by putting your bib number in a computer, which was a nice touch.

I highly recommend this race if someone needs Connecticut. For both the full and half-marathon there were only five hundred or so, of us. As an added bonus, Gwen and Joan live in Norwalk, Connecticut, a mere thirty miles north, so we were able to enjoy dinner after the race and a home-cooked lunch the following day.

After three days in Atlanta, during which our eighteen-mile training run was canceled by snow, we went to Lancaster, Pennsylvania, for another half-marathon. In addition to our individual goals, we had the team goal of both of us completing a half-marathon in all fifty states. Pennsylvania was going to be state number 20 for us. The other reason we picked Lancaster was that two close friends of ours, Linda and Greg, were going to do that race. Greg had shirts made for us with a Yoda saying, "Do or do not, there is no try," which I could truly relate with. For Linda, this was going to be her first half-marathon. Greg was an Ironman, so it would most likely be a walk in the park for him.

It was great for us too since we still needed to get in eighteen miles from the week before, so after we finished, we went back out and finished the race with Linda to get the extra training miles we needed. Win-win.

After our usual three nights in Atlanta, we were off to Olathe (pronounced, oh-LAY-the), Kansas. We loved it there and had a great race. Since it was so cold for the first four miles, I took my walk breaks every mile instead of my usual quarter- to half-mile. I started to warm up by then, so I transitioned to breaks every half-mile unless I was going uphill or downhill. The lack of big hills and what seemed like a lot of downhill portions helped a great deal.

I was very pleased with myself. As a matter of fact, I cut five minutes off my age group PR—in other words, this was the fastest I had run a half-marathon in the sixty to sixty-four age group. This was also the fastest I had run that distance in eight years.

They had two GU stops, so we both grabbed a handful at each of them. There was a vast variety of food options at the finish and eight different varieties of canned beer. As an added bonus, there was a booth that had CBD oil, lotion, cream, and tincture samples from a store just across the street.

In preparation for the full marathon in two weeks, I was going to let that PR stand and concentrate on my much slower marathon pace. It was going to be a bit tough since Catherine likes to run faster early, and I can't take the bait. This would be our first marathon in three years. I hoped it would be like riding a bike, but I doubted it.

One of the things we liked so much about Olathe was the number of nearby parks, paved sidewalks, and paths everywhere. I'm always noticing where we can run or walk when we drop in on a city, and Olathe does it right. As an added benefit, two of our racing buddies, Louann and Ernst, lived nearby and were able to join us for dinner.

After three uneventful days in Atlanta, we drove down the road to Snellville, Georgia, for our fifth half-marathons in six weeks. My daughter Mariah, came over to run the 5K. The very nice lady who puts on these races limits the field to about forty or fifty. This particular race, Run into Spring, was held in Lenora Park, where sixteen of us showed up for the half-marathon and another 19 for the 10 and 5Ks. Even before the race started, I knew I was going to win my age group since everyone else was younger than fifty.

The park was gorgeous, but I thought I was going to get bored since we had to do five laps around it for the half-marathon. Mariah hung with us for the first three miles, then ran ahead to get a shot of Catherine and me finishing the first lap. Surprisingly enough, the different sites around each turn kept my interest for the entire race.

The next weekend we were off to Wilmington, Delaware, for my fiftieth state where I had run at least a half-marathon. The weekend after that would our first marathon in three years, in Colorado.

I was using the same training program I had used for Mariah's first marathon when she was seventeen. I couldn't get her to do a training run longer than nine miles, but we did plenty of half-marathons. Something about the competition helped her push past the aches and pains of youth. Catherine and I did training runs of fourteen, sixteen, and eighteen miles, but mostly as add-ons before or after a half-marathon. I figured that, no matter what, every mile after thirteen was going to suck. Since I was only trying to finish before they rolled up the mats, I would struggle through.

I remember Mariah telling me at mile 18 that she had given up. While I was looking for transportation to the finish, a little old man shuffled past us. She looked at me and said, "Hell no, give me a minute."

We caught the man around mile 24 and I told him as we went by that he was the inspiration my daughter needed to finish the race. I think I made his day. I thought I was going to have one of those father-daughter moments of us crossing the finish line hand in hand, but that vision was shattered when Mariah turned the corner and saw the finish line and a lady who had passed us earlier in the race.

All I heard was, "See ya!" and she sprinted off to the finish. My fast-twitch muscles refused to cooperate to keep up, but it was great to have her achieve her goal. She won her age group in her first, which I guess was her motivation to run her second marathon a month later when she once again left me in the dust at the finish. She thought about being certified as a maniac by running three marathons in ninety days but thought better of it after completing her second one.

We arrived in Delaware on Friday for the Sunday race. The weather was frightful, with heavy downpours every thirty minutes. Our flight was an hour late due to storms in the area, but that was much better than what happened to a friend of ours, David, whose flight was canceled for no apparent reason—but he was still able to make it to the race.

I have mentioned before how we take planned walk breaks, in most cases every quarter-mile for about thirty seconds. David took it to the extreme and did a twenty-second walk break every twenty seconds. I thought it would drive me crazy, but I considered it—just not during our upcoming marathon.

The weather at the start was a perfect 52 and cloudy, but I was still worried about a possible downpour during the race. We started and finished in the historic Tubman-Garrett Park in downtown Wilmington, which was a ten-minute car ride from our hotel in Dover.

The race itself had some hills, but I really didn't notice them until I was cruising down them on the way back to the finish. The donut hole stop at mile 7.5 was a treat. I think all races should have downhill finishes. A goal of mine was to finish the half before the first marathoner, and I achieved that goal. I also achieved my goal of completing at least a half-marathon in all fifty states.

This experience had taught me how to be flexible with my goals. I always see the positive aspects to changing them as time goes on. My first running goal was to finish one marathon upright and with my dignity intact, and I have built from there. At one time, I had visions of completing a marathon in all fifty states, but after my sixty-fourth marathon, I decided that thirty-eight states plus DC as full Marathons and the rest as halves was good enough for me.

It was especially satisfying to finish up the fifty states here since this area brought back so many fond memories. I attended the University of Pennsylvania in West Philly and used to be responsible for flight operations there during my last three years at UPS. Back in my early flying days, I flew a route from Raleigh to Richmond to Wilmington, Delaware, mainly to bring up DuPont executives. Back then, in the early eighties, the plane was a fifteen-passenger, turbo-prop Beach 99. I'm sure now it's all corporate jets.

Catherine's nephew Stephen works for DuPont and lives in the area, so we were able to meet up with him and his fiancée, Lauren, for dinner after the race. It was great catching up for the first time in many years.

Now it was time to focus on my next goal: finishing sixty-five marathons by age sixty-five, in Fort Collins, Colorado. When we had done the half-marathon there two years ago, it had been snowing and in the twenties on race day. I was literally picking up clothes that others had discarded on the side of the road in order to keep warm.

The Fort Collins marathon started at the top of a mountain, eight thousand feet above sea level, so we would pretty much run downhill three thousand feet to the finish. When we did the Top of Utah in Logan, the race was downhill for the first eighteen miles, and I pulled a calf muscle and had to limp in the last eight miles. That downhill was steep, and I flew down it like a madman. It was diabolical how my mind would enjoy the downhill ride when my muscles were screaming for much-needed oxygen. I hoped that I had learned something from that experience. I thought I might have to try David's 20/20 walk breaks to keep things in check.

We usually arrived in a new place two days before the race, but in this case, we got there three days before the race to acclimate to the altitude. Running six half-marathons in seven weeks had taken its toll, especially on my right knee, so rest, hydration, and rehab were on the agenda. Leading up to this race. I didn't do the typical sixteen-week marathon training program where you do multiple long-distance training runs of sixteen miles or more. I had done sixty-four marathons already, so I knew that everything after mile 19 or 20 was going to suck, so why practice sticking a knife in my eye?

Instead, I used a foam roller three times a day with some CBD oil on the tender spots and took some supplements called Clear Lungs to help out. On race day, as it often does, my mind told me that four hours of sleep was plenty, so I was awake three hours before my alarm went off. All those years of flying planes at odd hours and getting phone calls in the middle of the night were to blame. I can usually function very well on four hours of sleep, but I knew I would wish I had more sometime during the marathon today.

To this day, I still ask myself why I run marathons, and I keep coming up with the same answer: Because I can. That sounds simple enough, but in reality, it was part of my DNA. Not the part about being a long-distance runner, but more the fact that I like to do things differently than anyone else. As I have mentioned elsewhere, less than 1 percent of the population has run a marathon, and fewer than 1 percent of commercial pilots are Black. Since I am both, that makes me an extremely rare breed.

It turned out that running a marathon was like riding a bike. I had been worried about how my body was going to react to our busy race schedule and the altitude; but all the hydration, GU, and supplements got me through. No major body part had any concerns over the 26.2 miles and my lungs were in their happy place the entire race.

The weather gods cooperated too even though it was a bit chilly at the start. The first thirteen miles were basically downhill with a few rolling hills to keep it interesting, but for me, it seemed like we were on a slight uphill for the next seven miles, even though the map didn't agree. We worked our way back to town mostly on a very nice paved trail.

I usually listen to music during races, but the sound of the nearby stream was ten times better than any song on my playlist. That lasted for about fifteen miles. I switched to music from then until mile 25, when I switched to a meditation session on gratitude. I incorporated the lessons of the meditation into what I was doing and thinking at the time.

I thought "I'm very grateful to be able to do this race and, especially, grateful to be able to do it with Catherine." Because of her Alzheimer's, there are some things she won't remember, but I was sure this race would not be one of them. This was her forty-sixth state and marathon number 79. It was my sixty-fifth marathon, a year and two months ahead of my goal of finishing sixty-five marathons by sixty-five.

Once again, Catherine and I crossed the finish line hand in hand and with huge smiles on our faces. The race announcer mentioned the fact that all couples finishing together must end with a big kiss, and we did not disappoint.

Overall, I was very pleased with our performance in Colorado. Our time was fifteen minutes faster than my previous marathon, three years ago in Prague and only a minute slower than my Boston Marathon time one month prior to Prague. I was actually looking forward to our next marathon and being right there with Catherine when she achieved her goal of finishing a marathon in all fifty states next May in Maine.

While we were in Colorado, we had dinner with a fellow runner, Joanne, who we had met three years before on Easter Island. We met her halfway between Fort Collins and Denver, where she lives, at a restaurant called the Twisted Noodle.

The next evening, we met up with Jacqui, who lived in Boulder and was our all-time favorite tour coordinator with Marathon Tours. She had just flown in from the London Marathon Tours trip two days prior, and it was great seeing her. The last time we had seen her was in Jerusalem, and we would see her again when we went to Patagonia. She was so very special to us—even though she didn't like cruising, she had gone to Antarctica because we were going.

Our next stop was San Diego to see Aaron and Kelsey for a few days and meet up with Ana, another runner who we met in Madagascar during our journeys. One of the things we love about our lifestyle is that we can meet up with friends from around the world in places around the world.

# CHAPTER
# 41

## The Beginning of the End

Live with no excuses, travel with no regrets.
—Oscar Wilde

At the start of our latest twenty-seven-day sojourn around Europe, for the first time in my thirty-seven-year aviation career and more than four years of running all over the world, I opted for a sleeping pill for the eight-hour flight over. My fear had always been that I would take the pill, an emergency would occur, and I would be of no use to help with the evacuation. I had also heard some pretty strange stories over the years about people who had taken pills inflight and then sleepwalking.

It actually worked out pretty well, with Catherine and I getting four hours of deep sleep. The prescribed medication only stays in your system for four hours, so by the time we started our descent into Paris, we were refreshed and ready to go. The next day we were back at the airport for our Air France flight to Rome.

We stayed at the cheapest Marriott I could find since we had already been to Rome several times over the years. It was a nice hotel, and there were many folks, like ourselves, who were going out on a cruise the following day. I counted six ships at the port, with ours being the smallest.

The fifteen-day cruise started out very well, especially since the Windsurf was our favorite ship, and we had met many of the crew before, either in the Caribbean or last year when we did this cruise in the opposite direction, from Lisbon to Rome.

The first seven days took us from Rome to Barcelona with stops in Portoferraio, Portofino, Italy; Monte Carlo, Monaco; and Cannes, Sanary-Sur-Mer, and Port Vendres, France. We usually didn't do excursions but we had some shipboard credit to use, so we did have a great excursion to Eze and Villa Rothschild. We're vista junkies and love visiting gardens around the world, and this tour had both.

This was a designated James Beard Foundation trip so there was a specialty executive chef and beverage expert on board, along with Claire who we had met on another James Beard Foundation trip last December. She coordinated all the activities, which included two fantastic wine tastings and complimentary wine one evening. My favorite was the Chenin Blanc, Alban de St. Pre Vouvray.

We love Barcelona, so even though this was our third trip there, we still had several places we wanted to visit. We set out on foot around 9:30 a.m. "All aboard" was 4:00 p.m., so I figured we had plenty of time to visit Park Guel and Sagrada Familia.

Even though the temperatures were in the nineties, most of the route we took was shaded. We love going to parks wherever we visit, and nature has a positive effect on people with Alzheimer's. Parc Guel is full of tiled animals designed by the famed architect Antonio Gaudi.

Gaudi's masterpiece, the Sagrada Familia cathedral, is simply outrageous. We visit it every time we go to Barcelona. It looks as if the builders over the years didn't really know what they wanted it to end up looking like, so they just kept adding spires and buttresses as they went along.

As we followed our Apple maps route back to the ship, I joked to Catherine about the reports of folks who ended off-roading in Denver while following turn-by-turn directions. We were only about one mile from the ship when it became clear that our route was taking us through a security area for the cargo ships.

We backtracked and noticed a railroad track that ran alongside the route. Looking at it, we decided it wasn't a viable solution. It was now 2:30 p.m., and with only ninety minutes till "all aboard, I was starting to worry about getting back to the ship on time. There was a fort up a huge mountain, though, and I figured if we made it up there, we could catch a cab in plenty of time.

So up we went. Judging by the dead seagulls on the road and others hovering overhead, it became obvious that this road wasn't used very often. I wasn't deterred, but when we got to the top, we quickly realized that this section was closed to the public and completely surrounded by fencing.

With time not on our side, we went back down to the guarded area and tried to explain to a man that we needed to get to our boat through their area. He didn't speak much English but made it very clear that we were not getting there the way Apple maps had routed us.

I remembered there being a bar about a half-mile back down the road, so Catherine and I started jogging back to the bar. I figured for twenty Euro I would easily get someone to drive us the final mile to the port. The reason we hadn't been routed that way was because it was along a very busy highway.

Unfortunately, no one at the bar spoke English and no one was willing to leave their beers to help us out. I kept replaying in my mind the Captain reminding those coming back to the ship for the next eight days not to miss the boat. We were now down to forty-five minutes, and no cabs were willing to come out to this remote area. We saw several people heading to the bus stop for bus number 21, which was scheduled to arrive in five minutes.

After ten minutes, we started trying to hitchhike. Then the bus finally arrived. When we got off the bus we ran to the port, with ten minutes to spare. After it was all over, we had walked seventeen miles nonstop for around six hours. On the cruise, we had done more than ten miles each day, even though we considered that we were taking some time off from a very active spring race season.

Over the next eight days, we made stops in Palma, Cartagena, Almeria, and Malaga, Spain. The highlight for us was the stop at the Rock of Gibraltar. As a matter of fact, this was a major factor in our picking this cruise. We were able to see the Rock off in the distance last year but it had always been on my list of places to visit.

With some more shipboard credit to spend, we went on another excursion while there. The whole history of the Rock was fascinating to me. Only thirty-four thousand people live there while another ten thousand drive over from Spain to work there. It's part of the UK, and its major industry is tourism, with an average of ten thousand people coming to visit most days. On average, they only have five hundred people who are unemployed.

We lucked out by being the only ship that arrived that day, so it was easy to catch the cable car up to the top of the Rock. Online betting is the second-biggest industry in Gibraltar. There are more than one hundred miles of tunnels, many of which you can't get to, but some of which lead to an area where the computers that track the online bets are housed.

The original reason to dig the tunnels was to transport two cannons to the top of the Rock to fend off the Spanish back in 1782. That planned changed when they realized they could make portholes inside the rock looking out and place many cannons along the Rock. They came upon this idea while trying to figure out how to supply air to the areas they were digging and blasting. As the plan progressed, they ended up building several hospitals in the Rock, along with areas to house airplanes and other military equipment.

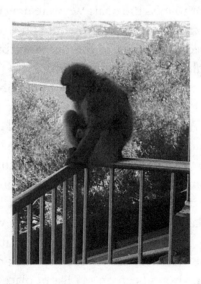

You can't forget the monkeys that also live there. Gibraltar is home to the only wild monkey population in the whole of Europe. Scientists believe that the Barbary macaques, the proper name of the Gibraltar monkeys, were introduced to Gibraltar by the Moors, who kept them as pets when they lived there between 700 and 1492.

The monkeys are well-protected and can come and go everywhere on the island. You have to be very careful, because they'll steal something from you, and then you have to trade that item for food. Despite the thieving monkeys, I was very happy to cross a visit to the Rock of Gibraltar off my life list.

The last day of the cruise was a sea day and was also my birthday. It was my first birthday at sea, which worked out well since I have a tradition of eating lobster on my birthday, and the chef was willing to accommodate. Birthday wishes from many passengers and just about all of the crew made it a very special day.

They kicked us to the curb in Lisbon, Portugal. After another Air Chance flight to Paris, we were waiting for a train to the village of Varennes-Sur-Fouzon when they turned out the entire airport and train station for about thirty minutes to investigate a bag that had been left near the Egyptair check-in counter. The train was on time, but we still had an hour-long cab ride to get to the villa that Gwen and Joan had rented for two weeks.

Sometimes I don't look into all the details of some of these treks Catherine and I go on, but as Oscar Wilde said, I travel with no regrets. When we got to Varennes-Sur-Fouzon, we were able to get in our first run in three weeks, making our way through and around the corn and fields upon fields of sunflowers.

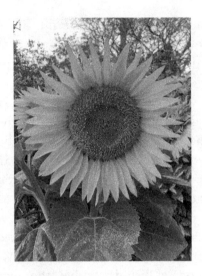

We enjoyed some fabulous food and got to see a magnificent church called Cathedral Sainte-Croix in Orléans, along with one of the largest castles in the world, Chateau de Chambord, clocking in at 450 rooms. The story goes that the design, including an amazing double helix staircase, was inspired by Leonardo da Vinci.

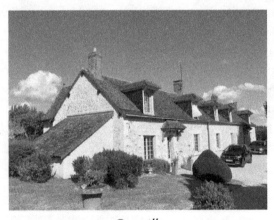

*Our villa*

We spent the last three days of the trip to Amsterdam. It was quite an adjustment to go from three weeks of temperatures in the '90s in France to the '70s in Amsterdam. I asked a long-time resident what was the best time to visit, and she said, "You can never tell since the weather has a mind of its own."

I'll close with the "live with no excuses" part of Oscar Wilde's quote. We chose to run all over the world, but it was time to bring this chapter in our life to a close. Five-and-a-half years of packing up and moving on was long enough. It had been a blast, but all good things must come to an end.

Why the change? It was a combination of factors, the first being that we needed to cut back on the cash burn rate. It had been averaging about $517 per day with a goal of $500 per day so I am satisfied, and we needed to adjust it to a more reasonable $200 a day. Airfare, cruising, and exotic tours had made up the bulk of our expenses, so we were planning to slow down to one Windstar cruise and one tour per year.

We had made 503 stops over 1979 days. We visited more than eighty countries, running a race in thirty-four of them. We averaged around fifteen races of all shapes and sizes a year. We would still be running and traveling the world, but not at the breakneck pace of moving from place to place every 3.93 days. Instead of going somewhere for a few days, we would probably spend more like a few weeks to a month.

Unfortunately, I did miss the birth of Shawn and Cassie's firstborn, Lily Ann, while Catherine and I were on our way to Patagonia, but with today's technology, it almost felt like I was there. I always say you can't do or see it all, but we have done our very best to try. As Catherine said, Lily Ann won't know that we weren't there, but this did bring us to another reason to slow down our pace of travel.

As my grandkids started to arrive and Cat's grands got older, it was time to spend more time with them. My oldest, Aaron, was getting married in February, and I was sure babies were in their future as well. It sounded more practical to come by and stay for extended periods of time.

With Catherine's family in the Louisville area; her daughter and grands in Bloomington; and Shawn, Cassie, and Lily Ann in Cincinnati; it made perfect sense to spend a month in the area. We liked spending time in Mexico, the Caribbean, and Florida during the winter months so it would be pretty easy to slow this pace way down.

Reason number three was that we had just about seen and done it all. I'm not a big fan of going back to the same place year after year, and we had only a few more places left on our life list, like Bali, the Maldives, the Fiji Islands, and India. We would still do our race thing, with Catherine only having three more states to get all fifty done. After that, it would be more of the half-marathon/10K/5K variety.

We had no excuse for this crazy lifestyle, but it was what we needed. My open-heart surgery and Catherine's early-onset Alzheimer's had taught us that life was way the hell too short. Running/walking was our passion, and we would continue to sightsee one step at a time. We looked at this grand adventure as a gift, and we were so blessed to be able to enjoy it in the way we had chosen for ourselves. First, though, we had to take our travel to a few more extremes.

# CHAPTER

# 42

## The Land of Fire and Ice

"Travel makes one modest. You see what a
tiny place you occupy in the world."

—Gustave Flaubert

Iceland is called the Land of Fire and Ice because it's a country of extremes, with glaciers and volcanic springs located next to each other. Located near the Arctic Circle between Greenland and the European mainland, it has several active volcanoes, including Eyjafjallajokull, Reykjanes, and Askja.

Due to its northern location, more land in Iceland is covered by glaciers than in all of Europe. Its capital, Reykjavik, is the world's northernmost capital. The country generally experiences volcanic eruptions twice every decade, which adds more lava to the landscape. Europe's largest waterfall, Gullfoss, is also located in Iceland.

As this phase of our lives of running all over the world neared its end, Catherine and I decided to visit somewhere we had once been before, back in 2013, when we ran a marathon in Reykjavik with Marathon Tours. All the locals from all over Iceland had come out to participate in one of the many races held that day, everything from a marathon down to a 5K and kids' run. Catherine still talks about all the burly guys giving rides on their motorcycles through downtown. It was truly a big deal for this island, and I got to see firsthand how tall Norwegians are. I had never had to look up to so many people in my life—even the women.

Here are some demographic facts about Iceland:

1. Iceland has the highest rate of female employment in the Organization for Economic Co-operation and Development (OECD), with more than 77 percent of women in employment compared to an OECD average of 59.6 percent.
2. The Icelandic fertility rate is also amongst the highest at 2.22 children per woman, well above the OECD average at 1.74 and above the rate that guarantees the replacement of the population.
3. In Iceland, 8.2 percent of children live in poverty, which is well below the OECD average of 12.7 percent.
4. Icelandic households are slightly smaller than the OECD average, with 2.57 persons per household, compared to an OECD average of 2.63.
5. The ethnic composition of Iceland today is 93 percent Icelandic. The largest ethnic minority is Polish, at 3 percent of the population.

Iceland reminded me of Switzerland when it came to the pricing of everything. Our thirty-minute cab ride from the airport was $150, dinner was $100, and the cruise we took around the country had the highest per day cost. I guess it was because everything had to come from somewhere else, and the transportation cost must be very expensive—that included our airfare.

I selected a Hilton hotel close to downtown rather than an off-brand Marriott which was much more expensive. Of course, the rooms weren't ready when we arrived, so instead of sitting around waiting in a very nice lounge area or spending thirty bucks apiece for a buffet breakfast, Catherine and I hit the streets to get our steps in.

In fifty degrees and what seemed like gale-force winds, we made our way downtown to a little coffee shop that was playing Pink Floyd on their very old record player. We were then off to Hallgrimskirkja

Church, which was a magnificent structure both inside and out. You can't miss it, since it towers above all other buildings in the area.

Our seven-night cruise would make five stops on its way completely around Iceland: Vestmannaaeyjar/Heimaey Island, Seydisfjordur, Akureyri, Isafjordur, and Grundarfjordur. We got upgraded to the Sorrento Suite, which included a bottle of Champagne and endless fruit.

During the "welcome back" reception, we won a bottle of Champagne for having the most cruises with Windstar. This was our twenty-second week cruising with them over the last five years. We certainly noticed a few crew members from before, including our cabin attendant, ship's doctor, and even the Captain. This ship, Star Breeze, was going into an $85-million per ship expansion project in October. This one plus two other power ships would be cut in half and a section would be added to expand its capacity from two hundred to three hundred passengers.

We had to back into the small port in Vestmannaeyjar. That was a first for me, and I was glad we were able to make it in there, especially since they had to bypass this port last time due to high winds. This place came to international attention in 1973 with the eruption of Eldfell volcano, when one-fifth of the town was destroyed during a six-month lava flow.

We were able to climb the seven hundred feet to the top of Eldfell, where we could get a great view of its five-thousand-year older brother, Helgafell, next door. The Eldheimar Museum was built around one of the mostly destroyed dwellings and gave a great history lesson about Eldfell and the eruption that created Surtsey Island back in 1963.

On our way back to the ship, we stopped by the Aquarium where we could get up close and personal with puffins wobbling and swimming around. They also had a video presentation on the relocation of two beluga whales from China to Iceland.

We had a partial sea day for our afternoon arrival at Seydisfjordur. The seas were a bit rough so we stayed in our suite almost the whole time at sea. We were able to get out and taste their local beer, El Grillo, when we arrived. That evening we enjoyed the local singers who came on board and gave us a very entertaining history lesson about the region. The next day we got in a nice, chilly, five-mile run plus a hike to a nearby waterfall.

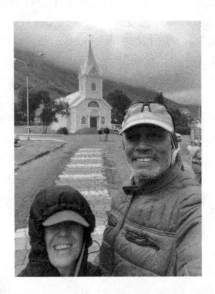

The two-mile cruise in and out of Seydisfjordur Fjord was magnificent and we enjoyed the way out in the whirlpool on the bow of the ship. Unfortunately it did get a bit rough on our way to Akureyri. Overnight we transversed the Arctic Circle and now have certificates to prove it. I actually didn't know it was a thing to do. I was still awake during that portion of the cruise and it was a "hold on" type of ride. Catherine, on the other hand, slept like a baby.

Akureyri was located in northern Iceland, only 60K from the Arctic Circle and within one of the deepest fjords in Iceland. While others went rafting or whale-watching, we were off to the botanical gardens to get our nature fix. Along the way, we stopped by Akureyrarkirkja, the church of Akureyri. Built in 1940, it's the symbol of the city and houses a 3,200-pipe organ.

We also visited the very avant-garde Museum and the more traditional Folk Museum. Along the way, we stopped to watch a young adult training session at an outdoor pool facility. I was impressed that they were swimming outdoors while we were all bundled up.

Isafjordur was our next-to-last stop, and it was time for us to go for another run. We had a half-marathon in Patagonia coming up in a month, so since it was chilly in Iceland, we got to try out what we probably would be running in Patagonia. We got all bundled up and put in a slow, solid six-mile run along the harbor and around the city.

My right knee was once again giving me problems, so ice twice a day was now the standard. It was kind of funny, since it started out hurting but got better as the miles went by—at least for a while. As the miles pass 10 or more, the knee started complaining. I refused to be one of those folks, who say to me that they used to run but had to give it up because of their knees.

We weren't sure what we were going to do in Grundarfjorour, a tiny port situated between a mountain range and the sea. The nearby mountain, Kirkjufell, forms a small peninsula. There was a national forest, but it was thirty-five miles away. There was also a lava field called Berserkjaheaun, but that was twenty-five miles down the road toward Stykkishólmur. Many passengers went for an Icelandic, sushi tour but that sounded a bit risky to me.

The ship had a town map that showed a gravel walking path that paralleled the mountain range. It was just what we needed to help digest breakfast and get us ready for lunch. As you entered the town from either end, there was a detailed aerial map of the town. We had a fun, leisurely walk, and even went off-roading to get a striking picture of the nearby waterfall.

The ship had a "future cruise coordinator" on board and I had my eye on a fifteen-night cruise that goes around New Zealand. It wasn't scheduled until January 2021, but I couldn't help myself. I put down $200 deposits for each of us. Maybe we could pair this up with a trip to Fiji, which was still on my life list.

Back in Reykjavik, we dropped our bags and went for a walk around the part of town we hadn't visited before. They have biking and walking paths, everywhere so it was really easy to get around the city. This time we found our way to the Perlan Museum, where they had an ice cave, a planetarium, and an outdoor 360-degree viewing area of the surrounding city.

Instead of going straight back to the hotel, as I often did, I got us some extra miles of walking by using my phone to find interesting, out-of-the-way spots to stop and see. This time it was the Hateigskirkja Church and Fjoltaekniskoli University.

Overall, we really enjoyed our ten-day trip. The quick cruise turned out better than I had expected, and it was nice to trade the oppressive summer heat and humidity of Atlanta for some fresh cool air.

As we left, we found out that Iceland had unveiled a memorial plaque to its Okjokull ice sheet, the first of the country's hundreds of glaciers to melt away due to climate change. Scientists see the shrinking of glaciers as one of many warning signs that the earth's climate is lurching toward dangerous tipping points. According to satellite images from the NASA Earth Observatory, the glacier appeared as a solid-white patch in 1986, but in an image from August 1, 2019, only small dashes of white ice remained.

A ceremony to unveil the memorial plaque was attended by scientists and locals at the glacier in west-central Iceland, which was no longer fulfilled the criteria to be classified as a glacier after melting throughout the twentieth century.

The inscription on the plaque, written by Icelandic author Andri Snaer Magnason, says: "Ok (Okjokull) was the first Icelandic glacier to lose its status as a glacier. In the next two hundred years, all our glaciers are expected to follow the same path." A message to future generations says, "We know what is happening and what needs to be done. Only you will know if we did it."

# CHAPTER

# 43

## This Is It, or Is It?

A mile of road will take you a mile. A mile
of runway will take you anywhere.

—Anonymous Aviator

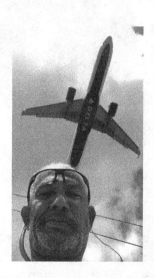

The forty-five-day extravaganza that closed out our five years of running all over the world started in the Delta Concourse F lounge with two friends, Sarah and Elayne. We first met them in Istanbul, and since then had done two other trips with them to Africa and Queenstown. They were on their way to do a marathon in the Medoc region of France, while we were heading to meet up with Marathon Tours in Santiago, Chile.

In Chile, we had a very nice three days in Santiago, including a sunny day touring the nearby mountain, San Cristobal Hill. We went up by cable car and down by funicular. The next day the sun gods did not cooperate as we traveled to Valparaiso for a day tour of the coast and the nearby, quirky town full of wildly colored housed and street art, including a famous mural of Jack Nicholson.

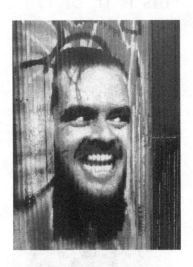

We also visited the tallest building in South America, the Gran Torre. Turns out they did a lousy job of planning, as they could only sell a third of the office space in the building due to lack of parking. On the way to the airport, we traveled under the river in an almost four-mile tunnel. Since they were late to the table adding a subway system, the ones they built are nearly six stories underground so as to not disturb the traffic and buildings above.

Our destination was the Rio Serrano resort in Torres del Paine, Chile. We were there to run the Patagonia half-marathon (named for the region of Chile, not the outdoor clothing brand many of you might know). There was a multitude of available activities including hikes, rock climbing, kayaking, horseback riding, and skiing, but we only did one: the afternoon trip to the west side of the Natural Park where we could see a glacier off in the distance. The views everywhere we turned were spectacular.

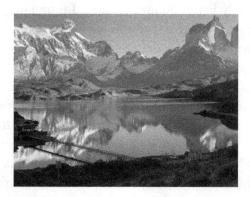

The resort, which used to be a hostel, was over the top. The staff was comparable to the outstanding crews on the Windstar cruise line, and there were food and drinks anytime we wanted it—on top of three-square meals as a group. Watching the chefs cook lamb over an open pit was quite an experience.

The temperatures in the forties during the day and high twenties at night took some adjusting to, partly because our trip was continuing on to Cape Town and the Seychelles Islands, and with fifty-pound bag restrictions, I simply couldn't carry all that was required. No big deal: multiple layers worked pretty well.

The Patagonia half-marathon had an 11:30 a.m. start. All told, there were nearly one hundred of us with Marathon Tours from all over the world. The toughest hills were between our start and the 10K start, but we all had to tackle the 1K mountain near the finish. The good thing was that what goes up must come down, so we all got to enjoy the ride and the scenery as we headed back down the mountain to the finish.

As we jogged around the grassy area just prior to the finish, we had to avoid horse crap and outright holes in the grass. This wasn't what I had expected, but I did manage to stay upright. The finish line was well stocked with lamb, hot dogs, pasta, and very cold beers.

Neither one of us placed in this race, but I did manage to come in fifth in my age group.

I basically walked up the hills and ran down them, and my right knee was not very happy about that idea. I found out, after all these years of running, that Advil works much better than Tylenol after the race, especially since my major complaint is pain from inflammation. I planned to give it a try before a race next time.

If you're a true adventurous type and don't mind being a bit chilled the whole time, then this race is perfect for you. Turning on the shower to heat up the bathroom prior to using it in the morning wasn't my cup of tea, but to each their own. We spent the day after the race enjoying the resort's lovely spa, pool, and massage, and the ride back to the airport was very pleasant. Since it was during the day, we got to see great views of the nearby mountains.

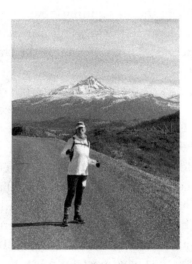

After landing back in Santiago, we went straight to the Holiday Inn near the airport. There was no sense in fighting traffic two more times for a short layover before a very long day ahead including a three-leg trip to Cape Town: the four-hour trip up and across South America to Sao Paulo Brazil, a four-hour layover, another nine-plus to cross the South Atlantic Ocean and Africa to Johannesburg, a ninety-minute layover, and a two-hour flight down to Cape Town.

Booking business class on South African Airways, which gave us the use of the lounges in both Sao Paulo and Johannesburg, made the trip somewhat enjoyable. We also took sleeping pills for the overnight flight, so after dinner and a movie, we both got at least five hours of sleep.

We arrived in the morning and our rooms at the Radisson Blu, our waterfront hotel in Cape Town, weren't ready, so we hit the streets for a refreshing two-hour walk along the waterfront and around the nearby mall.

The next day we met our guide for a day-long tour around Cape Town that included the famous Table Mountain, which had been formed three hundred million years ago. Another first was the 360-degree rotating cable car that we took up and back down. That evening we had a lovely dinner at a fantastic restaurant called Lily's. (I couldn't pass it up since it was the name of my new granddaughter.) Our second full day of touring took us down to the southernmost point of the peninsula, the Cape of Good Hope. We made some stops along the way and hiked along a gorgeous trail to get there. After lunch, we stopped by the sanctuary of African penguins, which I had not known existed.

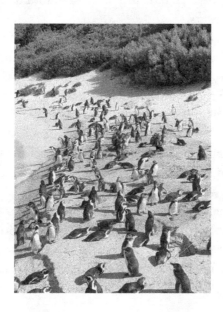

The next day was race day, and it was our first international 10K. I wasn't supposed to start doing that distance until I was seventy, but the only other races here were a trail 22K and the Marathon, so we opted for the 10K since I have a tendency to trip and fall on trail runs.

The course was perfect: we started and finished adjacent to the sports arena and ran along Beach Street right next to the water. At the turnaround point, we came up onto the seawall path, then back onto Beach Street for the finish. We had a bit of a hairy start trying to get around the many walkers who were ahead of our corral, but that just made it more challenging. Instead of taking walk breaks every quarter mile, we ran the entire race. Our time was decent, and my right knee cooperated fully.

For our three-day safari adventure in Port Elizabeth, Catherine and I stayed at Eagles Crag at the Shamwari Private Game Reserve with another couple from our group. I thought I had seen and done just about everything, but this place took the cake—literally. After all our travels, I could confidently say that Eagles Crag served the best carrot cake in the world. After a tour of the grounds, we were shown to our bungalow, which included a fully stocked bar, heated blankets, an outdoor jacuzzi, and both an indoor bathtub and indoor and outdoor showers.

After a quick bite to eat, we met up with head ranger Minolan, who was both very entertaining and extremely informative. There was not a question he couldn't answer, including the names of the elephants, when they were born, and to whom. If he couldn't answer on the spot, he would have the answer on the next game drive. The evening drive ended with our Jeeps being completely surrounded by a group of elephants. They were so close that I could have touched their outreached trunks that were taking a sniff of each of us. I got the feeling they were used to being around humans.

Minolan helped to alleviate my recurring fear of wild animals by telling me that it would be bad for business for a client to be injured and to trust him like I would a pilot. This was very helpful, since just telling myself that wild animals don't eat jeeps was no longer working.

The next morning it was up and out for a 6:00 a.m. game drive, which was chilly and exciting at the same time. The Big Five animals that everyone goes to see in Africa (Cape buffalo, elephant, leopard, lion, and black rhinoceros) were basically everywhere. After breakfast, we were back at it again, with a stop by the Born Free foundation where all sorts of injured animals were kept in their forever homes.

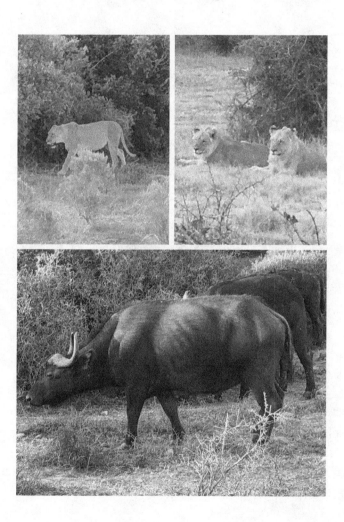

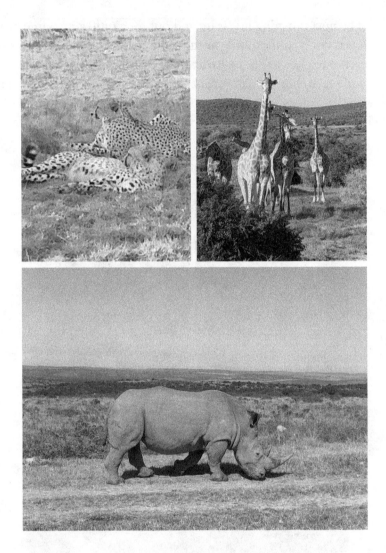

The evening ended with a drink break to end all drink breaks. We made our way to the top of a mountain for an awe-inspiring sunset with an open bar and snacks. Four others from our Marathon Tours group met us there for a toast.

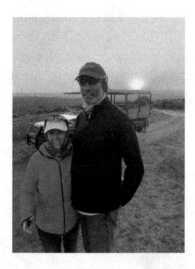

The next day we were still in search of the elusive leopard and a pride of lions, but instead, we met up with a group of elephants at the local watering hole—and that was a sight to behold. We did manage to locate a lion pride on our way to the Wildlife Rehabilitation Center, where they were doing important work in providing a pathway for injured animals back to the wild. They share some hopeful stories, but also sad ones such as the plight of the rhino. There was also a poster showing all the local species that have gone extinct.

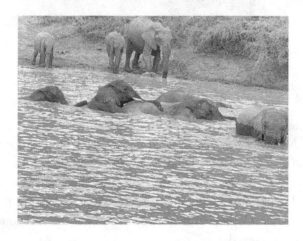

As we left, we passed a full-size mirror representing who is at fault for the loss of all these animals. The young lady who gave us the short tour was very passionate about her job, but it was a rather depressing tour. I walked away with the feeling that we were fighting a losing battle, especially when it comes to the poaching of rhino tusks.

The management at Shamwari, which translates to mean "friend," put the cap on our total wildlife experience with an evening featuring a multitude of starters by the outdoor bar area and at least eight tapas-style main courses around an open fire. It was a fitting way to end this somewhat overwhelming experience.

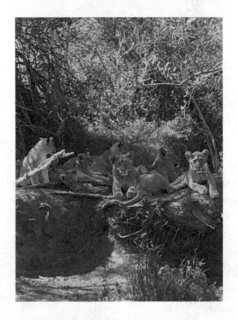

Catherine and I departed the next morning for the Seychelles Island of Mahe. Seychelles is a group of 115 islands located east of Africa and northeast of Madagascar, and 90 percent of the population lives on Mahe. We stayed at a branded Marriott called Le Meridien Fisherman's Cove. We were looking forward to spending a week someplace tropical and not having to get up and tour, catch a flight, or race every day.

Creole was the native language here, and everyone was so very friendly. We took very long walks in the first two days. On the second day, we followed several roads up into the mountains. None of them connected, so we had to come back down the way we went up. We manage to get in a run on the third day, but there were few sidewalks, so we had to do two loops of beach and street to get in four miles. We ended the day sitting beside the pool and taking in some much-needed vitamin D while gazing out into the Indian Ocean surrounded by the towering mountains.

This resort was just what we needed at that time. The impressive staff rotated around from place to place. There was a main dining area for breakfast and dinner, along with a specialty French restaurant for dinner and a bar where we caught the perfect sunsets while sipping a cocktail. They had a wide variety of gins so I tried one called Mom, which was infused with strawberries—one fruit that I couldn't find anywhere else while there.

None of the tourists looked like me or spoke English amongst themselves—although they could all speak English to the staff at the hotel. It turned out that most of them were from France and Germany.

The hotel wasn't very full, and the price was right for our week-long stay. They also tossed in free breakfast every day, a 20 percent discount for dinner, and had upgraded us to their best suite right on the water. The flowers were gorgeous and plentiful, and I understood why, since there was an on-again, off-again drizzle most days we were there.

I did learn the hard way that running on the beach is really bad for my knees and ankles. You see people running on the beach all the time, but the slightly slanted nature of a beach and loose sand underneath my feet wasn't good for my age. I bounced back pretty quickly, though.

After one night on our own back in Cape Town, we switched hotels and met up with our AMA Waterways group at the five-star Cape Grace Hotel for a fifteen-day Wine Enthusiast's tour. The location was right on the very vibrant waterfront. Those of us who had arrived the evening before took a tour of Robben Island, where

Nelson Mandela spent eighteen years in prison. All I can say is that it was a very depressing, but at the same time very informative, experience. I highly recommend it, but be aware that it's a thirty- to forty-five-minute ferry ride each way, and it can be very choppy.

We had an extremely elegant welcome reception that evening, and I could tell right away I was going to like this portion of our last forty-five-day trip. There had been a lot of moving pieces to putting this all together, but thirty days in, everything was going smoothly. The only problem was that we were now entering malaria-afflicted areas, so we had to start taking preventive meds.

The next day it was back down to the Cape of Good Hope to visit the African penguins, but this time an outrageous lunch was included at the Harbor House restaurant. Every now and then the waves crashed up against our huge glass windows while we were eating. After all that wining and dining at lunch, dinner was not necessary.

If that wasn't enough, we made a stop at a fabulous winery called Constantia Glenn, located on the other side of Table Mountain. The views were somewhat better than the wines, but the taste is in the tongue of the beholder. I heard they had a magnificent botanical garden close by, but that was one sight that we could not manage to squeeze in.

The plan for the next day was to meet up early, do the cable car tour of Table Mountain, and then move on to Glenelly Estate Winery in the Idas Valley. With the weather looking windy and rainy, we opted out and slept in. After a nice, long shower and leisurely breakfast, we caught an Uber and met up with the group for an 11:00 a.m. wine tasting. They had one red blend called Lady May that I really enjoyed.

From there we moved on to another over-the-top lunch. At a restaurant/winery called Longridge, they started us off with a welcoming toast of a very nice Rose Brut Champagne. We finished this feast at 3:30, so once again, dinner was not required. It was an hour-long bus ride back to the hotel, and most of us napped along the way.

The next morning, we were up and out at 5:00 a.m. for our flight to Johannesburg and on to Kasane, Botswana, where we had the strangest border crossing I had ever experienced. We all got in Jeeps from the airport. After a ten-minute drive, we pulled into a parking lot for the immigration building alongside the Chobe River, where we then got our passports stamped because we were leaving the country that we just arrived in.

We then got into tender boats and went down the Chobe River to another building to have our passports stamped for arrival into Namibia, which turned out to be our eightieth country visited. Back in the tender boats, we pulled alongside the Zambezi Queen, our home for the next four days.

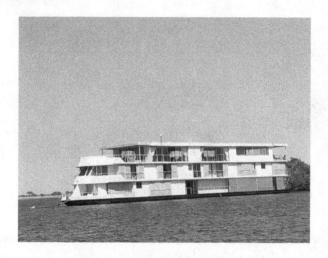

That evening, after we got some information about the ship from Captain John and watched a presentation on the area, dinner included endless local wine, beer, and spirits. Fortunately, we got to sleep in before our 10:00 a.m. safari by tender boat.

This type of safari was new to us. The concept behind it was that all animals have to drink water, so they would come to the river. However, due to high winds, some stayed in the bush so it wouldn't be as easy for predators to locate them.

There were 130,000 elephants located in this area, more than anywhere else in the world. We didn't see many new animals but did identify a wide variety of birds on this trip. There were crocodiles everywhere, and they told us that if we fell in the water, we shouldn't yell but should swim to the closest bank as fast as we could. If you had on a life jacket, the idea was to blow the whistle, since crocodiles hadn't evolved to the point where they understand that was the signal for a person overboard. I give them a few more years to figure that one out.

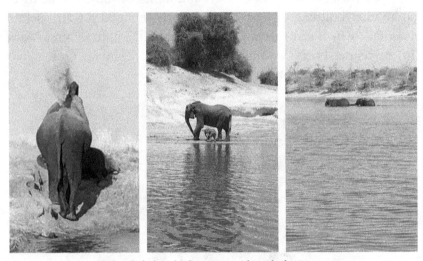

*Why did the elephant cross the Chobe River?*
Because the grass was greener on the other side.

The next day was a more traditional safari by Jeep in the Chobe National Forest, the second-largest national park in Botswana. Here we got up close and personal with both lions and lionesses. One was taking a nibble on a nearby elephant. I was also able to get a few pictures of some native birds. A trick I learned is to take a video then go back and freeze-frame the shot you want with a screenshot. Then you can edit the picture.

There were two unique aspects of this cruise line. First, when the ship was moored, they ran a power line in the water to an offshore generator that provided electricity to the entire ship. Second, most of the crew didn't stay on board at night. They used tender boats to transfer them back and forth to their tented homes nearby. The folks there learned English from a young age in the nearby school and had to go through a six-month training program before they were able to work on the ship. The crew belonged to the Kasenu tribe and worked one week on and one week off. I was glad to hear they didn't have to make the forty-five-minute high-speed tender boat ride each way each night.

The next day we visited the village of Kasenu, where we had the opportunity to donate money or clothes to the locals. I was happy to drop off some race T-shirts I no longer need. In this village, there were three families for a total of ninety people, and Catherine made the most of it by joining them for some traditional tribal dancing.

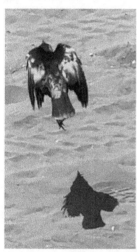 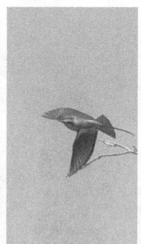 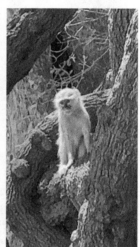

We finished off the evening with a flavorful, traditional African dinner with singing and dancing. They gave us a brief history of their tribe and we all stood while they sang their national anthem. Our resident wine expert, Paul, managed to get them to pull out the good wines. I enjoyed the Pinotage, while Catherine was partial to the Rose Champagne.

We spent the next morning doing the customs four-step: (1) tender boat from the ship to get our passports stamped as we left Namibia; (2) tender boat further down the river to get our passports stamped again entering Botswana; (3) short bus ride to get them stamped as we left Botswana; (4) another short bus ride to enter Zimbabwe. The last leg of the day was an hour-long bus ride to Victoria Falls.

After checking into the very impressive Victoria Falls Hotel, we all met for a steam train ride to the iconic Victoria Falls Bridge for a sunset viewing point of the hotel and the surrounding area. The train was built in 1905 when they hoped to lay a half-mile to a mile of track each day, and its seven-thousand-mile route runs from Cairo to Cape Town. Catherine and I enjoyed the climb in and out of the engine and a toast on the front of the engine. The sunset was somewhat impressive, but the tapas and wine-filled ride from and to the hotel made my day.

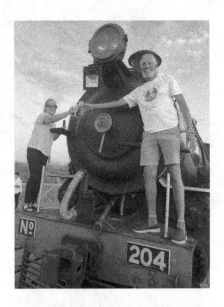

The next day was the real reason we were there: to see the famous Victoria Falls, one of the Seven Natural Wonders of the World. I had two thoughts about the Falls themselves: (1) Would they still be here in twenty years? (2) I'm glad we didn't come during the high season. There are seventeen viewing points but because of the low water due to a drought in the area, only fourteen were actually open.

Even with the water being low, there was a lot of mist in the air. I understood that that mist can be so bad that it can actually be hard to see the falls themselves. It was strange to think about all the money being spent just to see water run over volcanic rock.

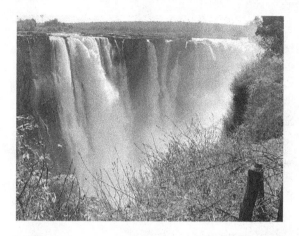

While others in our group were buying trinkets to take back home, we went for an extremely hot run. It was well-needed since it had been over a week since we had run or walked any real distance.

To complete the day, we went on a sunset cruise along the Zambezi River, where a historian gave a thirty-minute talk about the Falls and the man credited with discovering them, David Livingston (as in, "Doctor Livingston, I presume.")

There were two things I didn't like about the Falls area. The first was the fact that all the money that flows into the area from tourists didn't seem to make a dent in the level of poverty of the locals. Their local currency is a worthless bond note which many sell to tourists like they would any other trinket. The second was the continuous sound of helicopters overhead. I felt like I was on the set of MASH. All these helicopters were for folks to see the Falls from above, and the price they were charging was simply outrageous. By contrast, the locals were lined up around the block at the two local gas stations to get their allocation of gas.

This wasn't the longest trip we had taken over the five years of running all over the world, but it was by far the most expensive. It was my intention for this to be the grand finale, so no expense was spared. Over the forty-five days, we took eighteen flight legs plus numerous bus and van rides.

Flights

1. Atlanta–Santiago, Chile
2. Santiago–Patagonia
3. Patagonia–Santiago
4. Santiago–Sau Paulo
5. Sau Paulo–Johannesburg
6. Johannesburg–Cape Town
7. Cape Town–Port Elizabeth
8. Port Elizabeth–Johannesburg
9. Johannesburg–Seychelles
10. Seychelles–Johannesburg
11. Johannesburg–Cape Town
12. Cape Town–Johannesburg
13. Johannesburg–Kasane, Botswana
14. Victoria Falls–Johannesburg
15. Johannesburg–Kruger Natural Park
16. Kruger–Johannesburg
17. Johannesburg–Amsterdam
18. Amsterdam–Atlanta

I often joked that I flew more now as a passenger than I did as a pilot at UPS. I did fly way more in my early commuter days. I still remember sleeping in my uniform or in the airplane at night, waiting four hours for them to process the canceled checks I brought in from cities in the Carolinas.

Our dear friend Kayna once asked me how much time we spend in airports and on airplanes. Doing a rough calculation of an average of five hours of travel time for each of 485 destinations gives you 2,400 hours or 100 days, which was about 5 percent of our total time as nomads.

We mostly flew at least Business Class on this trip, and just about all the hotels were five stars. Some had amenities I had not experienced before—for example, all African toilets have air fresheners. One hotel had an electric blanket that was turned on during their turn-down service.

All in all, our experiences had been luxurious, if not purely over the top. Then came the stark contrast when we landed back in Johannesburg.

We stayed at the Fairlawn Boutique and Spa, which was located in what they referred to as the Beverly Hills section of Johannesburg. It wasn't far from where Nelson Mandela lived later in life, and of course, the group of twenty-five of us was picked up in a very nice bus and greeted with cool towels and mints.

All the homes and businesses had tall fences around them topped with two feet of electrified fencing. That was because somewhere between 30 and 40 percent of the population was unemployed. Along the roads, there were men sitting around hoping for someone to stop and pick them up for day work. It blew my mind to see such inadequacies with all the gold and other precious minerals found here over the years.

From the hotel, we made it to where Nelson Mandela lived most of his life as a free man. We took a short tour and heard a brief history of that home, located in the Soweto section of Johannesburg. It was still mostly segregated. It was hard to believe since apartheid had officially ended more than twenty-five years ago.

We moved on to an area called Kliptown, where we visited their youth program. They said that the level of poverty had shrunk in terms of total people affected over time, but it was still the case that twenty families in the area shared one of the port-a-potties lined up on the street. I rarely used those at race sites, but this was how these folks lived day in and day out. The youth program was a beacon of hope and had a very good success rate, but overall, it was a heartbreaking experience. If that wasn't bad enough, after lunch we made a visit to the Apartheid Museum.

I was flummoxed by all the sounds and sights there. They gave us two hours to go through the entire museum, but I could only handle ninety minutes. I'm unsure of what was the most shocking aspect of apartheid. Was it the fact that it happened in the first place, or the fact that it only ended twenty-five years ago? Visitors aren't allowed to take any pictures there, and I had to wonder why. I guessed there was still some well-deserved shame on their part.

The next day the group flew on to the Hoedspruit airport, which services Kruger National Park. Since most private game reserves are only capable of housing sixty to twenty people at a time, our group of twenty-five went to two different reserves.

We stayed at Makanyi, where the lodge used to be a private residence and had been converted into a public lodge four years before. For everyone else in our group, this was their first time living among wild animals, so of course, it was the best they had experienced. This was somewhere around our eighth such experience, so I'll just say that, even though this place was nice enough, it wasn't our favorite.

For example, while we were out tracking a lioness pride, our trackers went alone on foot without any weapons. Our rangers didn't seem concerned, but as the sun was going down, I thought it was simply crazy. Our rangers in Shamwari had been armed, and I was pretty sure these animals didn't differ much by location.

After three nights at Makanyi, we flew back to Johannesburg. This trip had more moving pieces than any other we had been on, but it went off without a hitch. We didn't even have any complications from the anti-malaria meds, and I only got bitten by a mosquito once—on our last day in Africa. (Most bars that we went to had a wide range of gins because some people don't take the meds and instead just drink a lot of gin for the quinine.) We even managed to get in a few runs, so hopefully, we were ready for a very hilly half-marathon that was our next destination.

Our evening flight was to one of our favorite overseas locations, Amsterdam. We finished up this forty-five-day extravaganza with a three-night stay there. Waiting for us back in Atlanta was my first grandchild, Lily. We flew her, Shawn, and Cassie to Atlanta since we wouldn't be in their area until after Thanksgiving. Mariah drove up from Athens and we had a great visit.

To circle back to the title of this chapter, we had several reasons why we needed to slow down, and some might think that one would be Catherine's battle with early-onset Alzheimer's. Some might think that our lifestyle was contrary to a prudent approach to how best to handle this disease, that those affected should have a routine in their lives. What we had done over the last five years was counterintuitive.

As I have explained many times in the past, these memories of running all over the world went into long-term memory. Right now, that part of her memory wasn't affected, so when she couldn't remember where the bathroom was in the hotel room, instead of getting frustrated, she could relish something exciting she did or saw earlier that day. Because of that, we will probably keep bopping around the world until we simply can't do it anymore.

Another benefit is our level of exercise and sleep. Even though we did bounce around in different time zones, regular exercise helped Catherine (and me) fall asleep, no matter where we were in the world. Being on many tours and interacting with various people as we move about forced us to socialize, which was a very good thing. Sitting around staring at each other isn't good for any relationship, and especially for those with Alzheimer's or their caregivers.

So to answer the question of the title was twofold. We would slow down but would keep going and not establish roots anywhere.

# CHAPTER
# 44

## The Finale—for Now

Every run holds both the promise of enlightenment and the threat
of embarrassment, the capacity to embrace us or punish us. Every
race has the potential to be a celebration or a humiliation.
—John "The Penguin" Bingham

After our last whirlwind trip to South America and South Africa,
we did our usual touch-and-go in Atlanta, then we were off to
Portland, Oregon, to do the Columbia Gorge Half Marathon once
again. It was fun to catch up with Kayna and others who live in the
area. The race went well, and Catherine was ready for her eighty-first
marathon in her forty-eighth state the following weekend.

From Portland, we went on to Seattle for a follow-up exam of
my repaired ileac artery. All looked good, and I would return the
same time next year. I would be on Medicare by then, and I wondered if it would pay for the expensive required testing.

Back through Atlanta we went, this time on to Boston where we
met up with Barb and Teri, Catherine's mom and sister for the drive
to New Hampshire for the marathon. After twenty years of running
as an adult, this would be the first time that I would not run a race
that I had signed up for.

The reason was that the race organizers had a very strict time
cutoff at the midway point of 2:30. I knew that I wasn't going to be
able to accomplish that, so I decided my efforts would be best utilized

if I supported Catherine and Teri. It was great to watch them take on this marathon, especially since it rained, sometimes very hard, with temperatures in the low forties.

There was a three-mile off-road section of the race that they had to run twice. The second time it had flooded out, so they had to endure ankle-deep water. That was just prior to the finish and explained why it took them so long to complete the last three miles.

With that race under her belt and with only two more left, we were off to Loreto, Mexico, for some much-needed rest and relaxation. Of course we ran after a week off.

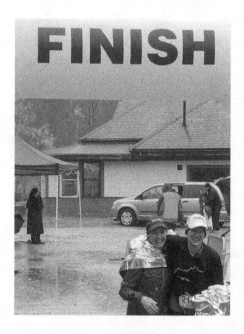

There was a half-marathon and various other races scheduled while we were there, but it rained cats and dogs for two straight days just prior to the race. Since we were in the desert, the streets ended up flooding, so the race was called off. We got a refund and were able to keep the shirts. When the water receded, I charted a 10K course for us to run, and we set out and accomplished our uncertified race.

Unfortunately that was where things started to take a turn for the worse. Catherine started complaining of knee pain. This was a first for her, and I really didn't think much of it. I started using the same method I used whenever my knee starts bothering me: ice it down, then relax and enjoy the Mexican sun.

From there, we were on to Indiana for Thanksgiving with Catherine's family. While we were in the area, we visited with Shawn, Cassie, and Lily Ann in Cincinnati, then headed to Bloomington to visit Christie and family. All during this time, Catherine was complaining more about pain in her knee (and other body parts). Since the temperatures were hovering in the thirties, I once again didn't give it much thought.

I figured it would all get better once we got to St. Kitts for our planned five-week stint there. The weather was perfect, and we both loved the island. At the same time, Catherine was once again experiencing short periods of delusions which she had had over the last year. She was complaining more and more about all-over body pains and was now extremely tired.

I did my research and looked at the possible side effects of her current medications and other supplements that I gave her. During her last Mind Center exam five months ago, they had suggested that I add Namenda, a drug that was similar to Donepezil and was often prescribed for folks who have moved into the moderate range of Alzheimer's.

It had a very strict protocol for dosing: I started out giving her 5 mg in the morning for a week, then 5 mg in the morning and 5 mg in the evening for a week. Then I stepped up to the final dosage of 10 mg in the morning and 10 mg in the evening.

I had tried several times in the past but could only get her to tolerate 10 mg in the morning. After referring to the doctors at the Mind Center, we decided to leave her on that dosage. While we were in Mexico, I had once again increased the evening dosage to 5 mg, and when we got to St. Kitts increased it once again to the recommended dosage of 10 mg in the morning and 10 mg in the evening.

Now that her symptoms were getting worse instead of better, I decided to take her completely off that medication since the common side effects were now aligning up with her complaints, including tiredness, body aches, and joint pain.

After only five days off the Namenda, I could see some improvement, even though she was still complaining of back-of-the-knee pain on both knees. We had been in St. Kitts for two weeks and had been walking more than five miles each day (and some days as much as ten miles) but hadn't run for over a month.

Catherine had also been going to the nearby hotel gym to ride the bike and elliptical trainer and do some swimming at the nearby Marriott Hotel pool. It was really hard to get Catherine to completely rest, especially since there has been so much research showing the advantages of intensive exercise on quality of life for those with Alzheimer's.

After two weeks off Namenda, she was doing somewhat better, but the pain in the back of both knees hadn't gone away. I was just hoping this wasn't the physical problems that arise with Alzheimer's. We got back to Atlanta in three weeks, we could consult with her doctors about Namenda, but in the meantime, I put together a training and travel plan for the next four months and hoped her body would cooperate with that plan.

If not, we would have to go with plan B: relish the success of her completing a marathon in forty-eight states plus DC and counting the other two states as half-marathons which she had completed last year.

We were able to get in two short runs during the final week in St. Kitts, and she seemed to be getting better over time. After we left St. Kitts, it was back to Atlanta for a short stay, then back to the cold northeast to visit both Catherine's and my family. We would start to increase our mileage over time. Over the last three months, we had put in a lot of training miles while at the same time enjoying ourselves with family. Aaron and Kelsey had a beautiful wedding back in Wilmington, North Carolina, where they first met. The weather there was great, so we ran just about every day.

From time to time, I like to do what I call "unscientific studies." One of them had to do with alcohol consumption and joint pain. As we were looking forward to January 2020, I ran across an article about "Dry January" and decided to give it a try.

It wasn't like I abused booze, but since we ate out all the time, I found myself having a beer/wine or two with dinner each night. No big deal, I thought. Being a pilot for all those years and being on call the majority of the time, I didn't drink much, if at all. There was an eight-hour "bottle to throttle" policy, so not knowing when you might have to fly didn't leave much time to partake. Also UPS, like all airlines, had a very strict alcohol- and drug-testing program.

When we first started our vagabond lifestyle, I did drink more than I cared to admit. That didn't last long since I also saw that it had a negative effect on our cash burn rate.

In case you haven't heard of it, the premise of Dry January is that if you can go for a month without alcohol, then you can go for the rest of your life. I wasn't sure if that was going to be my goal, but I was willing to give it a try for a month.

Surprisingly enough, it had very positive effects on my running performance. Not much in terms of speed, but more so with the level of effort I had to exert to maintain the same slow pace we were running. The most amazing finding was that I had far less joint pain than I had ever experienced in my twenty years of running as an adult. I mentioned it to others, some in the medical field, and they all responded that it was quite obvious since alcohol is a contributing factor to inflammation. Just one more thing to consider when it comes to pain management.

Not drinking was the proverbial no-brainer for Catherine. We all know that alcohol kills brain cells, so to keep as many healthy brain cells as possible, she usually had only one glass of Prosecco with dinner each night—any more than that was like someone else having five or more drinks in terms of mental impairment.

Dry January took me back to my flying days. As Catherine's caretaker, I thought it would be wise for me to always have my full mental capacity to better care for her. No one wants a pilot or surgeon who has had a drink or two just before surgery or flight—even if it was just to help them numb their knee pain.

The last hurrah for our vagabond lifestyle was a Windstar Cruises back in the warm Caribbean for fourteen days. Just prior to the start of the cruise, the entire world was turned on its head by the onset of the vicious COVID-19 pandemic. We disembarked in St. Maarten and flew over to St. Kitts for what was supposed to be two weeks.

Our saga of running all over the world came to a crashing halt. We still got in a lot of miles running or walking, but we instantly knew that our life as distance runners would forever be changed, and not for the better.

Soon a travel advisory came out discouraging Americans to travel outside of the US. Shortly thereafter, St. Kitts closed its borders. In the blink of an eye, the thought of traveling as we once did scared me to death.

We loved this tiny island of forty thousand inhabitants, but it simply wasn't the same without the daily cruise ship and weekly airline arrivals. The hustle and bustle was gone. Our favorite restaurants were closed. People at first didn't want to stop and talk, and eventually, you couldn't even see their friendly smiles behind their face masks.

I wasn't sure which scared me more, the virus or the simple fact that we were no longer able to come and go as we saw fit. There were no future trips to plan. Our only thought was how and when we would be able to get Catherine back to her family.

Curfews and lockdowns were now the norms. Every few days they would let us out to forage for food and supplies. Medical products and medications were now my concern. Did we have enough on hand? Could I have them sent from the States?

I started ordering and having things sent to our UPS box in Atlanta, with thoughts of exactly what day I would have to pull the trigger to have them sent to us here. Cargo was exempt from the closed borders.

You could tell that the Federation, as the government of St. Kitts called itself, was taking this very seriously and had plans for any and every eventuality. They were willing to cut off their livelihood, tourism, to save even one of their citizens from this terrible disease. When a TV reporter asked when the borders would be reopened, they simply said they didn't know and didn't care, since their major concern was to take care of their people.

I knew in a flash that we had to leave, for two reasons. First, if something were to happen to me, Catherine would be all alone here. With COVID closing so much of the world down, the hospitals weren't allowing visitors, and no one could fly in to help. With her condition, that wasn't something I was willing to risk. The second reason was that all Catherine could think about was being with her family. The lack of socialization was really getting to her. The US was getting hit hard by the virus, but at least there we could be near loved ones who could care for her.

They say you should always put your oxygen mask on first, and I am a firm believer in that principle, but you still have to put the mask on for those that you love and care for. I started looking for private charter flights off the island. Using social media, I found that the local airline was putting together a flight for any US citizens who wanted to go back to San Juan. I had booked a flight to leave later in the week, but now that I knew that flight would not be operating, my sole mission was to get on the flight to San Juan, which left the next day.

While we were in St. Kitts, I listened to a book called This Naked Mind: Control Alcohol, Find Freedom, Discover Happiness & Change Your Life by Annie Grace while we ran and walked whenever we could. I had listened to numerous books during our travels, but this was the first one that I actually listened to twice.

My thought process was that, with the success of Dry January and with us going back to the States where the virus was prevalent, I needed to boost my immune system just in case I did become infected. As a Black man over sixty with a history of heart trouble, I already had three strikes against me when it came to being prone to die from the virus. So, as an early sixty-fifth birthday present to myself, I was inspired to give up alcohol for good.

"Surreal" is an understatement when it comes to describing our three-day trek back to Jeffersonville, Indiana, where it had all started over five years ago. Before we could join twenty-four others on a Silver Airways flight out of St. Kitts, our cabbie had to get written permission from the Police Commissioner to come pick us up since a twenty-four-hour lockdown was still in effect. That document, which he had to display at all times, had written instruction about how he was to interact with us.

At the airport, the airline had a form for us to sign stating that we didn't have any indications of being infected by the virus. Everyone there was masked and gloved up. Every passenger on the flight had to pay double since the plane was flown in empty because the border was still closed.

The protocol in San Juan was unexpected but very understandable. All the personnel screening us were in full hospital garb, including face masks and full-face shields. First, they took our temperature, then we waited six feet apart to answer intake questions so that we could leave the airport. They were especially concerned with my overall health since I was sixty-four years old.

We opted to stay at a Marriott near the airport. It was one of their best resorts on the island, but it was completely empty. None of the services were available, and the adjacent beach was completely empty too. The only other people we saw during our twenty-hour layover were the few employees working there.

The next day our Delta jet only had forty passengers, ten of whom had come from St Kitts the day before. Box lunches and water were the fare in first class, and all of us were in masks—except for the pilots, for some strange reason. As a matter of fact, I didn't see a single pilot wearing a mask the entire time we made our way back to Indiana.

Once again, we were back to our home hotel in Atlanta, the Renaissance Gateway, except this time, we were the only ones there. It was so sad not to see all the smiling faces that used to greet us when we arrived, asking where we had been and wishing they could stow away in our bags.

The next morning, we went by the UPS Store, which was classified as an essential business. Our box was full of mail and supplies I had ordered online over the last month. Next, we dropped off items at our storage unit that we wouldn't need for the foreseeable future. There was no telling when we would need cruise clothes once again.

On our afternoon flight to Louisville, there were more people in first class than there were in coach. I never thought I would see a passenger load like that in my lifetime.

When we got back to Jeffersonville, we did a self-imposed fourteen-day quarantine at the TownePlace Suites Hotel, just a few blocks from the condo we left to start this crazy nomad lifestyle. I didn't know where we would go from there, but I must admit it was nice to run and walk around our old neighborhood.

The two marathons we had planned for Catherine in May were canceled, so after our quarantine was over, we found an Airbnb in downtown Louisville, where we stayed for a month. That was as long as we could stay put, though. We flew back to Atlanta for my annual doctor's visit and Catherine's four-month follow-up appointment with the Mind Center, then back to Louisville for a week, and on to Bloomington to see Catherine's daughter.

In spite of everything, Catherine still wanted to run marathons in Maine and Rhode Island, so in late August, we were on the road again, with a destination of Portland, Maine. But first, we had to take a COVID test in Louisville no more than seventy-two hours prior to our arrival. We found a site that was able to post our negative results just before we got to Boston.

Our flight was at the maximum capacity Delta was allowing: 70 percent in coach with no occupants in the middle seats, and 50 percent in first class. Everyone was required to wear masks unless they wanted to be kicked off the plane and banned from the airline for life. Just to be safe, we also wore goggles.

It helped our peace of mind that I know how effective air filtration systems on airplanes are—and they were changing their filters twice as often as they used to. The air goes out at your feet and clean air comes in overhead, so with our overhead fans turned all the way up, our air was cleaned as often as if we were in a COVID ward at a hospital.

After being cooped up for months, of course, we had to do some socially distant visits with Marathon Tours cohorts, both in Boston and Portsmouth, New Hampshire. None of the friends we met up with had traveled yet, but they could all understand why we had decided that the risk of traveling was worth the reward of running and seeing people like them.

Only eighteen out of the fifty registered runners showed up to the race in Portland. For the marathon, we had to do seven loops around nearby Back Cove Lake on hard-packed dirt. Even though I ran at a very slow pace, this was the most consistent race I had run in a long time. I achieved another personal record since it was my first marathon over the age of sixty-five. I had been alcohol-free for more than four months, and Catherine hadn't had a drink for two months, and I didn't think it was a coincidence that neither of us had any knee pain during the race. Once again, we crossed the finish line hand in hand, and the day after, we both felt so great we thought we could go for another run.

We had proved to ourselves that if we couldn't run all over the world, we could at least run around the country. To complete Catherine's 23-year quest to run a marathon in all fifty states, on October 25th, 2020, we traveled to Narragansett, Rhode Island.

The city and state only allowed 225 participants, and we once again had to provide a negative COVID test result no more than 72 hours prior to entry into the state. My sister Gwen and sister-in-law Joan drove over from Connecticut for the occasion, and our new best friends from our Myanmar trip two years ago, Rick and Lisa, were also there.

Lisa, who had run more than 260 marathons, provided the mental support before and during the race, while Rick handled the nutritional and logistical support by car. It was a bit chilly and windy at the start, with a "feels like" temperature of 39 degrees. We chose the 6:30 AM early start, so it was still dark out, but we wanted the extra time to make sure we finished. And we did, hand-in-hand as always.

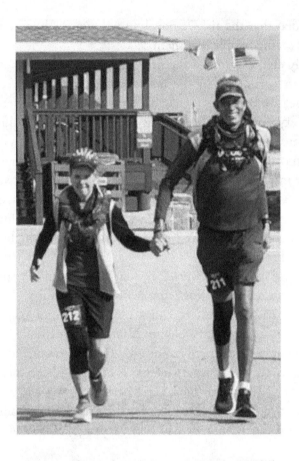

A representative from the 50 States Marathon Club was there to certify Catherine's amazing accomplishment. (Her finisher's Trophy was waiting for her back in Atlanta.) To continue the celebration, we visited our timeshare in Puerto Vallarta, Mexico, for two weeks. They were having a promotion for their grand reopening, so we were able to get an extra week free. Next stop was Aruba for two weeks, since they were one of the few places that would allow U.S. citizens on their shores.

Because we were still vagabonds at heart, we planned a two-week Windstar cruise of the Caribbean in February, but there was no telling if that would operate. We also set a new goal: to run half-marathons in all 50 states. We'd done 23 of them so far, which left us plenty of room to roam. With no timeframe set to achieve this goal, we would just take it one step at a time.

With quarantine, testing requirements, and social distancing, traveling and racing wouldn't be the same as it had been for the past five years; but they would still be possible. As I planned for our life as COVID nomads, I thought about what made all the expenses, inconvenience, and health risks worth it; and I landed on this anonymous piece of advice: "Talk with people who make you see the world differently." We did that every day as we ran all over the world, and no amount of social distancing would keep us from making new best friends every time we hit the road. As long as we were both able to put one foot in front of the other, travel would continue to enrich our lives, change our hearts, open our minds, and allow room for empathy to grow.

# APPENDIX

I f you've read this far, you know that I love numbers. Here are some facts and figures that summarize our five years of running all over the world.

**Domestic Flights**

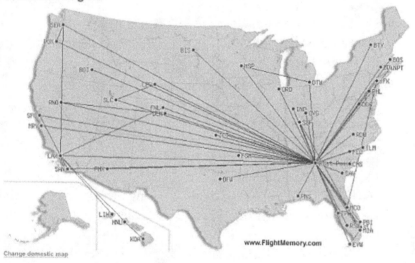

www.FlightMemory.com

Change domestic map

*Cities and countries we have visited (a few
are from my pilot life at UPS)*

Note: The number after each country signifies life expectancy.

1. King George Island, Antarctica
2. Saint John's, Antigua and Barbuda (73)
3. Buenos Aires, Argentina (75)

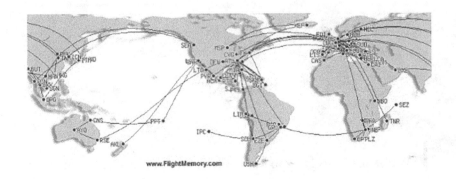

4.  Oranjestad, Aruba (76)
5.  Sydney, Cairns, Ayers Rock, Australia (81)
6.  Vienna, Austria (80)
7.  Nassau, Bahamas (72)
8.  Bridgetown Barbados (77)
9.  Brussels, Belgium (80)
10. Belize City, Belize (73)
11. Hamilton Bermuda (80)
12. Kasane, Botswana (54)
13. Rio de Janeiro, Sao Paulo, Porto Alegre, Campinas, Bebedouro, Brazil (73)
14. Tortola, British Virgin Islands (78)
15. Paro, Punakha, Bhutan (68)
16. Phnom Penh, Koh Chen, Oudong, Kampong Tralach, Kampong Chhnang, Prek Kramer, Siem Reap, Cambodia (63)
17. Montreal, Toronto, Canada (81)
18. Santiago, Patagonia, Ushuaia, Easter Island, Chile (78)
19. Beijing, Hong Kong, Xian, Taipei-Taiwan, China (73)
20. Bogota, Colombia (72)
21. San Jose, Costa Rica (79)
22. Rovinj, Split, Dubrovnik, Hvar, Croatia (76)
23. Havana, Cuba (780
24. Limassol, Cyprus (78)
25. Prague, Czech Republic (77)
26. Copenhagen, Denmark (79)

27. Roseau, Dominica (75)
28. Santo Domingo, Dominican Republic (72)
29. Quito, Ecuador (75)
30. Cairo, Luxor, Aswan, Edfu, Kim Ombo, Egypt (73)
31. San Salvador, El Salvador (71)
32. Helsinki, Finland (80)
33. Paris, Lyon, Marseille, Arles, Avignon, French Polynesia, Nice, Medoc, Cannes, Sanary-Sur-Mer, Port Vendres, France (81)
34. Cologne, Munich, Berlin, Germany (80)
35. Athens, Gythion, Monemvasia, Katakolon, Nafplio, Santorini, Mykonos, Patmos, Crete, Greece (80)
36. Guatemala City, Guatemala (70)
37. Port-au-Prince, Haiti (58)
38. San Pedro Sula, Honduras (72)
39. Budapest, Hungary (73)
40. Reykjavik, Vestmannaaeyjar/ Heimaey Island, Seydisfjordur, Akureyri, Isafjordur Grundarfjordur Iceland (81)
41. Dublin, Galway, Ennis, Ireland (79)
42. Tel Aviv, Jerusalem, Gaza City, Israel (81)
43. Rome, Venice, Senna, Florence, Luca, Pisa, Milan, Lake Como, Amalfi, Sicily, Sorrento, Lipori, Giardini Naxos, Capri, Portofino, Portoferraio, Civitavecchia, Sardinia, Italy (82)
44. Kingston, Jamaica (72)
45. Tokyo, Kyoto, Japan (83)
46. Dead Sea, Petra, Amman, Jordan (80)
47. Nairobi, Masai-Mara, Kenya (54)
48. Antananarivo, Toliara, Morondava, Madagascar (65)
49. Johor Baharu, Malaysia (74)
50. Fort-de-France, Martinique, overseas department of France
51. Mexico City, Guadalajara, Playa del Carman, Cabo San Lucas, Cancun, Acapulco, Puerto Vallarta, Loreto, Mexico (75)
52. Monte Carlo, Monaco (80)
53. Kotor, Montenegro (73)

54. Casablanca, Tangier, Morocco (71)
55. Yangon (Rangoon), Mandalay Bagan, Inle Lake, Myanmar (Burma) (66)
56. Amsterdam, Oranjestad-Aruba, Curacao, Netherlands (80)
57. Auckland, Queenstown, New Zealand (80)
58. Chobe River, Namibia (52)
59. Managua, Nicaragua (71)
60. Oslo, Bergen, Sognefjord, Flam, Norway (80)
61. Panama City, Panama (75)
62. Lima, Peru (72)
63. Lisbon, Porto, Portugal (78)
64. Basseterre, Saint Kitts, and Nevis (70)
65. Singapore, Singapore (81)
66. Bratislava, Slovakia (75)
67. Cape Town, South Africa (54)
68. Seoul, South Korea (80)
69. Madrid, Malaga, Almeria, Cartagena, Ibiza, Tarragona, Barcelona, Spain (81)
70. Stockholm, Sweden (81)
71. Geneva, Switzerland (82)
72. Mahe, Seychelles (74)
73. Bangkok, Thailand (69)
74. Port of Spain, Trinidad and Tobago (69)
75. Istanbul, Cappadocia, Kuşadası (Ephesus), Turkey (72)
76. Dubai, United Arab Emirates (77)
77. Edinburgh, Scotland, London, Anguilla, Hamilton-Bermuda, British Virgin Islands, Lerwick, Stornoway, Kirkwall, Invergordon United Kingdom (80)
78. All of the United States (78)
79. Vatican City, Vatican City
80. Ho Chi Minh City (Saigon), Cai Be, Sa Dec, Tan Chau, Hanoi, Ha Long Bay, Vietnam 73
81. Victoria Falls, Zimbabwe (54)

We have visited more cities in Italy than any other.
Countries Where We Have Run a Race

1. USA 2000-2020
2. Montreal, Canada 2006
3. Athens, Greece 2011
4. Paris and Medoc, France 2012/2015
5. London, England 2012
6. Stockholm, Netherlands 2012
7. Reyjakavic, Iceland 2013
8. Barcelona, Spain 2014
9. Berlin, Germany 2014
10. Tokyo, Japan 2015
11. Rome, Italy 2015
12. Beijing, China 2015
13. Copenhagen, Sweden 2015
14. Akers Rock, Australia 2015
15. Brussels, Belgium 2015
16. Dublin, Ireland 2015
17. Istanbul, Turkey 2015
18. Tele Aviv and Jerusalem, Israel 2016/2018
19. Mexico City, Mexico 2016
20. Prague, CR 2016
21. Easter Island and Patagonia Chile 2016/2019
22. Nairobi, Kenya 2016
23. Amsterdam, Netherlands 2016
24. Havana, Cuba 2016
25. King Georg Island, Antarctic 2017
26. Antananarivo, Madagascar 2017
27. Petra, Jordan 2017
28. Queenstown, New Zealand 2017
29. Limassol, Cyprus 2018
30. Geneva, Switzerland 2018

31. Paro, Bhutan 2018
32. Yangon, Myanmar 2018
33. Cairo, Egypt 2019
34. Cape Town, South Africa 2019

Trips We Have Done with Marathon Tours and Travel

1. Paris, France 4/2012
2. London, England 4/2012
3. Stockholm, Sweden 7/2012
4. Reykjavík, Iceland 8/2013
5. Hamilton, Bermuda 1/2014
6. Berlin, Germany 9/2014
7. Medoc, France 9/2015
8. Dublin Ireland 10/2015
9. Istanbul, Turkey 11/2015
10. Boston, Massachusetts 4/2016
11. Prague, Czech Republic 5/2016
12. Easter Island, Chile 6/2016
13. Napa to Sonoma, California 7/2016
14. Nairobi, Kenya 7/2016
15. Havana, Cuba 11/2016
16. King George Island, Antarctica 3/2017
17. Fianarantsoa, Madagascar 6/2017
18. Napa to Sonoma, California 7/2017
19. Petra, Jordan 8/2017
20. Queenstown, New Zealand 11/2017
21. Jerusalem, Israel 3/2018
22. Paro, Bhutan 5/2018
23. Bagan Temple, Myanmar 11/2018
24. Patagonia, Chile 9/2019
25. Cape Town, South Africa 9/2019

# ABOUT THE AUTHOR

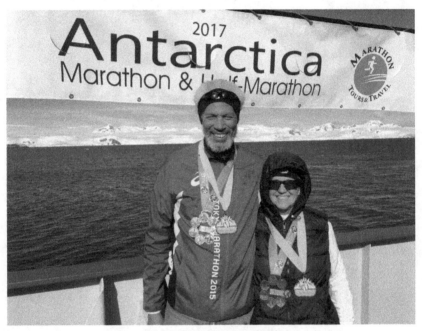

Antarctica, March 2017

Anthony L. Copeland-Parker was a professional pilot/manager for thirty-seven years, the last twenty-seven with United Parcel Service. His last job had him managing pilots and flying B757/767-type aircraft all over the world. When he retired, he began writing his blog, PlayHard-HaveFun.com. Since then, he and his partner Catherine have traveled to eighty-two different countries. They have run at least a half-marathon in thirty-five countries and on all seven continents.

CPSIA information can be obtained
at www.ICGtesting.com
Printed in the USA
JSHW041338180721
16752JS00001BA/1